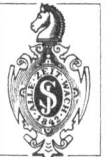

Peter D. Phelps · Glyn A. S. Lloyd

Diagnostic Imaging of the Ear

Second Edition

With 314 Figures

Springer-Verlag
London Berlin Heidelberg New York
Paris Tokyo Hong Kong

Peter D. Phelps, MD, FRCS, FRCR, DMRD
Consultant Radiologist, Walsgrave Hospital, Coventry and Consultant Radiologist, Royal National Throat, Nose and Ear Hospital, Gray's Inn Road, London WC1X 8DA, UK

Glyn A. S. Lloyd, MA, DM, FRCR
Formerly Director, Department of Radiology, Royal National Throat, Nose and Ear Hospital, Gray's Inn Road, London WC1X 8DA, UK and Consultant Radiologist, Moorfields Eye Hospital, London EC1, UK

ISBN-13: 978-1-4471-1726-1   e-ISBN-13: 978-1-4471-1724-7
DOI: 10.1007/978-1-4471-1724-7

British Library Cataloguing in Publication Data
Phelps, Peter D.
    Diagnostic imaging of the ear.
    1. Man. Ears. Diagnosis. Radiography
    I. Title   II. Lloyd, Glyn A. S.   III. Phelps, Peter D.
    617.8'0757

Library of Congress Cataloging-in-Publication Data
Phelps, Peter D.
Diagnostic imaging of the ear/Peter D. Phelps and Glyn A. S. Lloyd. – 2nd ed.
    p.   cm.
    Rev. ed. of: Radiology of the ear. 1983.
    Includes bibliographical references.

    1. Ear—Diseases—Diagnosis.   2. Temporal bone—Imaging.   3. Temporal bone—Magnetic resonance imaging.
I. Lloyd, Glyn A. S.   II. Phelps, Peter D.   Radiology of the ear.   III. Title.
[DNLM: 1. Diagnostic Imaging.   2. Ear Diseases—diagnosis.   WV 210 P541r]
RF123.5.I4P44   1990
617.8'0754—dc20
DNLM/DLC
For Library of Congress   89–21768
                                                                      CIP

Softcover reprint of the hardcover 2nd edition 1990

First edition published as *Radiology of the Ear* by Blackwell Scientific Publications, Osney Mead, Oxford
Second edition 1990

2128/3830–543210   Printed on acid-free paper

Foreword to the Second Edition

Over the past six years, there have been conspicuous developments in the applications of imaging technology to the examination of the ear. There has, therefore, been a demand for this new edition of the book which Dr. Peter Phelps and Dr. Glyn Lloyd brought out in 1983.

The developments in imaging technology have been primarily twofold. First, far better imaging can now be obtained with computerised tomography (CT). Secondly, there has been the successful introduction into clinical practice of magnetic resonance imaging (MR). Thus we now have two superb, but complementary, imaging techniques for the examination of the ear and of the auditory and vestibular nervous pathways – CT for hard tissues, MR for soft tissues. These two techniques are of particular importance to our own area of interest, since nowhere else in the body is a 3-dimensional perspective so necessary.

The phenomenon of nuclear magnetic resonance was discovered independently by Bloch and by Purcell over 40 years ago. For this work, they fittingly received the Nobel Prize in 1952. The phenomenon involves the interaction of the nucleus of a selected atom, e.g., hydrogen, with an external magnetic field and with an external radiofrequency oscillating electromagnetic field, which is changing as a function of time at a particular frequency. MR needs to use field gradients in order to obtain structural information. The imaging slice needs to be defined by either a selective irradiative process or by applying an alternating field gradient. Thus the magnetic imaging technique avoids the use of ionising radiations. Yet, as this book shows, it produces superb images to which imaging using ionising radiations can only aspire.

With these developments in clinical morphology handled by doctors such as Peter Phelps and Glyn Lloyd, the clinician interested in aural malfunction will feel securer in his diagnosis. He will, therefore, read this new edition with appreciation.

May 1989

R. Hinchcliffe

Preface

This book is based upon a previous work published in 1983 (*Radiology of the Ear*). Since that date, the most important advance in the imaging of the petromastoid has been the application of magnetic resonance scanning, especially when combined with the use of the recently introduced paramagnetic contrast agent, Gadolinium DTPA. Although computerised tomography remains the dominant investigation in this field, magnetic resonance is becoming increasingly important. The account which follows is an attempt to summarise present knowledge in this division of otorhinolaryngology imaging.

The format of the chapters has been retained from the original work, with an initial account of imaging techniques and normal anatomy followed by chapters on congenital ear disease, trauma, inflammatory disease and neoplasia. Acoustic neuroma is given a separate section and there are two final chapters on vertigo and otosclerosis.

The authors are deeply indebted to their surgical colleagues for cooperation and help in the preparation of the text and their readiness to allow access to clinical material. In this respect, we are particularly indebted to Professor Ronald Hinchcliffe, who has written the Foreword. We are greatly indebted to Dr. Hermann Wilbrand of Uppsala, Sweden, for some line drawings and to Drs. Anthony Lloyd and David Beale, Consultant Neuroradiologists at the Walsgrave Hospital, Coventry, for several radiographs, including many of the angiograms and MR scans. The neuroradiologists of the National Hospital, London, willingly advised and provided some much appreciated case material. Professor Leslie Michaels and the Department of Histopathology at the Royal National Throat, Nose and Ear Hospital, provided us with most of the histological sections. We are grateful to Messrs. SR Mawson and H Ludman as well as Edward Arnold (Publishers) Limited for Figs 2.1, 2.2 and 2.4; to Mr. JA Ballantyne for allowing us to reproduce Figs 5.5, 5.6, 5.7 and 5.8 and to Mr. JM Stansbie for various alterations and for reading the proofs. The medical illustration departments in Coventry and at the Royal National Throat, Nose and Ear Hospital in London provided several of the diagrammatic illustrations and we are most grateful to Miss Jinette Newns and Mrs Ann Barraclough for typing the manuscript.

We also wish to thank the Editors of the following journals for permission to reproduce illustrations which have already appeared in previous publications: *British Journal of Radiology*, *Clinical Radiology*, *Clinical Otolaryngology*, *Acta Radiologica*, *Annals of Otology*, *Journal of Laryngology and Otology*, *Advances in Oto-Rhino-Laryngology and Neuroradiology*.

May 1989

Peter Phelps
Glyn Lloyd

Contents

1 Radiological Methods of Investigation of the Petrous Bone and Mastoid Process

The radiological imaging of the petromastoid involves plain radiographs in standard projection, pluridirectional tomography, computerised tomography (CT) and magnetic resonance imaging. Angiography has a minor subsidiary role.

Plain X-ray Examination

The need for maximum radiographic detail and contrast is more necessary in the petromastoid than in most other parts of the body, as the structures examined are small and pathological changes may only produce minimal radiological signs. High energy X-ray tubes with a fine focus (0.3 mm or less) are an advantage so that enlargement techniques can be applied where necessary. Also essential is the use of a skull table, which keeps the film and the incident X-ray beam central and allows small cones to be used. Satisfactory mastoid films can be obtained with an upright or table-top Potter–Bucky grid, but a specialised skull unit lightens the burden of the radiographer and ensures standardisation of technique, when a large volume of mastoid radiography is undertaken.

Generally the projections to be described in the following pages will be based on the use of this type of skull table. There are now, however, advanced skull units available, such as the Orbix (Siemans), Arco Universal (CGR), and Pentodiagnost (Philips), which allow the X-ray tube to be adjusted to any point on the surface of a sphere. The x-ray film is located opposite and perpendicular to the central beam and the part of the skull to be investigated is positioned in the centre of the sphere. With the skull immobilised in the supine position, accurate angulation in three reference planes is easily reproduced, and there is constant magnification and no distortion of the radiographs. The head has, however, to be extended from the fixed supine position for a base view and the advantages of the fixed reference planes are forfeited if a special table is not used or if the examination is not performed with the head supine. Mathematically-accurate positioning can be achieved using the reference planes. A full description of the technique has been given by the Swedish authors Radberg and Thibaut (1971).

We use the first four of the following basic projections for almost all conventional radiography of the temporal bone. The two that show both sides on one film are standard skull views with the field size reduced. For the following description, the base line is the orbito-meatal line from the outer canthus of the eye to the centre of the external auditory (acoustic) meatus.

Lateral View

Schuller (1905) introduced a lateral projection, which avoided overlap of the opposite mastoid process and this principle is still used to-day. Since the petrous bones are symmetrically placed on both sides of the skull, a true lateral results in superimposition of the two sides. It is, therefore, necessary to angle the incident ray, or alternatively the skull, in order to prevent superimposition. The greater the tilt the more the attic (epitympnaic recess) and

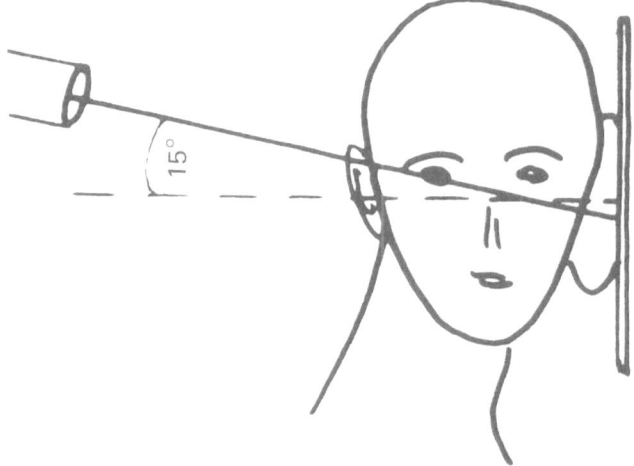

Fig. 1.1. The position and incident ray for a lateral view of the mastoid. The caudal inclination of the beam prevents superimposition of the mastoid process.

antrum will be thrown clear of the mass of bone around the labyrinth, but this is offset by increased distortion. As shown in Fig. 1.1 the lateral projection of the petromastoid is obtained by placing the head in a true lateral position and angling the tube caudally 15°, thus preventing superimposition

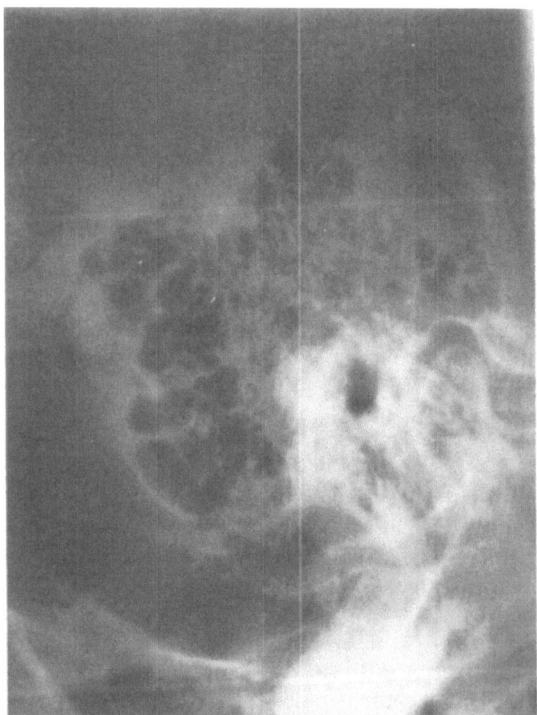

Fig. 1.2. A lateral view of the mastoid showing normal air-cell system. In this projection there is superimposition of the internal and external meatus.

of the mastoid processes. The incident beam is centred 5 cm above the uppermost external auditory meatus. The angled lateral view (Fig. 1.2) results in a superimposition of the petrous bone on the mastoid and the internal and external auditory canals are also superimposed. The view also allows assessment of the degree of pneumatisation of the mastoid, the state of translucence of the air cells, the position of the lateral sinus and its relation to the tegmen tympani. The attic, aditus and mastoid antrum are also visible. In practice, this view is used principally to show the state of the mastoid air cells and for the surgeon to assess how much room there is between the external auditory meatus and the middle fossa dura above, and the lateral sinus behind, when making an approach to the mastoid antrum (See Chap. 7). Erosion of the attico-antral region, and of the bony bridge formed by the outer attic wall, can be shown but only when this is extensive.

Oblique Postero-anterior View (Stenvers Projection)

In this view, the whole length of the petrous bone is demonstrated by placing it parallel to the X-ray film with the incident ray passing at right angles to it. When a skull table is used the patient sits erect facing the film. With the radiographic base line horizontal, the sagittal plane of the skull is rotated through 35 degrees and tilted 15° away from the side to be examined (Fig. 1.3). The incident ray is inclined at an angle of 12° cranially and is centred on a point 2 cm medial to the mastoid tip. A radiograph in Stenvers position (Fig. 1.4) should demonstrate the petrous tip and internal auditory meatus, the semicircular canals and middle ear cleft. Erosion of the petrous tip and widening of the internal (acoustic) meatus (IAM) may be shown on this projection, although the changes are generally better demonstrated by conventional tomography or CT. Plain X-ray evidence of bone erosion in the antrum in the presence of a cholesteatoma is best shown on this projection.

Half-axial (Towne's) View

The classical position for a Towne's projection is shown in Fig. 1.5. The reversed Towne's view (Fig. 1.6) should be used whenever possible; the radiation dose to the eyes in the classical position may be as high as 8 mSv per exposure (Lloyd et al. 1979). The radiograph in the Towne's projection (Fig. 1.7) shows the IAM and middle ear. Enlarge-

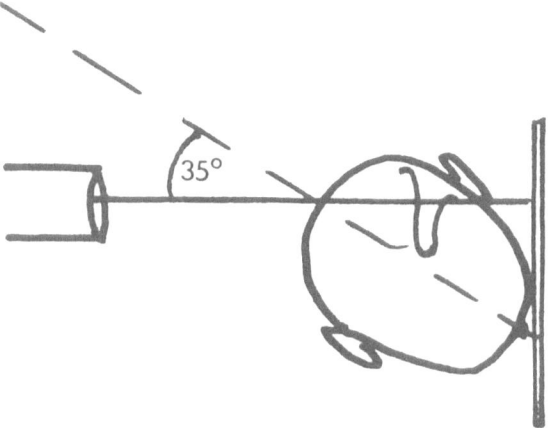

Fig. 1.3. The necessary position for Stenver's view. Essentially, the head is placed so that the petrous bone lies parallel to the film.

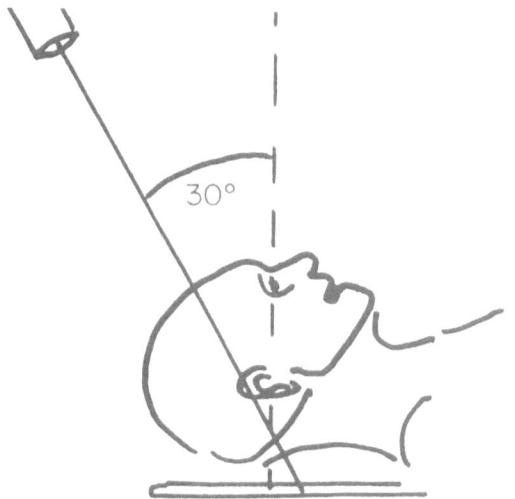

Fig. 1.5. Line drawing to illustrate the position for a classical Towne's view.

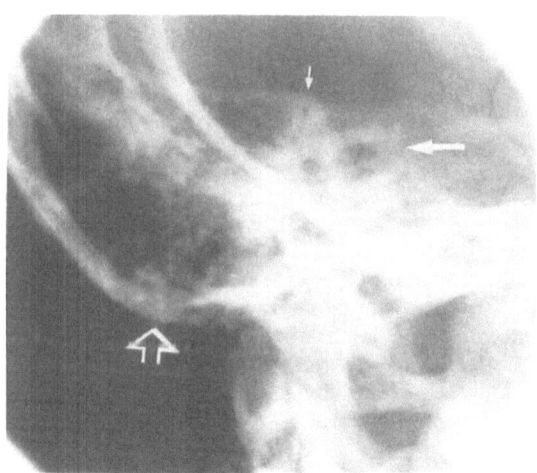

Fig. 1.4. A normal Stenver's projection. IAM (*large arrow*), superior semicircular canal (*small arrow*) and mastoid tip (*open arrow*).

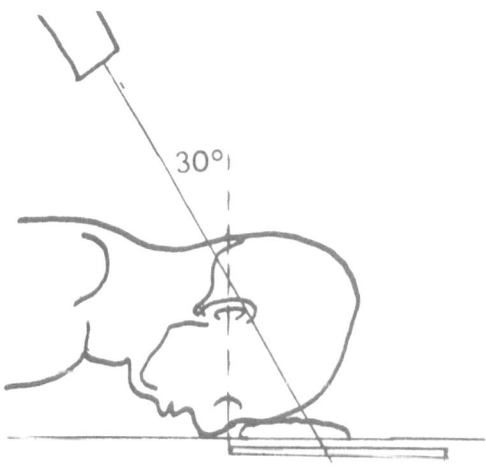

Fig. 1.6. Reversed Towne's view. Whenever possible this projection should be used instead of the classical Towne's view (Fig. 1.5) to reduce the radiation dose to the eyes.

ment and erosion of the attic and antrum can be seen in this view, and it is possible to identify the lateral spur or scutum, which may be eroded by a cholesteatoma.

Axial or Submento-vertical View

This is an important item in the X-ray examination of the ear and no plain X-ray study is complete without it. The radiographic position is illustrated in Fig. 1.8. In the classical position, the base line is

parallel to the film and the incident beam centred at a point mid way between the angles of the mandible. If the centring point is too far anterior or the head insufficiently extended, the angle of the jaw is projected over the middle ear and obscures it. To avoid this, a centring point slightly lower than the one illustrated in the classical position is recommended. The radiograph (Fig. 1.9) demonstrates the middle ear, the external and internal auditory meatus and the Eustachian (auditory) canal. The plan view of the middle ear provides the best plain X-ray assessment of its air content and degree of

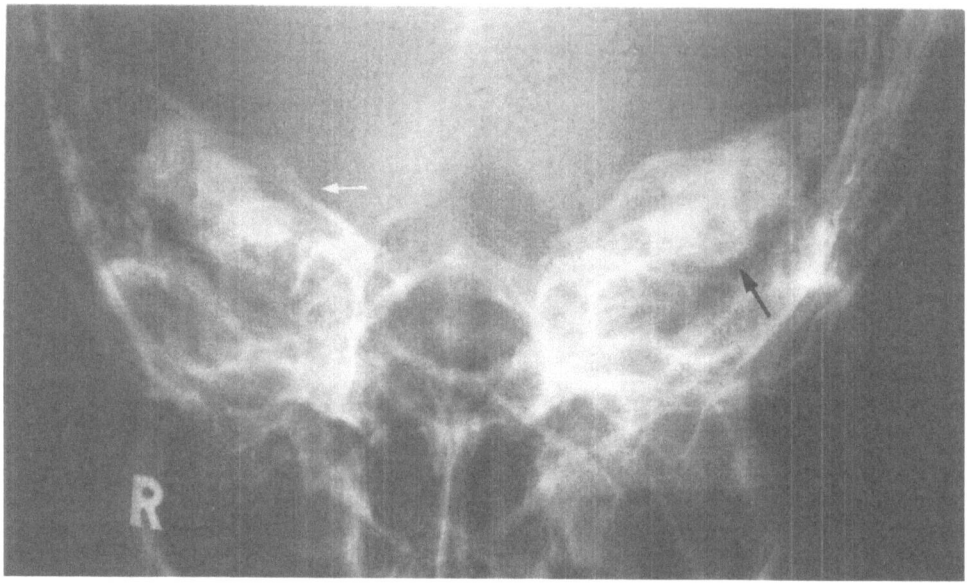

Fig. 1.7. Normal Towne's projection. The *white arrow* points to the IAM and the *black* to the cochlea.

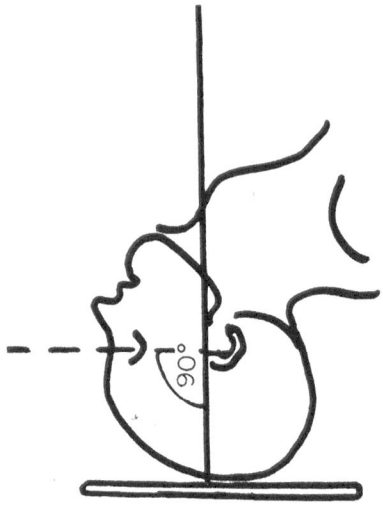

Fig. 1.8. The position for a standard submento-vertical view. The base line is parallel to the film and the incident beam is centred at a point midway between the angles of the mandible.

translucence and of the ossicular chain: the head of the malleus, the body of the incus and the cartilage space of the incudo-mallear joint are clearly visible. The cochlea should be identified on this view and the condyle of the mandible is demonstrated in its long axis.

Transorbital View

This is the best view of the IAM if tomography is unavailable. To avoid radiation to the eyes a postero-anterior position is preferred for this projection and macrography is an advantage. The position is illustrated in Fig. 1.10. With the orbito-meatal line at right angles to the film, the tube is angled 5–10° caudally, centring between the orbits. The petrous pyramids are thus projected through the orbits.

View for the Jugular Foramen

This view is used when a glomus jugulare tumour is suspected. The radiographic position is similar to that of an occipito-mental view of the paranasal sinuses. With the mouth open and a low centring point, the patient is placed in the postero-anterior position with the orbito-meatal line elevated 45° and the central ray directed in the mid line at the level of the internal auditory meatus (Fig. 1.11). The jugular fossae are thus projected through the open mouth.

In normal circumstances when pluridirectional tomography or CT is readily available, the views described above are all that are needed for adequate plain X-ray of the petromastoid: if further investigation is required then the radiologist should employ CT.

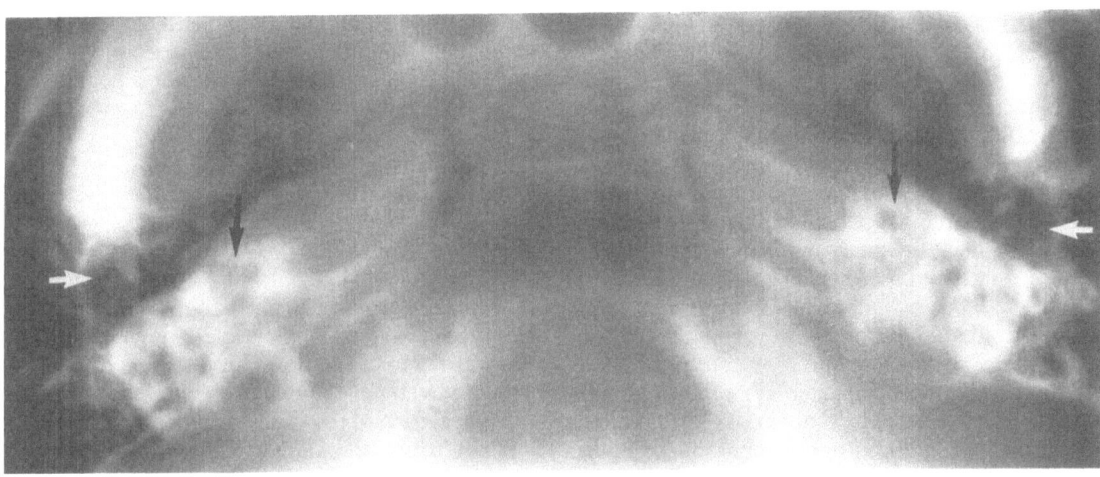

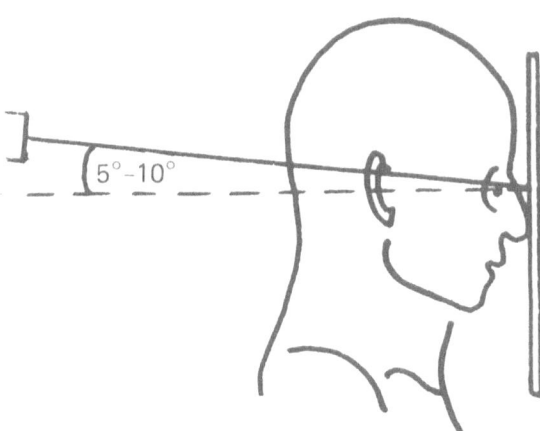

Fig. 1.9. Normal submento-vertical or base projection of the petrous bones. Middle ear cleft and ossicles (*white arrows*); cochlea (*black arrows*).

Fig. 1.10. The radiographic position for the transorbital projection of the petrous bones.

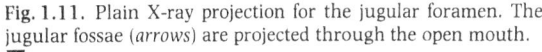

Fig. 1.11. Plain X-ray projection for the jugular foramen. The jugular fossae (*arrows*) are projected through the open mouth.

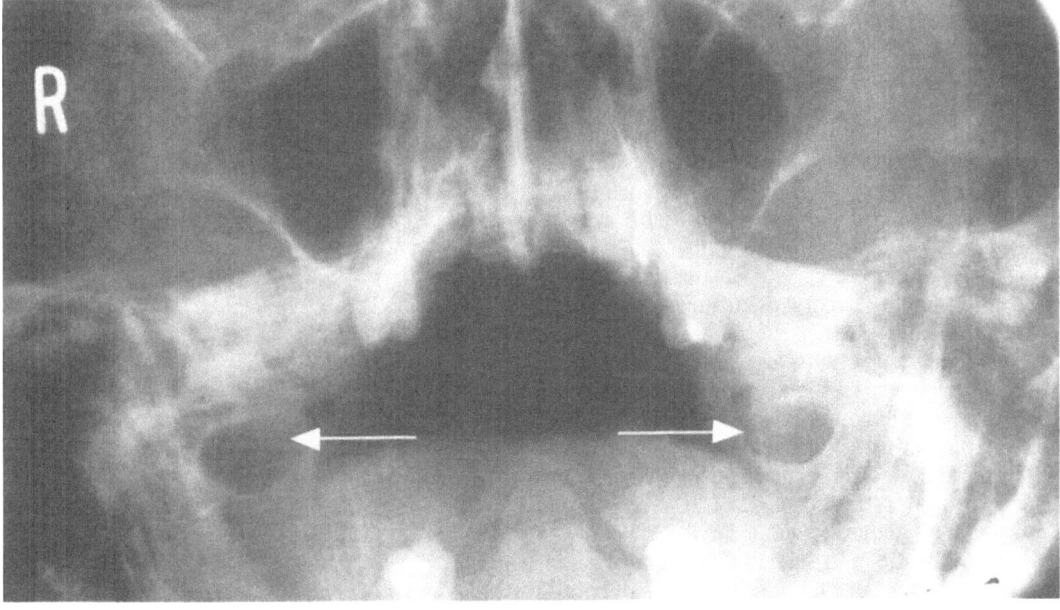

Pluridirectional Tomography

Pluridirectional tomography became available to the radiologist in the early 1960s with the introduction of the Philips Massiot Polytome. This revolutionised the radiological investigation of ear disease. The hypocycloidal movement available with this machine gives five times the blurring capacity of an equivalent linear tomograph and it can produce sections of 1-mm thickness with minimum loss of sharpness and an angle of tube swing of 48°. Other machines using a spiral movement of the tube are available and produce a comparable blurring capacity and tomographic sections which differ very little from those produced by the Polytome.

General Considerations

The essential prerequisite for good quality hypocycloidal tomograms is to produce radiographs of high definition and high contrast. The latter quality is especially important since the thin section tomograms and high blurring capacity of the Polytome produce sections of inherently low contrast. A satisfactory screen/film combination should be chosen to achieve these results without incurring a high radiation dose per exposure. The faster rare-earth intensifying screens reduce radiation and kilovoltage to a considerable degree at the expense of lower film definition, and in practice a compromise is necessary between film quality and the speed of the screen/film combination. A focal spot size of 0.3 mm is used and the grid is removed.

Correct exposure and good beam collimation are also necessary to achieve satisfactory petrous bone tomography. A slit beam collimator is generally satisfactory since this allows both petrous bones to be tomographed on the same film. Alternatively, simultaneous separate coning of the petrous bones can be arranged on the same film with a two-hole mask. Apart from enhancing the quality of the radiographs produced, careful collimation has the added advantage of reducing unneccessary radiation to the patient. Since the report of Chin et al. (1970) much attention has been given to protecting the lens and cornea of the eye during tomographic procedures to the temporal bone. These authors showed that, in full hypocycloidal tomography of the temporal bones in the antero-posterior position, the cornea may receive a dose of 10.5 rad. These exposures are generally considered to be unacceptably high and it is essential to modify radiographic technique to reduce eye dosage. This should

include the use of lead eye shields for lateral and axial tomography. In this way three-plane hypocycloidal tomography of the temporal bone can be achieved for as little as 2.7 mSv to the cornea.

Coronal Sections

These are taken with the subject lying prone and the orbito-meatal line at right angles to the film and table top. For routine examination tomographs are obtained using the hypocycloidal movement of the tube at 2 mm separation of the sections. These should cover the full extent of the labyrinth from the apical turn of the cochlea to the posterior semicircular canal and allow comparison between the two sides. Four or five films are usually sufficient to show IAM, labyrinth, oval window (fenestra vestibuli), ossicles and the descending portion of the facial nerve. Any radiologist with an interest in otology must be thoroughly familiar with coronal and base sections of the ear and able to recognise the level at which any section is taken.

There are two sections in the coronal plane that are important and must be recognised: these pass through the centre of the cochlea and vestibule respectively (Fig. 1.12). The cochlear cut shows the modiolus or central bony spiral as a "curl", while above the cochlea is the pit for the genicular ganglion of the facial nerve. The ossicle shown in the middle-ear cavity is the malleus (Fig. 1.13). The vestibular cut, 3 or 4 mm posteriorly, shows the oval window and also the full length of the IAM. The ossicle is the incus and sometimes the stapes may be demonstrated (Fig. 1.14). The outer attic

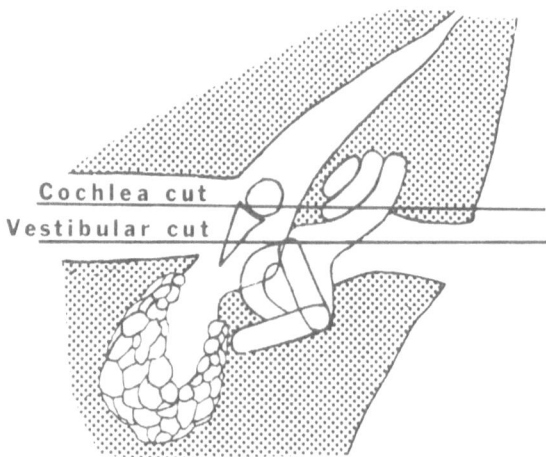

Fig. 1.12. Important sections in coronal tomography of the ear (From *A Textbook of Radiological Diagnosis*, H K Lewis, London.)

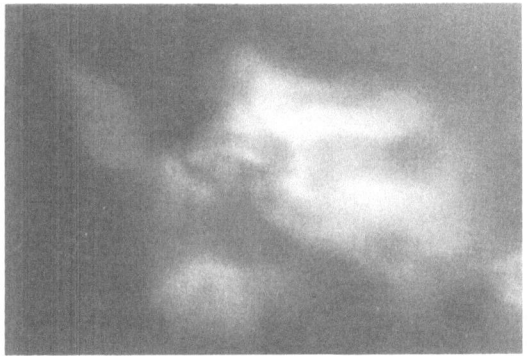

Fig. 1.13. Normal coronal section taken through the plane of the centre of the vestibule on the right side.

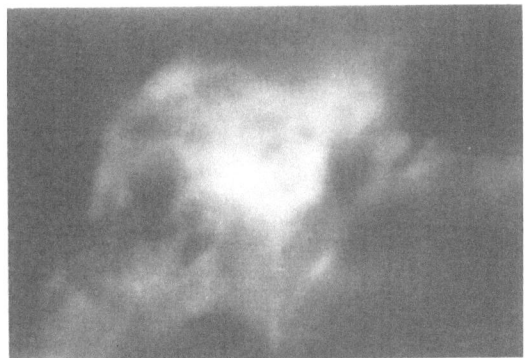

Fig. 1.14. Normal coronal section taken through the plane of the centre of the cochlea on the left side.

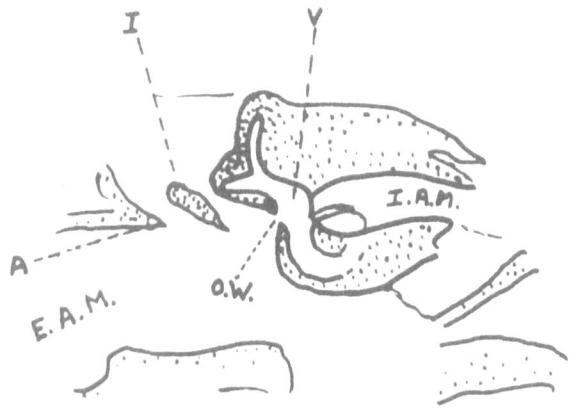

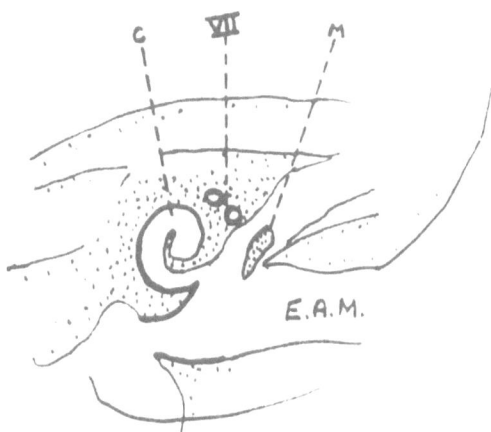

Fig. 1.15. Diagrammatic representation of the vestibular and cochlear cuts as shown on coronal section tomograms. V, vestibule; I, incus; OW, oval window; IAM, internal auditory meatus; M, malleus; C, cochlea; EAM, external auditory meatus; VII, facial nerve; A, the spur.

wall, which forms the roof of the deep part of the bony external auditory meatus is, because of its appearance, called the "spur". The carotid canal and jugular fossa are shown in the cochlear and vestibular cuts which are represented diagrammatically in Fig. 1.15.

Modified Coronal Sections

Zonography

As an alternative to the evaluation of the internal auditory meatus by coronal hypocycloidal tomography, thick section tomography or zonography using a circular motion of the tube can be employed (Lloyd and Wylie 1971). This is an easy and useful screening test for the exclusion of bony changes in a cerebello-pontine angle tumour, when a large number of patients are examined for sensorineural deafness. Sections are made with 10–12° angle of tube swing at 0.5-cm intervals. Usually 2 or 3 zonograms suffice to give adequate visualisation of the IAM on both sides. The result is, in effect, a superior version of the transorbital view described in the section on plain X-ray technique (Fig. 1.16).

Lateral Hypocycloidal Tomography

The head is placed in the true lateral position for sections in the sagittal plane. The sections are made at 2-mm intervals through the petrous pyramid, middle-ear and external auditory meatus, depend-

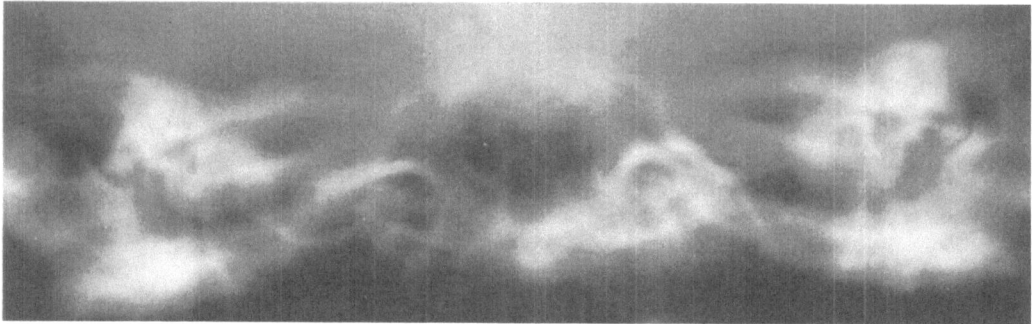

Fig. 1.16. Normal coronal zonogram showing the petrous bones and internal auditory meatus.

ing on the site of pathological change. This has the advantage to the otologist of visualising the anatomy in the same way as it presents itself through the surgical approach to the ear. Lateral tomography is particularly important because of the difficulties encountered with CT scanning in the sagittal plane. Such CT images must be obtained either with the patient in an uncomfortable position or by reformatting from axial slices, when much spatial resolution is lost; this is the result of intrinsic distortion and partial volume averaging as well as motion, which may occur not only during scanning but also during the inter-scan time.

The labyrinth is not well visualised, but the following anatomical structures can be usefully demonstrated, listed in order from lateral to medial:–

1. The external auditory meatus and tegmen tympani forming the roof of the middle ear cavity. These are usually involved in longitudinal type fractures

2. Sections through the middle ear will demonstrate the bodies of the malleus and incus, resulting in an image which has been likened to the appearance of a "molar tooth". The head of the malleus and the body of the incus combine to represent the crown of the tooth, the handle of the malleus forming the anterior root, and the long process of the incus the posterior root. The crown should normally appear as a solid shadow. Any disruption of this image, either in the form of separation of its two components or their misalignment, indicates a dislocation. Divarication of the roots of the image also indicates displacement of the incus.

An improved version of the lateral projection of the ossicles has been described by Naviez and Cornelis (1973). They point out that since the handle of the malleus and the long process of the incus incline medially in the lower part, the

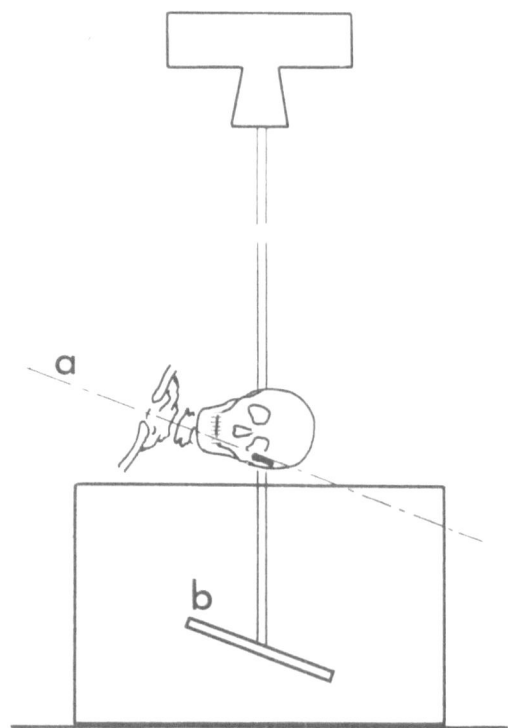

Fig. 1.17. Technique for lateral tomography of the ossicles. The X-ray film b is angled to correspond with the plane of the ossicles a.

plane of the tomographic section needs to be inclined accordingly. This can be achieved either by tilting the patient's head as described by these authors so that the ossicles are parallel to the table top, or by maintaining the head in the true lateral position but tilting the X-ray film to correspond with the plane of the ossicles (Fig. 1.17). In either case a better anatomical

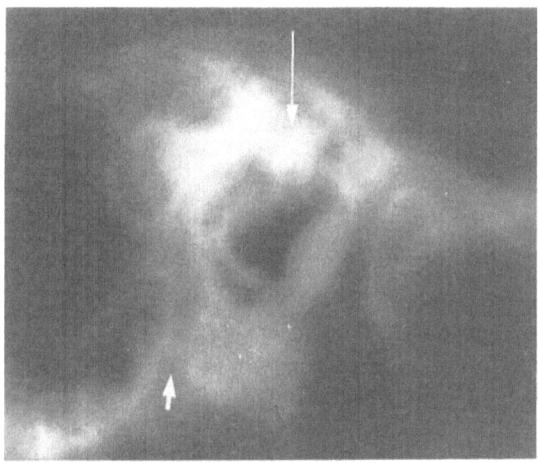

Fig. 1.18. Lateral tomogram. The *long arrow* shows the bodies of the ossicles appearing as a "molar tooth". The *short arrow* points to the stylomastoid foramen.

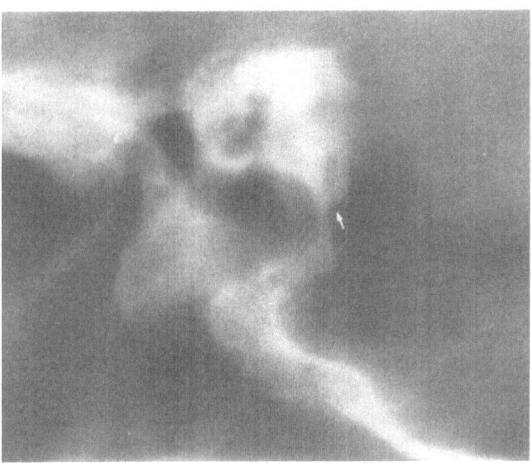

Fig. 1.20. The *arrow* points to the external aperture of the vestibular aqueduct. Note also the close proximity of the smoothly outlined jugular fossa in this patient.

representation of both incus and malleus is obtained than that provided by tomography in the true lateral projection

3. Descending facial nerve canal and second bend (Fig. 1.18). The normal canal widens as it approaches the stylomastoid foramen

4. Sagittal sections through the jugular fossa and carotid canal are a most important part of the examination to differentiate glomus tumours and other vascular masses and anomalies in the middle ear (Phelps and Lloyd 1986). A smoothly outlined jugular fossa with an intact spur or crest of bone separating it from the carotid canal

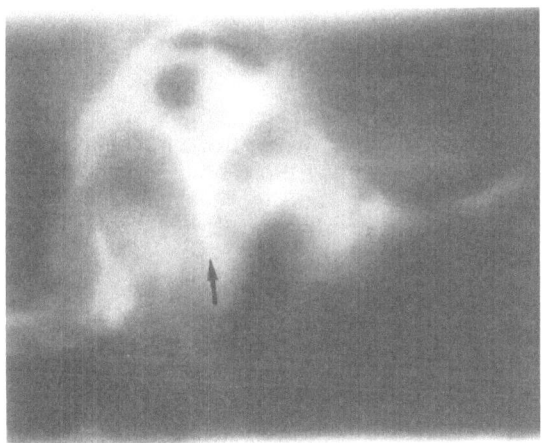

Fig. 1.19. Crest of bone between the jugular fossa and carotid canal.

(Fig. 1.19) virtually excludes a glomus jugulare tumour but not a glomus tympanicum or a high jugular bulb

5. The vestibular aqueduct is another important structure best demonstrated by lateral tomography (Fig. 1.20). The rather variable course of the vestibular aqueduct means that further sections in a slightly off-lateral position may be required (Stahle and Wilbrand 1974). This usually means elevating the chin of the patient about 20° if the underside temporal bone is being examined. The key to the correct level for identifying the vestibular aqueduct is the crus commune of the superior and posterior semicircular canal

6. Cross-sectional views of the internal auditory meatus give a better assessment of the degree of expansion than tomograms only in the coronal plane

Computerised Tomography

Computerised tomography is the representation of a tomographic section of an object based on X-ray transmission measurements through the volume of this section or "slice". It is developed from multiple absorption or attenuation measurements made around the periphery of the object (a scan). CT scanners use a highly collimated X-ray beam but the radiographic film of conventional imaging is replaced by a battery of ionisation detectors which enables the required information to be obtained with the maximum dose efficiency. The small volume (voxels) of tissue for which an attenuation value is derived have a cross-sectional area normally less than 1 mm^2 and a depth equal to the thickness of the slice, which may be from 1 to 12 mm, depending on the machine and the type of examination. The picture elements (pixels) are a two-dimensional reconstruction in the scan plane displayed as a greyscale picture on a television monitor. Computerised mathematical techniques are required to give accurate determination of the attenuation values at all points of the matrix within the section.

The success of CT has been due to the great sensitivity of the method for very small changes in X-ray attenuation. This is known as contrast resolution, which is the ability of an imaging system to visualise relatively large objects of low contrast with their backgrounds (1% or less). Image noise is the main limiting factor to the detectability of low contrast objects.

The ability of CT to show intracranial lesions was its first and most important contribution to diagnostic imaging, and for the otologist the premier role of CT is still the demonstration of intracranial complications of suppurative ear disease, such as brain abscess, and the intracranial extension of tumours of the petrous temporal bone such as glomus and acoustic neuroma. Normal brain scan techniques with contrast enhancement are required.

Rapid advances in scanner technology with a real increase in the number of detectors and a reduction in slice thickness allowing smaller pixel size have greatly improved spatial resolution, which may be defined as the ability of a CT scanner to show small details of high contrast (10% or more) in relation to their background. The quality of the CT image, however, depends on a complex relationship between radiation dose, spatial resolution, contrast resolution and noise. Noise is the mottling or granularity which affects the image when there is insufficient information from the detectors available for assessment. To some extent, therefore, there is a trade-off between optimum contrast resolution and optimum spatial resolution; (raising the radiation dose to unacceptable levels still only partially overcomes this problem). In practice, most scanners have two options for image production, called standard resolution for optimum density discrimination, as when demonstrating brain tumours, and high resolution for fine detail, especially small bony structures in sinus and temporal bone. With the new rotate-only scanners, it is possible to obtain images in both soft tissue and bone resolution from the same raw data, but inevitably the reprocessing increases the length of the examination.

High Resolution Thin Section CT

Since the introduction of high resolution thin section computerised tomography, CT has become the optimum imaging technique for the study of the temporal bone. The bony portions of the petromastoid are depicted with approximately the same resolution as with complex motion tomography, but the better radiographic contrast, freedom from spurious shadows outside of the slice and fewer problems with soft tissue silhouetting, make the pictures easier for the non-expert to interpret, as well as being much easier to reproduce as illustrations. It is, however, the ability of CT to depict the soft tissue components within and adjacent to the temporal bone that has provided the major advance in imaging of the ear. Contrast enhancement of masses may be helpful in the diagnosis, but generally tissue characterisation, in the middle ear particularly, has been disappointing and relies on the anatomical configuration and situation of a soft tissue mass. Thus a profound knowledge of temporal bone anatomy is mandatory for the interpretation of these sectional images.

Limiting Factors for High Resolution CT

Twenty years ago the demonstration of fine detail in the ear was considered the ultimate achievement of polytomography. In some respects the same is now true of high resolution CT and a brief consideration of some of the limiting factors of this technique for examining regions such as the middle ear seems desirable:

1. Partial volume averaging is a phenomenon that occurs with CT when the dimensions of the object being imaged are smaller than the slice thickness and the individual voxel. Non-representative attenuation values may be generated when all the densities within an individual voxel are averaged to produce a single attenuation coefficient. Bone or air in a voxel depicting soft tissue will significantly raise or lower the averaged attenuation reading of that voxel. This leads to blurring of the margin of the object when it is oblique to the plane of the section

2. Soft tissue silhouetting is the silhouetting of small dense structures which may occur when soft tissue densities such as normal adjacent

Thin plate of bone a 2 different planes to the tomographic section

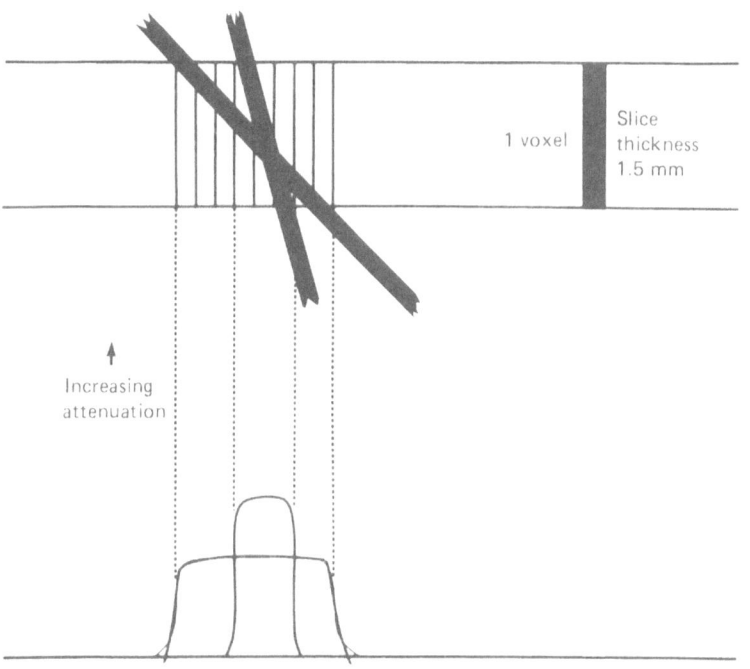

Problems with partial volume averaging and soft tissue silhouetting   b

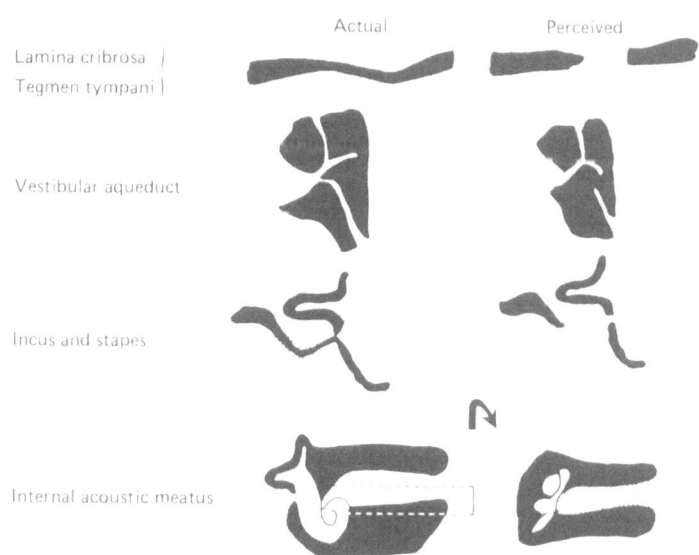

Fig. 1.21 a. The difficulties of imaging a thin plate. At certain angles to the X-ray beam the plate will appear thicker than it should and averaging of attenuation values may mimic soft tissue. **b** Some practical aspects of problems with CT imaging in otolaryngology. Thin bony plates may not be demonstrated and may be thought to be eroded or dehiscent. Small canals may not be shown, and may be considered to be obliterated. A soft tissue mass surrounding thin bony structures may obscure the bone detail, as in a cholesteatoma around the incudo-stapedial joint, and partial volume averaging may suggest a soft tissue mass within the internal canal at air meatography. (From Scott Brown's *Otolaryngology.* Vol I, Basic Sciences, Chapter 17.)

brain, haemorrhage, tumour or fluid envelope are contiguous with a structure usually bordered by air. The difference in density between the structures and the background density may be insufficient for their visualisation. This phenomenon is, of course, an even greater problem with the low contrast images of polytomography, and is important in the evaluation of particular abnormalities in conjunction with soft tissue masses or small erosions. Some practical aspects of these two phenomena are demonstrated in Fig. 1.21

Other Problems with CT of the Temporal Bone

1. Partial volume averaging or "Hounsfield" artefact. Dark bands crossing the posterior cranial fossa between the petrous pyramids may obscure a small neuroma in the cerebello pontine angle
2. Patient movement artefacts
3. Dental filling and other high density artefacts. These are mainly a problem with coronal sections, but may be avoided with appropriate gantry tilt and scout view

Radiation Dose

The first essential of CT scanning of the head is that it should be performed with the least amount of radiation to the eye lens and cornea. This is particularly important in high resolution thin section CT scanning because of the high radiation levels used. These can be considerably higher from CT than from properly performed hypocycloidal tomography with lead eye-shields or with the patient in the prone position (Phelps 1987). The subject of radiation to the eyes has not been adequately discussed in most recent textbooks, but it is important because of the multiple sections that are used to study the temporal bone, and therefore the need to keep the eye lens out of the direct beam of X-rays as far as possible on the standard base sections. This can be difficult despite the use of scout views with cursor lines and the tilting gantry of the machine. Using thermoluminescent discs on the corneas of a phantom we recorded a figure of 13 rads for 20 sections 1.5 mm thick as recommended in one textbook for an extended examination of the ear. The anthropological base line runs from the roof of the external auditory meatus to the lower orbital margin. Sections in this plane can be used to study the lower part of the petrous temporal bone without

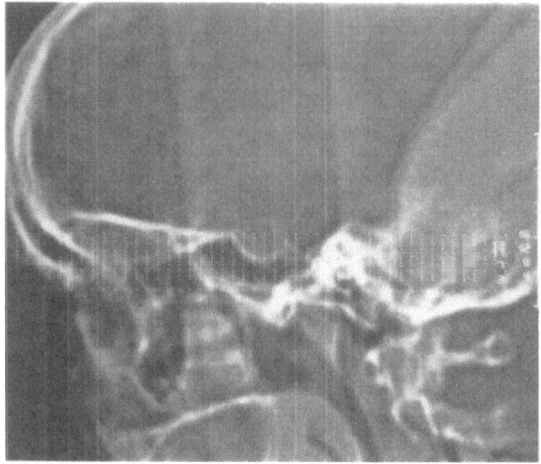

Fig. 1.22. Lateral scout view showing scan planes for a routine base section of the petrous temporal bone.

too much orbital irradiation, but for most examinations of the ear we recommend a plane at 30° to the base line parallel with the roof of the orbit so that the globe is mostly below the sections. The scout view for our standard investigation of the petrous bone is shown in Fig. 1.22. Multiple assessments using the thermoluminescent discs (TLDs) were made with the discs placed on the eyelids of patients. Although only rough estimates can be made we are confident that the dose to the cornea is between 0.9 and 1.8 millisieverts.

The radiographic base line orbito-meatal line is drawn from the centre of the external auditory meatus to outer canthus of the eye. It therefore passes through the centre of the globe and should not be used for base CT sections.

The best discussion of radiation in temporal bone imaging is probably by Curtin (1986). He considers that no specific dosage can be predicted for a CT scan in general. The variables include geometry of the machine, efficiency of collimation, thickness of slice and number and overlap of slice. While it is generally agreed that a dose approaching 200 rads is necessary for the formation of cataracts, this level would only be approached if multiple investigations were undertaken. Nevertheless, monitoring of radiation dosages with thermoluminescent discs placed on the eyelids is recommended, and careful consideration of dosages, particularly in children, advised.

Our machines are capable of 1 or 2-mm sections and for most purposes a thickness of 2 mm is adequate. Localised ossicular disruptions and densitometric measurement of otospongiotic foci (see below) are reasons for using the thinner sections.

We believe that accurate localisation and monitoring by a radiologist are mandatory for such examinations to avoid unnecessary pictures outside the area of interest. For the same reason we do not believe in reformatting techniques which necessitate many "extra" sections to obtain adequate images in other planes. We prefer pluridirectional tomography for lateral views (see above) as the spatial resolution is far superior to reformatted sagittal sections.

Normal CT Scanning of the Temporal Bone

Our routine CT studies of the petro-mastoid use thin sections in the high resolution mode or "bone algorithm". These are viewed on a wide window setting of 3000 or 4000 HU. Contrast enhancement is almost never used if lesions are confined to the petrous pyramid.

Sections in the base plane start just below the external auditory meatus and show the basal turn of the cochlea and round window niche; the mid-modiolor section shows the individual coils of the cochlea and incudo-stapedial region; the section through the vestibule shows the lateral semicircular canal. The last sequence ends with a slice showing the superior and posterior semicircular canals at right angles to each other. Sections at the level of the vestibule best show the internal auditory meatus. The head of the malleus and the short process of the incus are also shown at this level. The three parts of the facial nerve canal can be identified, although the base plane is least satisfactory for the descending portion, which is seen in cross-section behind the middle ear cavity. Although the crura of the stapes may be seen an adequate demonstration of the oval window is not obtained in the base plane. Six of the most important base sections are shown in Fig. 1.23. They should be compared with the anatomical slices shown in Fig. 2.7.

Coronal sections are obtained in the head-hanging or chin-up position to supplement the base views if required (Fig. 1.24). Sections 1 or 2-mm thick are obtained as near as possible in the coronal plane aided by gantry tilt. The radiation dose to the eyes from coronal sections is very low as they are not in the X-ray beam. The sections are very similar to those for the standard study on the polytome which may have to be done if the patient cannot maintain the position for coronal CT.

The six most important coronal sections are shown in Fig. 1.25. They begin at the level of the carotid canal and curl of the central bony spiral of the cochlea. The malleus is well shown at this level.

Further back the section at the level of the vestibule shows the internal auditory meatus as well as the stapes and oval window. Further back still, at the most prominent part of the lateral semicircular canal, the pyramidal eminence is shown between facial recess and sinus tympani. The descending facial canal and jugular fossa are assessed and the examination finishes at the posterior semicircular canal although further sections may be necessary to show the mastoid antrum and aircells.

Reformatted Images

Reformatted images can be obtained from multiple thin contiguous base sections. Reformatted images can be made in any plane but the quality is always inferior to a direct examination and depends on two factors:

1. The number of sections and therefore the amount of raw data available for the reconstruction process
2. Absolute immobility of the patient while these sections are being obtained

We have found reformatting most useful for the study of elongated structures such as the facial nerve (Fig. 1.26).

Soft Tissue Studies in Regions Adjacent to the Petrous Temporal Bone

For suspected abnormalities in the posterior or middle cranial fossae or infratemporal region, the regime of investigation is different. Thicker sections, usually 4 or 5 mm, are obtained on standard resolution to maximise density discrimination and intravenous contrast enhancement is usually required and is always necessary if the presence of an acoustic neuroma is suspected (see Chap. 9).

Intravenous Contrast Enhancement

The standard procedure is to inject 50 ml of iodine-containing contrast medium, but for very vascular tumours such as glomus tumours a rapid infusion of 250 ml is preferred, enabling the lesion to be enhanced in the vascular phase, i.e., with the contrast actually in the blood vessels rather than in the later extravasion phase with the contrast mainly in the extracellular spaces. This phase is more important for intracranial lesions. We rarely perform rapid sequential (dynamic) scanning for evaluation of vascular lesions although in some circumstances

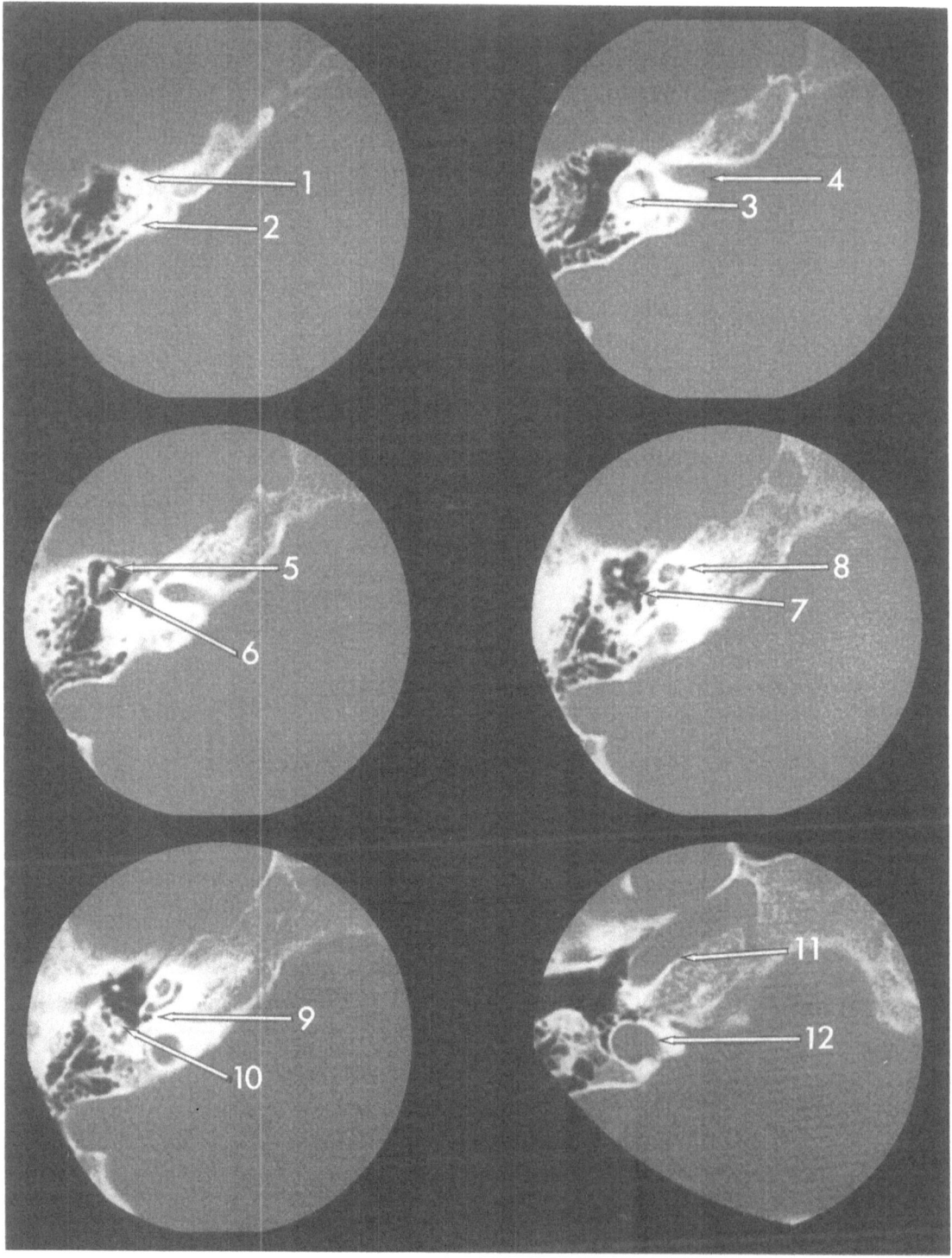

Fig. 1.23. Six basal CT sections of the middle and inner ears: 1, superior semicircular canal; 2, posterior semicircular canal; 3, lateral semicircular canal; 4, internal auditory meatus; 5, malleus; 6, incus; 7, stapes; 8, cochlea; 9, round window; 10, pyramidal eminence; 11, carotid canal; 12, jugular fossa.

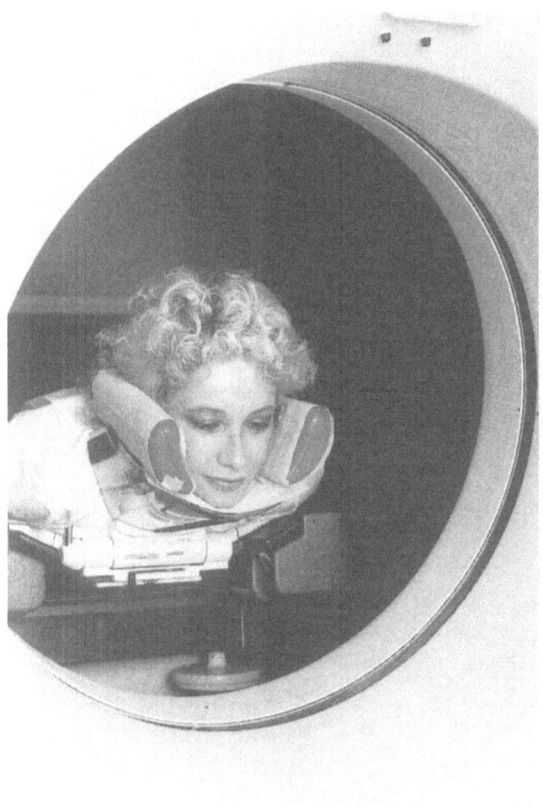

Fig. 1.24. Position for coronal sections.

the air to pass through the foramen magnum and into the cerebello-pontine angle. The first section is made at the level of the internal auditory meatus and, if air is demonstrated within the meatus, the examination is terminated (Fig. 1.27).

The seventh and eighth cranial nerves and the loop of the anterior inferior cerebellar artery can usually be recognised (Fig. 1.28). Air may enter the medial aperture of the cochlear aqueduct – a feature of negligible importance so long as this is not thought by the observer to be the porus of the internal auditory meatus.

Air meatography can be performed on an out-patient basis. However, although it seems free of any serious complications, there is a significant incidence of unpleasant side effects. The best analysis of these has been made by Greenberger et al. (1987), who found 72% of 84 patients to have prolonged headaches and other ill effects for a variable time after the procedure. They now recommend 24 h post-injection bed rest.

Other intrathecal contrast agents are rarely used in otoradiology. Large extra-axial masses in the posterior cranial fossa are not satisfactorily demonstrated by air CT studies and, if not clearly defined on the enhanced CT scan and magnetic resonance is not available, they are best outlined by a positive intrathecal enhancing agent such as Iopamidol (Niopam), which can show the relation of the tumour to the brainstem. An example of this is a cholesteatoma of congenital origin in the cerebello-pontine angle (Fig. 7.11).

helpful information can be obtained in such a manner.

Air Meatography: the demonstration of the contents of the internal auditory meatus and cerebello-pontine angle

Air CT meatography, otherwise known as gas cisternography is a simple and effective procedure which at present is the only sure way to demonstrate a small intrameatal acoustic neuroma other than the use of Gadolinium enhanced magnetic resonance (see Chap. 10); it is also the only certain way to exclude a neuroma, by outlining the normal nerves in the meatus. The patient lies on his side on the scanner table with the ear to be examined uppermost; a lumbar puncture is performed and cerebrospinal fluid sent for differential protein estimation. The patient is positioned at a sufficient spinal gradient to allow 3 ml of air introduced via the cannula to pass into the cervical region. After 2 min the head is elevated momentarily, to allow

Magnetic Resonance

Sectional magnetic resonance pictures in the region of the skull base are a valuable adjunct to CT, provided suitable scanning parameters are chosen to produce optimum signal strength and contrast, and to enable the lesion to be distinguished from surrounding structures. Bone produces a negligible signal on MR scans and so both the bone of the petromastoid and the air in the middle ear cleft and mastoid cell system appear as black areas on the scan, devoid of any of the bone detail so well demonstrated by conventional tomography and high resolution CT scan (Fig. 1.29). Thus, only soft tissue structures within the petrous temporal bone are imaged and this can be an advantage for the demonstration of the cranial nerves passing through the skull base, as the nerve itself will be shown, not the canal in which it lies (Fig. 1.30). In contrast to

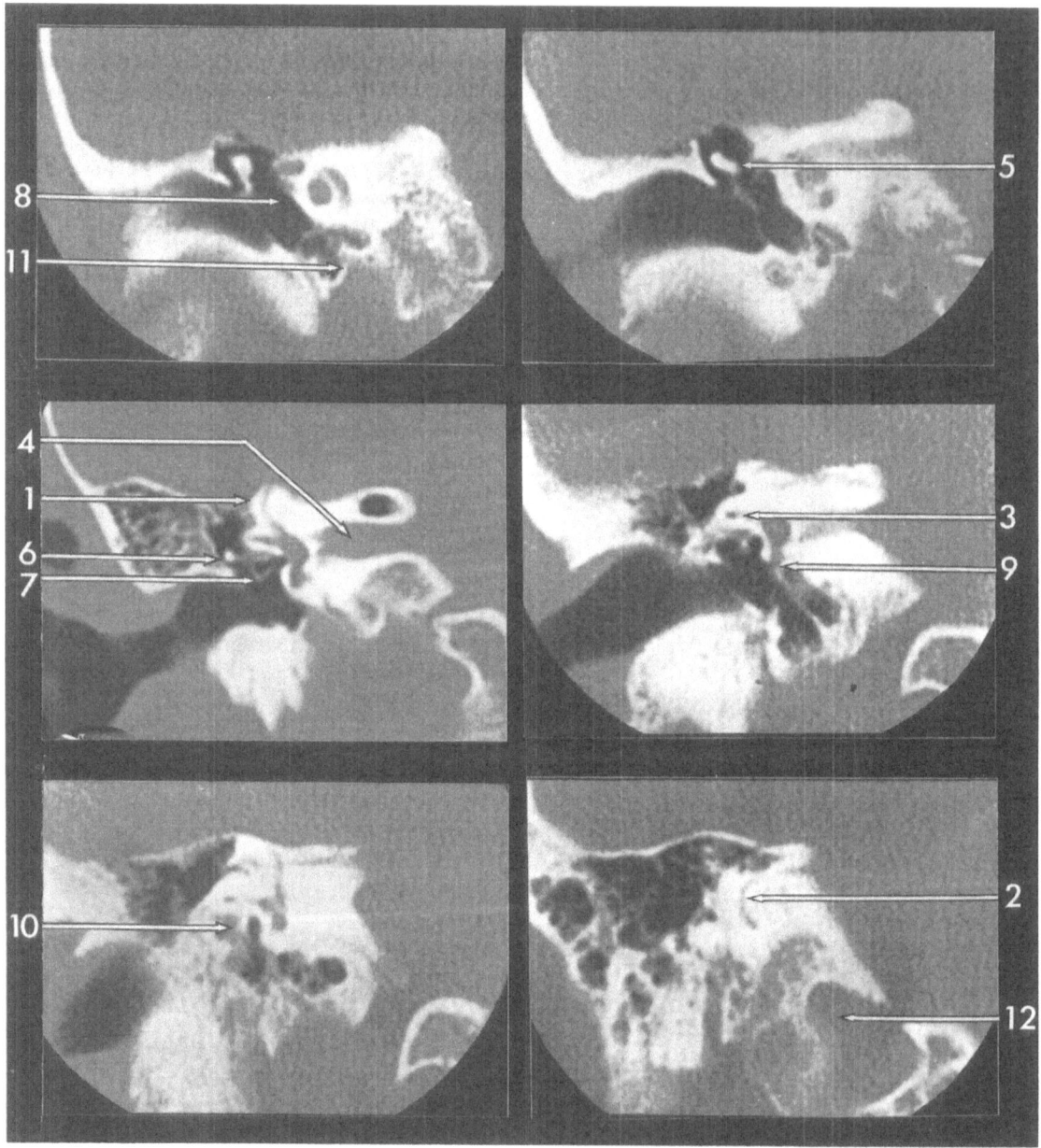

Fig. 1.25. Six important coronal sections with labelling as in Fig. 1.23.

the absence of signal from compact bone, marrow spaces which are very variable in extent but occur mostly in the petrous apex, give an intense signal because of their high fat content, particularly on T_1-weighted images.

Superior density resolution without contrast enhancement, absence of artefacts, and the poten-tial for three-plane imaging mean that MR is already replacing CT for the demonstration of masses in the posterior cranial fossa. Intra-axial masses are particularly well shown.

Cerebrospinal fluid in the cerebello-pontine angle and internal auditory meatus behaves like intra-ventricular fluid having a low signal intensity on

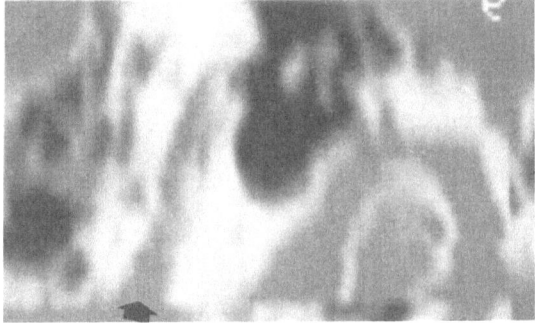

Fig. 1.26. Reformatted lateral view showing the external meatus, temporo-mandibular joint and descending facial nerve canal (*arrow*).

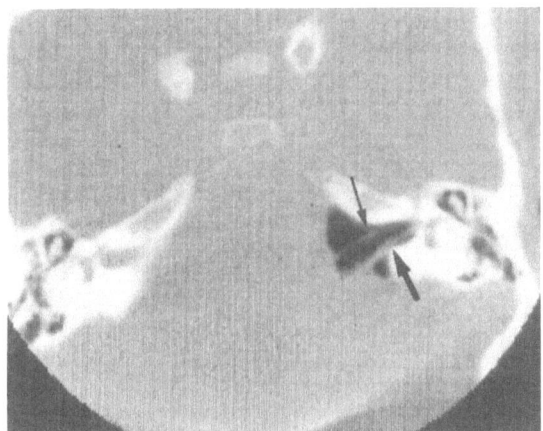

Fig. 1.27. Air CT meatogram. The *large arrow* indicates the VIIIth nerve, the smaller the VIIth nerve.

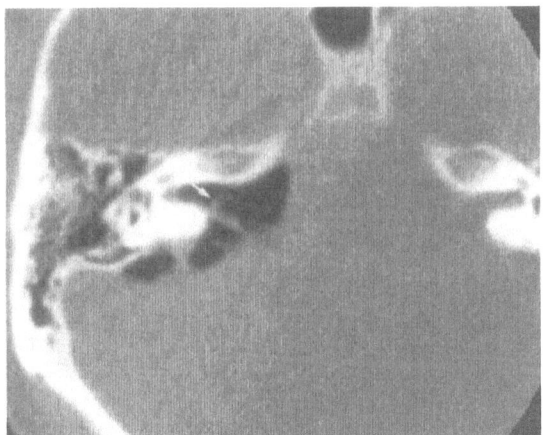

Fig. 1.28. Air CT meatogram. The *arrow* points to the loop of the AICA in the IAM.

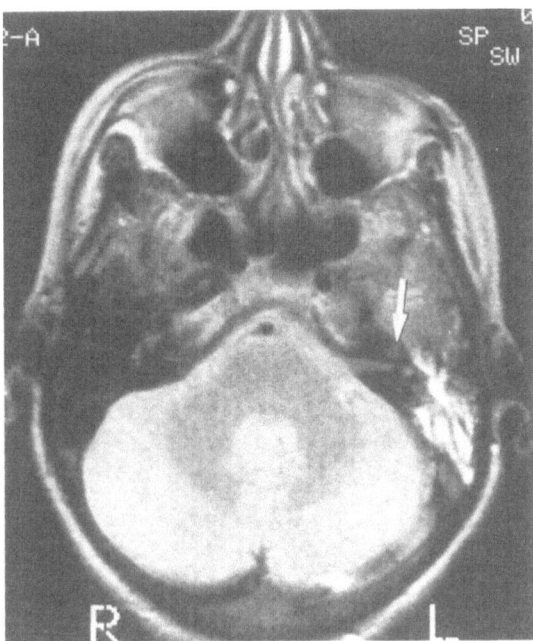

Fig. 1.29. Base of skull T_2-weighted MR scan. The bright signal is from a serous otitis in the left mastoid. Compare with the lack of signal from the other normal side, note the less bright signal from marrowfat in the petrous apices and basisphenoid and the differentiation of white from grey matter in the cerebellum. The arrow points to the cochlea.

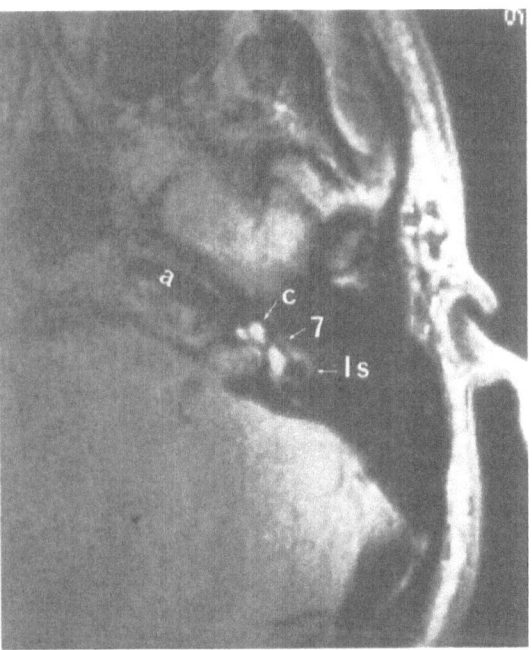

Fig. 1.30. Normal MR of the petrous bone with surface coil, a, carotid artery; c, cochlea; 7, second part of the facial nerve; ls, lateral semicircular canal.

T_1-weighted spin echo sequences (Fig. 1.31) and a high signal on T_2-weighted spin echo sequences using a long time to echo. Thus, on the latter, the CSF appears similar to positive contrast CT cisternograms. Problems in identifying small intrameatal tumours and the use of Gadolinium DTPA will be considered in Chap. 10. Flowing blood gives no signal and thus vessels normally appear black. Magnetic resonance is therefore very useful for the initial demonstration of aneurysms and vascular malformations.

Special surface coils placed on the side of the head can greatly improve spacial resolution and even enable the individual nerves to be identified in the

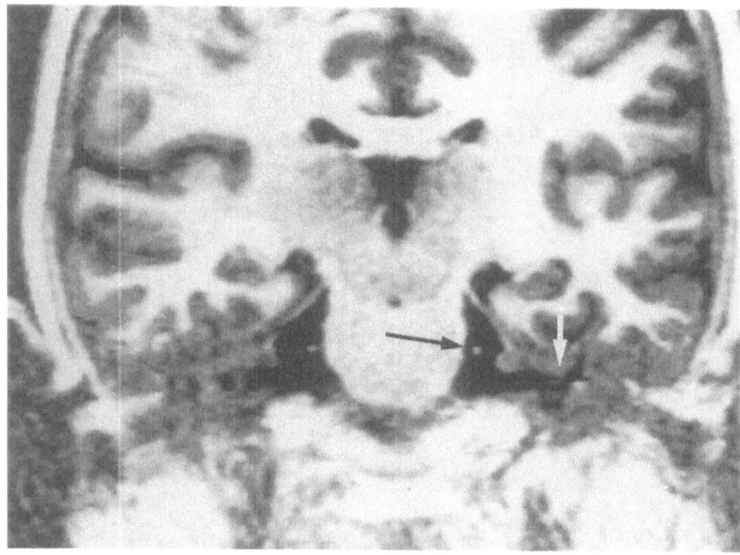

Fig. 1.31. A coronal inversion recovery MR section through the IAMs. On this most T_1-weighted protocol of all, the CSF appears black as do the fluids in the labyrinth (*white arrow*). The *black arrow* points to the trigeminal nerve.

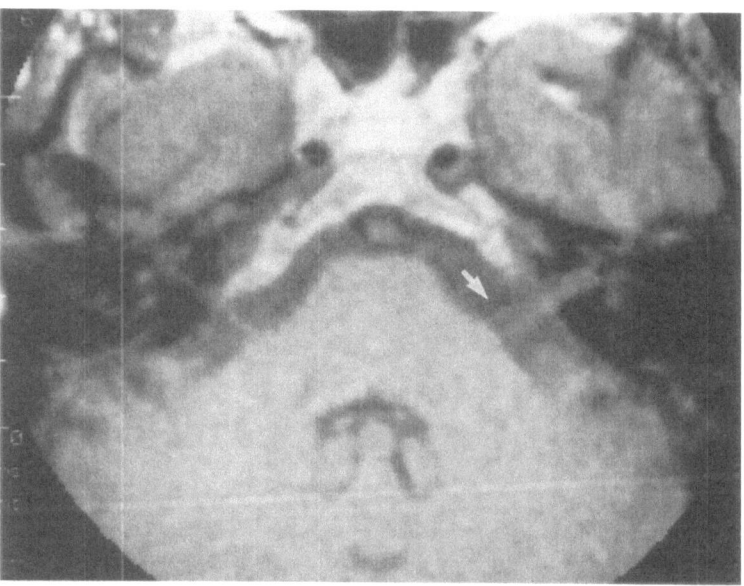

Fig. 1.32. Base short spin echo T_1-weighted MR image showing the nerves in the cerebello-pontine angle (*arrow*).

internal auditory meatus. However, surface coils have two major disadvantages;

1. There is progressive diminution of signal strength away from the coil, making comparison between superficial and deep structures difficult
2. Comparison with the opposite side is not possible

As spatial resolution improves and thinner sections can be obtained, it becomes possible to identify individual nerves in the cerebello-pontine angle, thus decreasing the likelihood of signal from normal nervous tissue (Fig. 1.32) being misinterpreted as representing the presence of an acoustic neuroma.

Angiography

The success of computerised tomography and, more recently, of magnetic resonance in demonstrating the position and extent of lesions in the petrous temporal bone, has meant a progressive reduction in the need for angiography, which now has a minor role. Except for the recently developed digital vascular imaging, almost all angiography of the head and neck is now done by catheterisation of the femoral artery, followed by manipulation of the tip of the catheter into the appropriate vessel under fluoroscopy control. High resolution image intensification together with rapid automatic film changing and advances in catheter technology have led to selective and super-selective examination of the area of interest. Angiography is now used principally in cases of cerebral ischaemia and of intracranial haemorrhage, and in the diagnosis of aneurysm and angiomatous malformations. It still has a role for vascular tumours, particularly glomus jugulare; and there has recently been an increased therapeutic application, particularly in the treatment of glomus tumours. The types of investigation may be listed as follows:

1. Arch aortography. This is used – although rarely now – for the demonstration of the major vessels of the neck
2. Common carotid injection
3. Internal carotid injection. This is used mainly for intracranial lesions
4. External carotid injection. This is used principally for lesions of the face, and for demonstrating the blood supply of meningiomata. Super-selection of branches of the external carotid, particularly the ascending pharyngeal and the maxillary artery, are important for

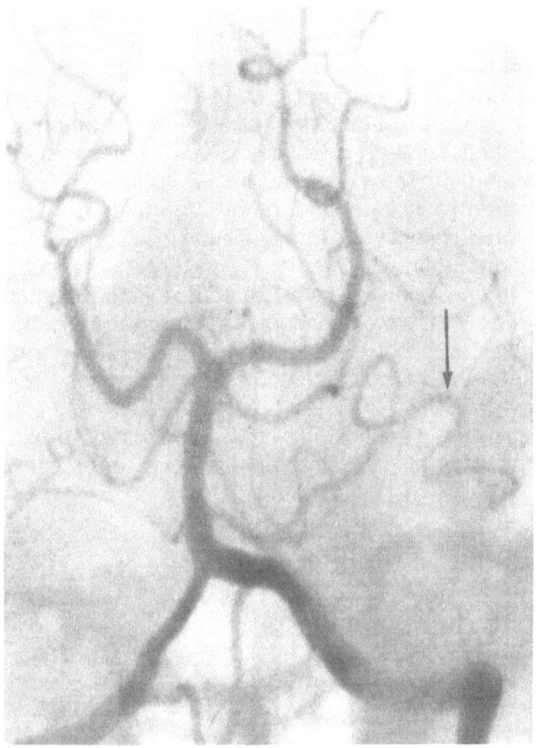

Fig. 1.33. Preoperative vertebral angiogram. The arrow points to the loop of the anterior inferior cerebellar artery, adjacent to the porus of the left IAM. On this side the AICA is larger than the PICA, an unusual variant.

embolisation techniques. Anastomoses with the internal carotid supply can also be demonstrated
5. Vertebral angiography. This was formerly used for diagnosing lesions in the posterior cranial fossa. Although it is no longer used in the diagnosis of acoustic neuroma, this type of examination is considered necessary preoperatively by some surgeons for showing the vascular architecture (Fig. 1.33)
6. Retrograde jugulography. This is occasionally used to confirm the diagnosis of a glomus jugulare tumour and to show its lower limits. The sigmoid sinus and the jugular bulb can often be shown in the venous phase of a carotid angiogram, and also by magnetic resonance

Digital Angiography

Digital subtraction angiography (DSA) is a modified form of the subtraction technique used in vascular imaging. The essential difference between DSA and photographic subtraction lies in the digitisation of the video signals from an image intensifier television system. This is followed by subtraction contrast enhancement and reconversion to analogue signals, which are subjected to further enhancement by windowing and greyscale manipulation – methods similar to those used for viewing CT images. In some systems image enhancement is performed digitally and the resultant data are subsequently converted into analogue form for the television display.

It was hoped initially that intravenous digital subtraction would completely replace intra-arterial procedures, but such techniques necessitate large doses of contrast agent, and have been largely unsuccessful.

The main applications of intravenous DSA are in the study of the extracranial cerebral arteries, of certain intracranial lesions, such as large aneurysms, and of arterio-venous malformations; and in the diagnosis of cerebral venous sinus disease. A good review of the subject and the advantages and disadvantages of both intravenous and intra-arterial DSA is given by Dawson (1988).

Intra-arterial DSA allows a low concentration of contrast medium and finer catheters to be used, reducing the risk of arterial damage. The rapid subtraction with real time display and the ability to study selected frames make this an ideal preliminary to interventional techniques, although the inferior resolution for small vessels can be a problem. The efficacy of embolisation and any alterations of flow which might take place can be immediately assessed, although at present the intra-arterial techniques (Fig. 1.34) appear more satisfactory than

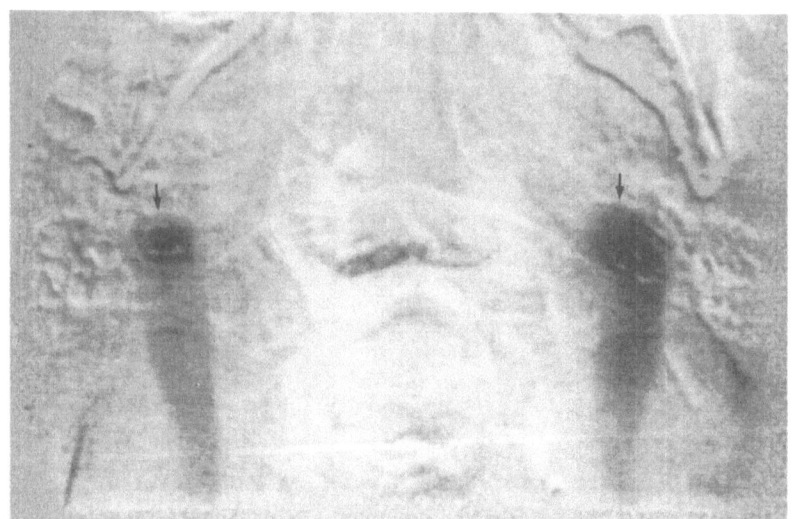

a

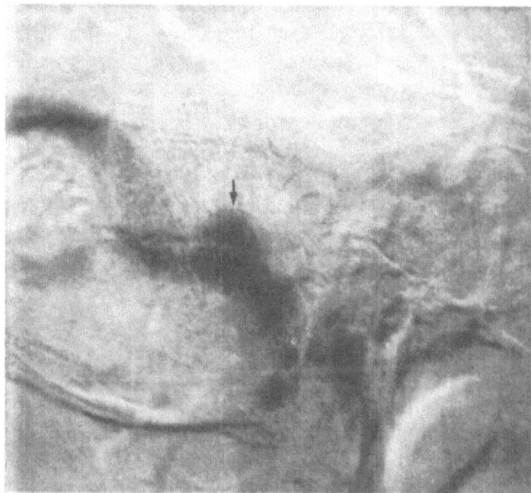

b

Fig. 1.34 a, b. Digital subtraction angiography in coronal (a) and lateral (b) planes showing the normal jugular bulb (*arrow*).

the intravenous ones, and are especially useful for children, where strict limitation of contrast dose is necessary.

Embolisation Techniques

Embolisation is a technique of intravascular occlusion in which catheters are selectively manipulated into a pathological vascular territory for the purpose of injecting occlusive or embolic agents. Detachable balloons have been used to obliterate large vascular fistulae, and a great variety of embolic agents – such as gelfoam, silicone spheres, tantalum powder and various chemical agents – have been used to obliterate feeding vessels of tumour, usually as a prelude to surgery. Super-selective catheterisation is an essential preliminary. Occlusion of the nidus of the lesion, and not merely of the feeding pedicle, should be performed; and the distal migration of the emboli to the venous circulation, and beyond it, must be prevented. Such procedures should be carried out only in a few specialist neuroradiological centres.

References

Chin FK, Andersen WB, Gilbertson DH (1970) Radiation dose in petrous tomography. Radiology 94:623–627

Dawson P (1988) Digital subtraction angiography. Clin Radiol 39:474–477

Curtin H (1986) In: Vignaud J, Jardin C, Rosen L (Eds) The ear: diagnostic imaging. Masson, Paris, p 101

Greenberger R, Khangure MS, Chakera TMH (1987) The morbidity of CT air meatography: a follow-up of 84 patients. Clin Radiol 38:535–536

Lloyd GAS, Du Boulay GN, Phelps PD, Pullicino P (1979) The demonstration of the auditory ossicles by high resolution CT. Neuroradiology 18:243–248

Lloyd GAS, Wylie IG (1971) Zonography of the petrous temporal bone. Br J Radiol 44:940–945

Naviez JP, Cornelis G (1973) L'étude radiologique de la chaîne ossiculaire en profil incline préétudié. Acta Otolaryngol Belg 27:488–491

Phelps PD (1987) Computerized imaging of the ear. Editorial. Clin Otolaryngol 12:401–404

Phelps PD, Lloyd GAS (1986) Vascular masses in the middle ear. Clin Radiol 37:359–364

Radberg C, Thibaut A (1971) Supine skull radiography with orbix. Solna, Sweden, Elema Schonander.

Schuller A (1905) Die Schadelbasis in Rontgenbild. Lucas Grafe u Sielern, Hamburg.

Stahle J, Wilbrand H (1974) The vestibular aqueduct in patients with Ménières disease: a tomographic and clinical investigation. Acta Otolaryngol 78:36–48

2 Anatomy and Development of the Ear

Anatomically the ear is usually divided into three parts:

1. The external ear, consisting of the auricle or pinna and the external auditory meatus
2. The middle ear, which is a vertical cleft continuous via the mastoid antrum with the network of mastoid air cells
3. The inner ear, comprising the organs of hearing and balance embedded in the dense bone of the petrous pyramid

Development in the Embryo

The primitive otic vesicle or otocyst of ectodermal origin undergoes a tortuous differentiation from the fifth to the ninth week to become the membranous labyrinth (Fig. 2.1), while the surrounding mesoderm develops into cartilage and eventually forms the hard bony labyrinthine capsule. At the same time the tubotympanic recess situated between the first and second branchial arches (an extension from the primitive pharynx) becomes involved anterolaterally with the developing ear capsule. In this way the tympanic cavity and proximal part of the Eustachian tube are included in the petrous temporal bone. Further differentiation of the middle ear around the branchial arch elements from the twelfth to the twenty second week gives rise to the ossicles (Fig. 2.2) and further extension of the cavity to the mastoid antrum and air cells. The first ectodermal branchial cleft forms the external auditory

meatus and where this meets the middle ear cleft, the eardrum (tympanic membrane) is formed. Arrest of these processes is often a feature of congenital malformations.

The Temporal Bone

The temporal bone is formed by the fusion of four morphologically distinct parts: the squamous, petromastoid, and tympanic portions and the styloid process. The squamous forms part of the floor and lateral wall of the middle cranial fossa. The petrous pyramid projects forwards and inwards at 45° to the sagittal plane, forming the boundary between the middle and posterior cranial fossae. The enclosed labyrinth is of adult size at birth. The dense bone of the labyrinthine capsule is almost avascular and has no capacity to form new bone, a factor of importance in the healing of fractures involving the bony labyrinth. The mastoid portion of the temporal bone is at first flat and the stylomastoid foramen, through which the facial nerve emerges, lies immediately behind the tympanic ring. As air cells develop, the lateral part of the mastoid portion grows downwards and forwards to form the mastoid process. Hence the stylomastoid foramen comes to lie on the undersurface of the bone. The tympanic ring is formed in membrane and is an incomplete circle, deficient above. It comes to form the medial two thirds or bony part of the external auditory meatus. The styloid process is developed from the cartilage of the second branchial arch.

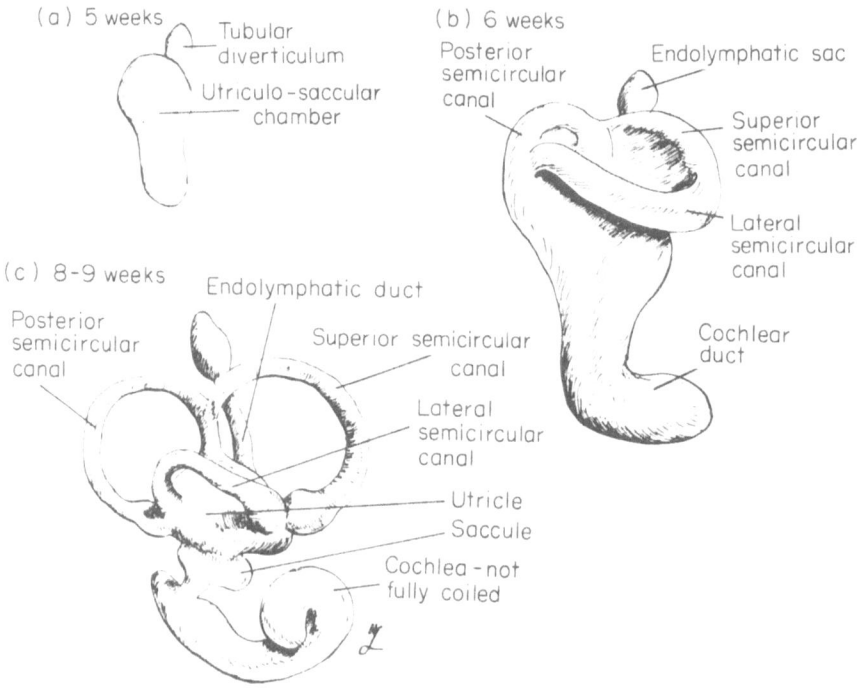

Fig. 2.1. Development of the labyrinth of the inner ear. (From Mawson and Ludman 1979.)

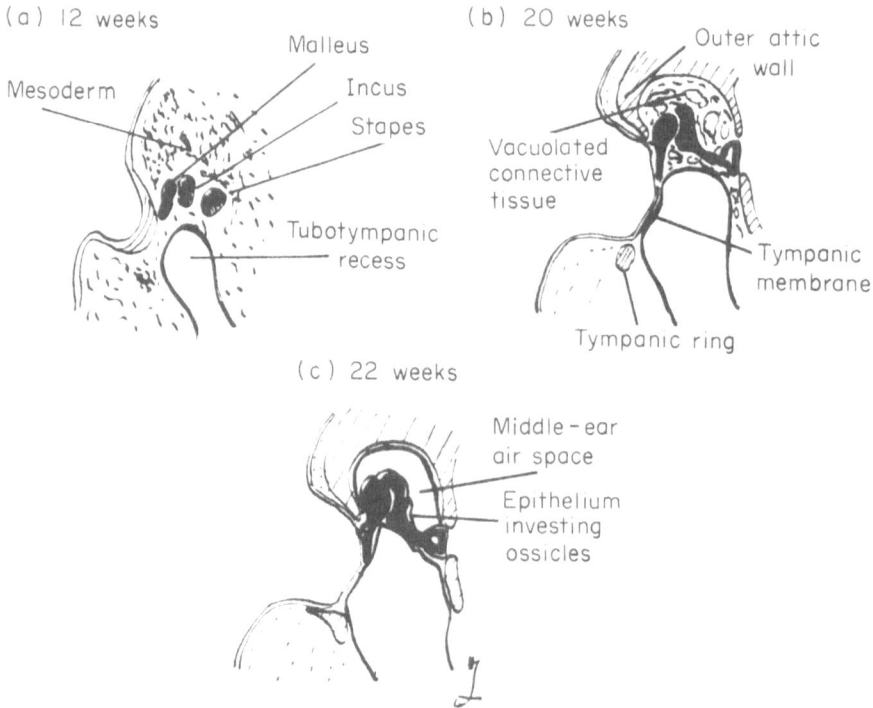

Fig. 2.2. Development of the middle ear. (From Mawson and Ludman 1979.)

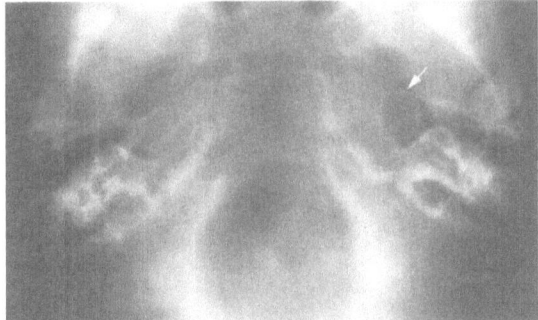

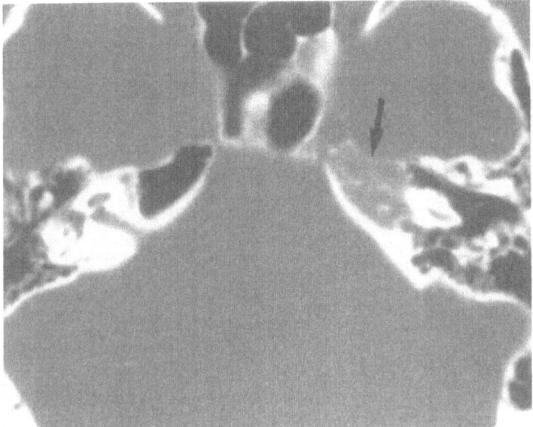

Fig. 2.4. Base CT shows a giant air cell in one petrous apex and bone marrow in the other (*arrow*). Bone marrow contains much fat and this gave a strong signal on an MR scan, which was mistakenly thought to be a unilateral abnormality.

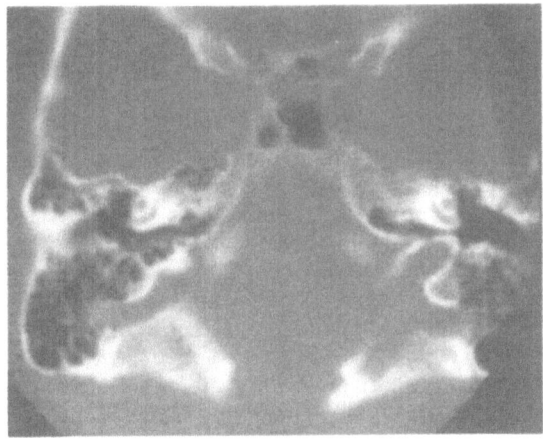

Fig. 2.3. a Normal plain SMV radiograph shows a unilateral giant aircell in the petrous apex (*arrow*). b. Base CT section shows asymmetrical pneumatisation of the petrous apex but also chains of air cells under the labyrinth.

Pneumatisation of the Mastoid

The mastoid antrum is invariably present at birth but it is only with the onset of crying and breathing that the mucoid material in the middle ear cavity and Eustachian tube becomes replaced by air. The mastoid air cells are then developed as outgrowths budding from the mastoid antrum. The cells invade the mastoid process. Pneumatisation of the petrous pyramid may occur. While the onset of pneumatisation is generally agreed to be soon after birth and completion is not expected for at least 2 years, this is by no means the rule, and acute mastoiditis may occur in infants aged under 1 year. There is also great variation in the degree of pneumatisation and 20% of mastoids never become fully pneumatised. Whether this is the result of individual variation dependent on the genetic pattern or whether it is due to arrest by pathological processes is still the subject of much debate. Generally three types of definitive mastoid are recognised:

1. Cellular, where air cells are large and numerous
2. Diploic, where air cells are small and less numerous and where marrow spaces are also present
3. Sclerotic (or ivory), where cells and marrow spaces are absent

It is generally believed that a sclerotic mastoid is the end result of infective processes leading to osteitis of the cellular septa. There is much histological evidence for this (Friedman 1974), although whether infection or failure of aeration due to blockage of the Eustachian tube can interfere with mastoid pneumatisation is less certain.

Pneumatisation of the petrous pyramid occurs in about 35% of the population. This is frequently asymmetric and 4% of people have giant air cells of variable size and shape (Dubois and Roub 1978) (Fig. 2.3). These air cells were often mistaken for pathological processes on conventional imaging but can now be readily identified by high resolution CT. Rather more of a problem is the marrow fat which is usually present in the petrous apex. The bright MR signal on T_1-weighted images may, if asymmetrical, suggest an apical lesion (Fig. 2.4).

The Inner Ear

The dense bony capsule of the labyrinth is clearly demonstrated on radiographs in the neonatal

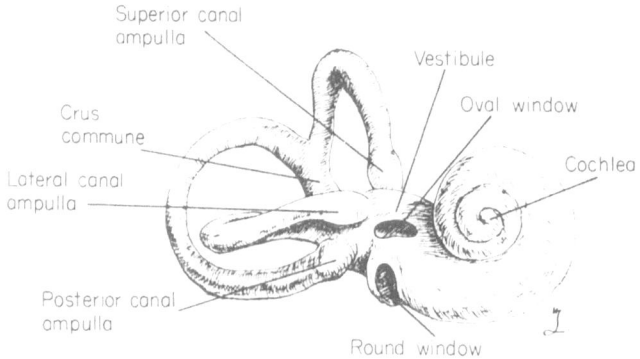

Fig. 2.5. The bony labyrinth. (From Mawson and Ludman 1979.)

period, before it becomes partially obscured by
further ossification of the surrounding petrous
pyramid. The vestibule forms the central portion;
situated between the lateral termination of the
internal auditory meatus (IAM) and the tympanic
cavity, it communicates in front with the basal turn
of the cochlea and behind with the five openings of
the semicircular canals (Fig. 2.5). The three semicircular canals lie at right angles to each other, and
each completes about two thirds of a circle. The
ampulla is a slight dilatation at one end, which
contains the sensory organ. The posterior canal lies
approximately parallel to the posterior surface of
the petrous pyramid. The superior canal runs at
right angles to the long axis of the pyramid and its
highest part forms the arcuate eminence on the
superior aspect of the petrous bone. The horizontal
or lateral semicircular canal bulges into the medial
wall of the attic and antrum. The cochlea lies anteriorly with its apex directed anteriorly and laterally.
The bony canal of the cochlea makes two and a
half turns around a central bony spiral called the
modiolus, in the base of which is situated the spiral
ganglion of the cochlear nerve.

The IAM extends from the medial aspect of the
labyrinth, from which it is separated by the lamina
cribrosa to open onto the postero-medial surface of
the petrous bone at the cerebello-pontine angle. It
contains the nerve and part of the blood supply to
the inner ear. The nerves are the components of the
VIIth and VIIIth (vestibulo-cochlear) cranial nerves;
the facial nerve antero-superiorly, the cochlea nerve
antero-inferiorly and the two vestibular nerves
behind.

Cochlear Aqueduct

The cochlear aqueduct is a narrow channel running
in a slightly S-shaped curve from the basal turn of

the cochlea near the round window in a medial
caudal direction, to end in an infundibular opening
in the anterior division of the jugular foramen. It
connects the subarachnoid space with the perilymphatic space of the inner ear. Its course and
length are correlated to the pneumatisation of the
pyramid, and also to the volume of the jugular
fossa. These two factors influence the radiographic
reproduction of the cochlear aqueduct, especially
on CT in the base projection, and to a lesser degree
on pluridirectional tomography (Muren and Wilbrand 1986). These authors found that the narrowest part of the bony canal had a mean diameter
of 0.14 mm. The aqueduct runs parallel to the IAM,
and therefore the medial part can be readily identified on coronal or base sections. The narrow lateral
part is, however, in our experience rarely if ever
shown extending to the basal turn of the cochlea in
adults (Fig. 2.6).

Vestibular Aqueduct

The vestibular aqueduct extends from the medial
wall of the vestibule to the outer opening in the
posterior surface of the petrous pyramid, and has
the shape of an inverted "J". The proximal segment
of the aqueduct, formed by the short limb of the "J"
extends upwards, medially and posteriorly close to
the crus commune, and then turns to run downwards posteriorly and medially to form the long
limb of the "J". Generally the best projection for
demonstrating the aqueduct is the lateral, but the
proximal segment and the bend or isthmus are very
narrow, and now reliably demonstrated on sectional imaging. There is considerable variation in
the course between individuals, depending on the
degree of surrounding pneumatisation. There have
been comprehensive descriptions of the radiographic anatomy of the vestibular aqueduct, par-

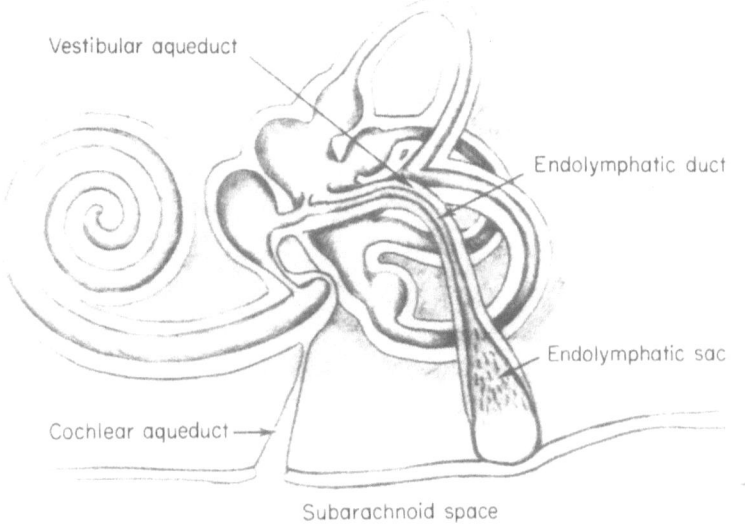

Fig. 2.6. The labyrinth and the cochlear and vestibular aqueducts. (Courtesy of Dr HF Wilbrand.)

ticularly by the Uppsala school (Wilbrand et al. 1974). The significance of the vestibular aqueduct in relation to vertigo will be considered in Chap. 10.

The geometry of the CT scanner is such that the base or horizontal plane is the natural one for sectional imaging with the patient in the supine position. It is fortunate, therefore, that this is also the natural plane for histological sectioning and so a ready comparison can be made between CT and histology sections (Fig. 2.7).

The Middle Ear Cavity

The external and middle ear, which make up the conducting mechanism of hearing, are also contained within the temporal bone. The middle ear cleft comprises the middle ear, the Eustachian tube, the mastoid antrum and cells. The antrum is always present in normal ears although it may vary considerably in size. The middle ear cavity is situated between the labyrinth and the eardrum but extends beyond the limits of the latter and is, therefore, divided into three parts; the hypotympanum, the mesotympanum and the epitympanum or attic. The cavity is continuous with the Eustachian tube in front and the aditus and mastoid antrum behind. On the posterior wall is the pyramidal eminence which surrounds the stapedius muscle (Fig. 2.8). It can be recognised on coronal section imaging as a small "blob" on the section just posterior to the one that shows the oval window. In congenital

malformations, the presence of the pyramidal eminence is a good indication that the facial nerve follows a normal course.

There are several important structures on the medial wall of the middle ear cavity (Fig. 2.9). From the top downwards, these are the lateral semicircular canal, then the canal for the second part of the facial nerve (Fallopian canal). The tensor tympani is a long slender muscle arising from the walls of the bony canal lying above the Eustachian tube. From its origins, the muscle passes backwards into the tympanic cavity where it lies on the medial wall, a little below the level of the facial nerve. The bony covering of the canal is often deficient in its tympanic segment, where the muscle is replaced by a slender tendon. This enters the spoon-shaped processus cochleariformis where it is held down by a transverse tendon as it turns through a right angle to pass laterally and insert into the medial aspect of the upper end of the malleus handle (Fig. 2.10). Below are the openings of the oval window (fenestra vestibuli) and round window (fenestra cochleae) with the promontory formed by the basal turn of the cochlea in front. The roof of the attic and antrum is a thin plate of bone, the tegmen tympani, above which is the dura of the middle cranial fossa. Under the floor of the middle ear lies the jugular bulb.

The internal jugular vein, posteriorly, and the internal carotid artery, anteriorly, are both closely related to the inferior aspect of the middle ear cavity and separated from it by thin plates of bone (Fig. 2.9). A dehiscence may be present and the

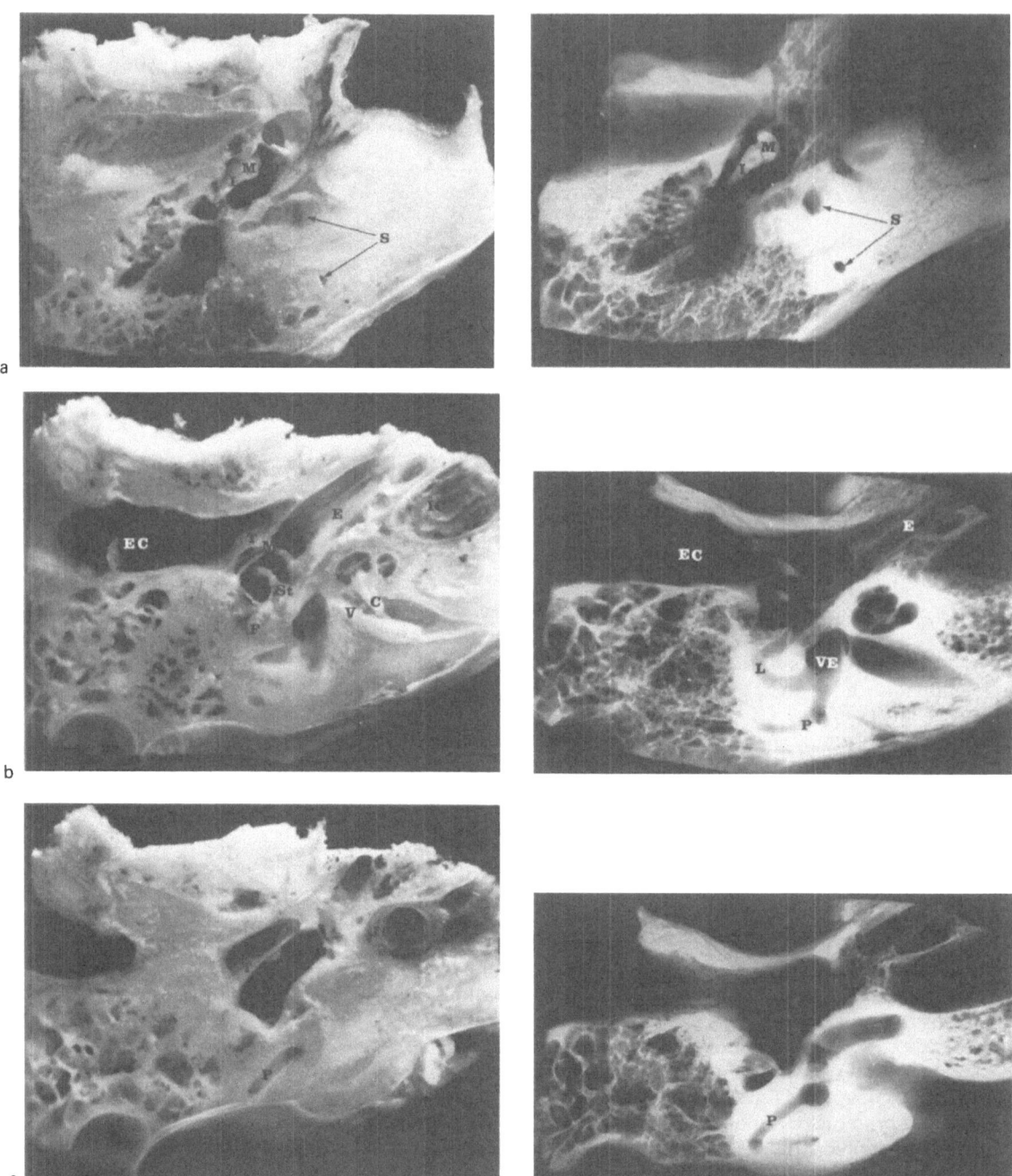

Fig. 2.7. a–c. Microslices through the normal temporal bone. The left-hand photograph is of the gross specimen of the particular slice. On the right is the X-ray of that slice. **a** Microslice passing through the attic region of the middle ear and showing incudomalleal joint. **b** Microslice to include mid-modiolar region of cochlea and showing stapes. The tendon of the stapedius muscle may be seen on the gross photograph, attached to the posterior crus of the stapes. **c** Microslice taken through the basal coil of the cochlea and hypotympanym. C, cochlear branch of eighth nerve; E, Eustachian tube; EC, ear canal; F, facial nerve; I, incus; IC, internal carotid artery; L, lateral semicircular canal; M, malleus; P, posterior semicircular canal; S, superior semicircular canal; St, stapes; T, tympanic membrane; V, vestibular branch of VIIIth nerve; VE, vestibule. (From Michaels 1987.)

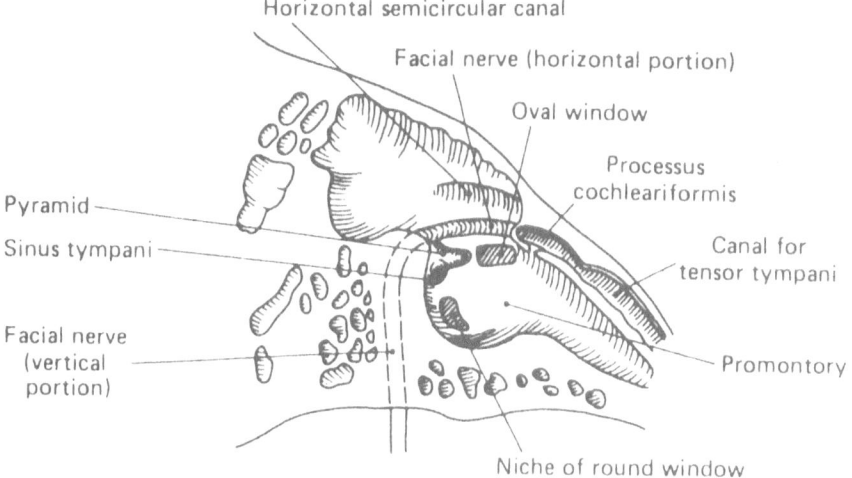

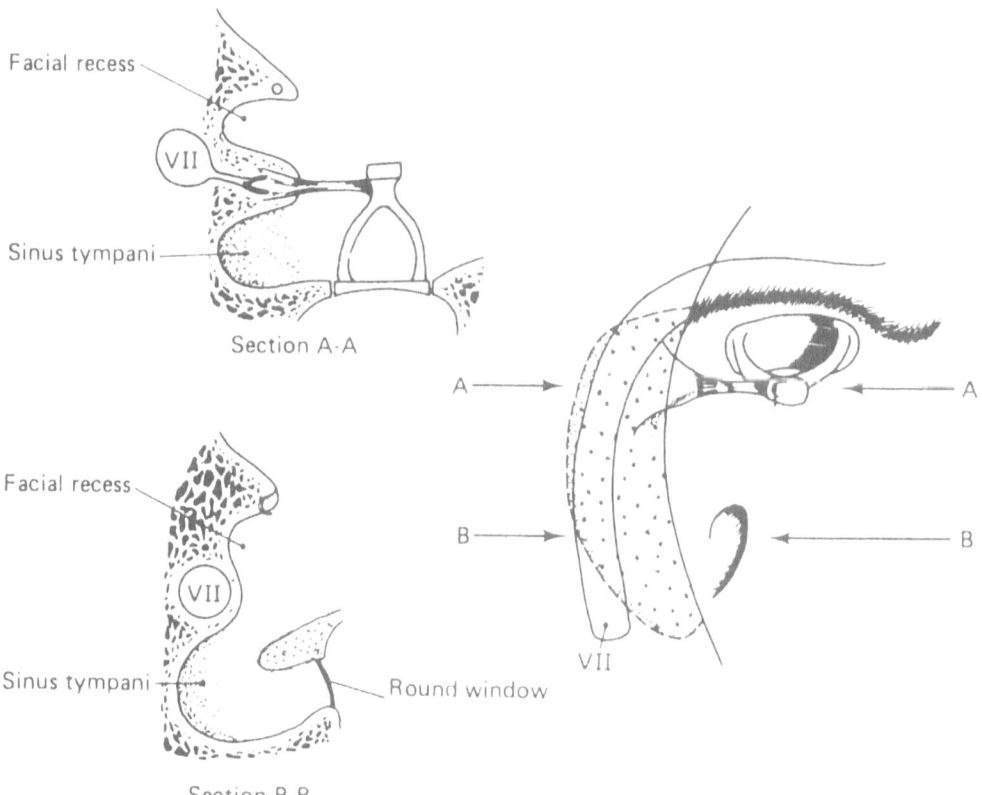

Fig. 2.8. The facial recess and sinus tympani at different levels in the middle ear. Section AA is at the level of the pyramidal eminence and stapes and section BB at the level of the round window where the facial recess and sinus tympani are more shallow. (From Wright (1987) Scott Brown's *Otolaryngology*, Butterworths, London, with permission.)

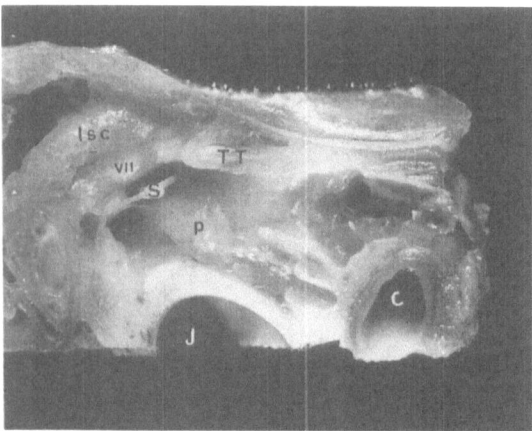

Fig. 2.9. The medial wall of the middle ear cavity. lsc, lateral semicircular canal; VII, second part of the facial nerve canal; TT, tensortympani; S, stapes; P, promontory; J, jugular fossa; C, carotid canal. (From Wright (1987) Scott Brown's *Otolaryngology*, Butterworths, London, with permission.)

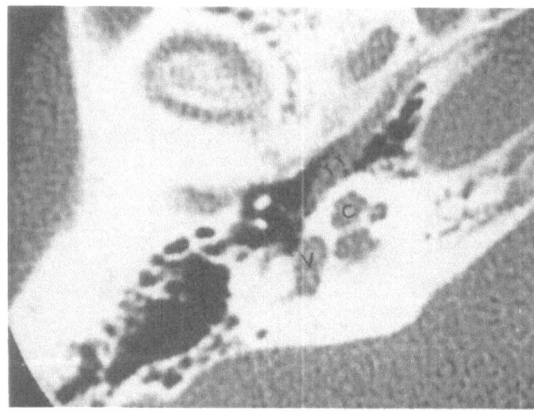

Fig. 2.10. Base CT section through the coils of the cochlea (C) showing the tensortympani muscle (TT) inserting into the head of the malleus. V, vestibule.

vessel is then at risk of being damaged by surgical interference.

The Carotid Canal

In the adult, the internal carotid artery enters the petrous bone through the carotid canal, which lies just medial to the styloid process. Initially, the internal carotid ascends vertically and anterior to the tympanic cavity, then bends sharply anterior and

medial, passing inferior to the Eustachian tube. It then goes through the foramen lacerum and exits into the cranium at the junction of the petrous apex and the basisphenoid. The internal carotid artery lies in close proximity to the tympanic cavity and Eustachian tube. It is usually well covered with bone, although there is said to be dehiscence in 1% of the population (Glasscock et al. 1980). However, these authors were quoting Myerson et al. (1934) who, in a study of pneumatisation, found "pin point" dehiscences in two specimens of 100 pairs of temporal bones. It would seem to us that the incidence of significant congenital bone defects over the carotid artery in the middle ear is considerably less than 1%.

In the human embryo, the carotid circulation is formed from the paired dorsal aortae and their arches. The first and second aortic arches involute early and form the primitive mandibular and hyoid arteries. Just adjacent to the hyoid artery is the third aortic arch, which evolves into the internal carotid artery. In the 6–7-mm embryo, the stapedial artery branches off from the hyoid artery, reaching its largest size when the embryo is 12–15 mm in length. At this time, the stapedial artery forms a connection from the internal to the external carotid through an anastomosis with the middle meningeal. Shortly after this stage, the stapedial artery atrophies, leaving the obturator foramen of the stapes.

Stapedial artery remnants are occasionally noted during routine stapedectomy, although they are rarely of significant size. When present, the stapedial artery courses from the foetal hyoid artery to pass across the promontory and through the obturator foramen of the stapes. The vessel then turns sharply anteriorly and enters the facial Fallopian canal. Usually the persistent stapedial terminates in anastomosis with the trigeminal artery.

Aberrant Internal Carotid Artery

Anomalies of the intrapetrous portion of the carotid artery are very rare and range from simple dehiscence to a soft tissue mass in the middle ear with a foramen in the posterior hypotympanum (Fig. 2.11). If the ascending part of the artery is more posteriorly placed than usual, with a very acute bend, it is probably more likely to be dehiscent (Fig. 2.12), although the crest between the carotid and the jugular bulb will be intact. In more severe aberrations a soft tissue mass will be shown in the middle ear by CT, but the important differentiating feature on coronal CT is absence of the normal carotid canal and a laterally and more posteriorly placed vertical canal (Fig. 2.13). These features

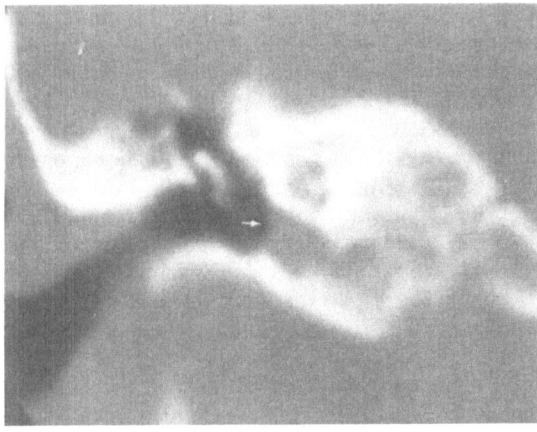
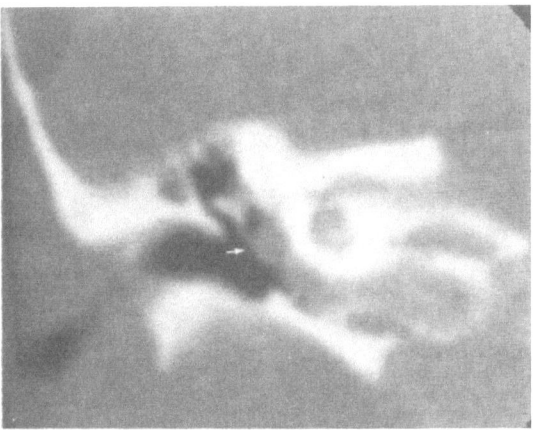

a   b

Fig. 2.11 a, b. Coronal CT sections of two patients with exposed carotid arteries in the middle ear (*arrow*); **a** A mild aberration with dehiscence of the medial wall of the middle ear below the cochlea (*arrow*). There was no confirmation by surgery or angiography but the tympanogram showed characteristic pulsations; **b** A more severe aberration of the internal carotid artery which appears as a soft tissue mass in the middle ear cavity.

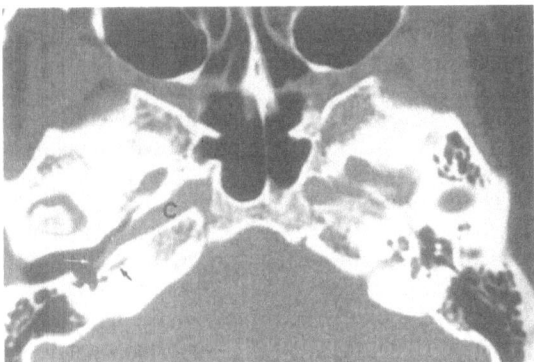
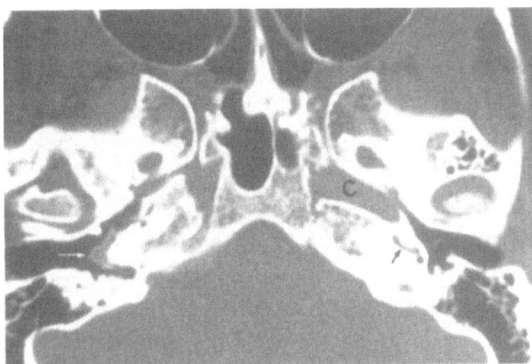

Fig. 2.12. Base CT sections showing the intrapetrous carotids (C). The *white arrow* points to the exposed artery in the middle ear cavity. The *black arrow* indicates the basal turn of cochlea. Note the hypoplasia of the aberrant carotid.

need to be confirmed by angiography, and there should be no attempt at surgical intervention.

We have recently examined by thin section, high resolution CT, three patients with an aberrant internal carotid artery, situated in the middle ear cavity. All were diagnosed with confidence by their CT appearances and although confirmatory angiography was obtained, in retrospect this proved to have been unnecessary. All three showed the characteristic abnormality of the carotid canal and a soft tissue mass in the hypotympanum associated with distinctive erosion and flattening of the promontory. One of these cases had a persistent stapedial artery arising from the acute bend in the carotid (Fig. 2.14). It was, therefore, very similar to the case described by Guinto et al. (1972), but subsequent review of the CT only showed evidence of this

branch on one base view showing the vessel in cross section. Other indications of a stapedial artery described by these authors were not apparent: the foramen spinosum could not be identified with certainty on either side and the Fallopian canal for the second part of the facial nerve was only marginally wider than the canal on the other side. However, modern angiography with subtraction delineates these small vessels with ease.

Jugular Fossa

The jugular foramen is really a short canal housing the jugular bulb, which is formed from the sigmoid

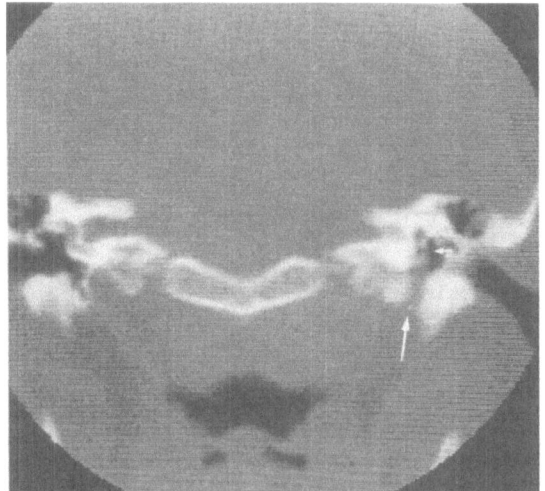

a

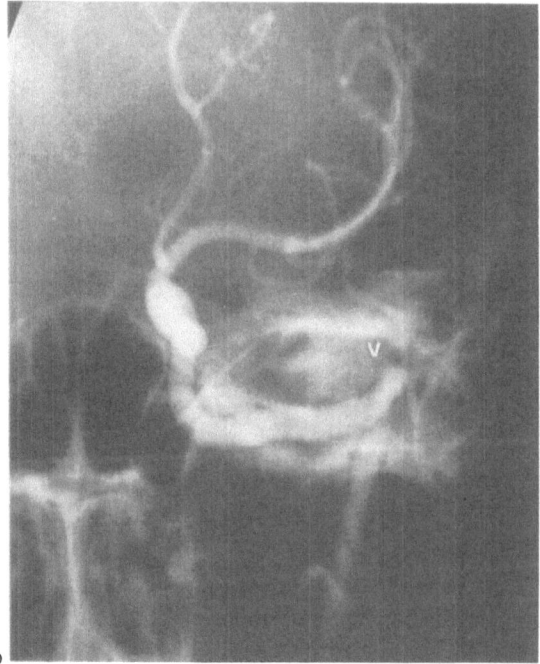

b

Fig. 2.13 a. Coronal CT scan showing the posteriorly placed ascending carotid canal (*large arrow*) at the level of the round window (*small arrow*). Compare with the opposite normal side at the level of the basal turn of cochlea. **b.** Internal carotid angiogram confirms that the artery lies lateral to the vestibule (V) in the middle ear.

and inferior petrosal sinuses. The foramen is bounded medially by the occipital bone and laterally by the temporal bone. A giant jugular foramen needs to be distinguished by its clear-cut margins from a pathologically expanded one.

The anatomy has been comprehensively reviewed by Graham (1975), who quoted dissections by other authors showing the jugular bulb extending above the inferior rim of the annulus in 6% of specimens, and a similar percentage showing dehiscence in the bony floor of the middle ear cavity.

When the jugular bulb is small it is separated from the floor of the middle ear by a comparatively thick layer of bone which is usually compact bone, but may contain air cells. Anteriorly, the bulb is in close relationship to the internal carotid artery but with the IXth, Xth and XIth cranial nerves between. A spur or crest of bone separates the jugular fossa from the carotid canal at the skull base (see Fig. 1.19). When the jugular bulb is very large it can extend up into the mesotympanum with only a thin bony covering, which is easily damaged by instrumentation (Fig. 2.15). Such a high jugular bulb can cause conductive deafness by blocking the round window niche or by interfering with the incudostapedial part of the ossicular chain. When there is dehiscence of the bony covering, the exposed jugular bulb is at even greater risk of inadvertent surgical penetration. Whereas the sigmoid sinus is covered by two layers of dura and the internal jugular vein has a tough adventitia, the jugular bulb has a very thin wall (Glasscock et al. 1980).

The soft tissue mass of a dehiscent jugular bulb is well shown by CT, especially in the coronal plane (Fig. 2.16) and by retrograde jugular venography and magnetic resonance. Whether progressive enlargement of the bulb ever occurs is uncertain, but at least two cases of slow expansion of a jugular bulb have been reported (Graham 1975). Sometimes a diverticulum from the bulb may extend up behind the IAM (Fig. 2.17) and a widened jugular fossa may even extend up to the superior surface of the petrous pyramid. Jahrsdoerfer et al. (1981), besides reviewing previous reports of jugular bulb diverticula, describe surgical exploration of a case in which "the endolymphatic duct was seen to splay over the surface of the diverticulum and be obliterated by it". It was felt that this resulted in endolymphatic hydrops and the typical symptoms of Ménière's disease of which the patient complained.

The most recent work on the high jugular bulb and diverticulum was by the Uppsala School (Wadin and Wilbrand 1986). The radioanatomy of the temporal bone was investigated in plastic or silicone casts of 245 tomographically examined temporal bone specimens. Fossae above the lower border of the round window were classified as high ones. The frequency of high fossae, including those situated both medially and laterally, was 24%; they were more common in the right than the left temporal

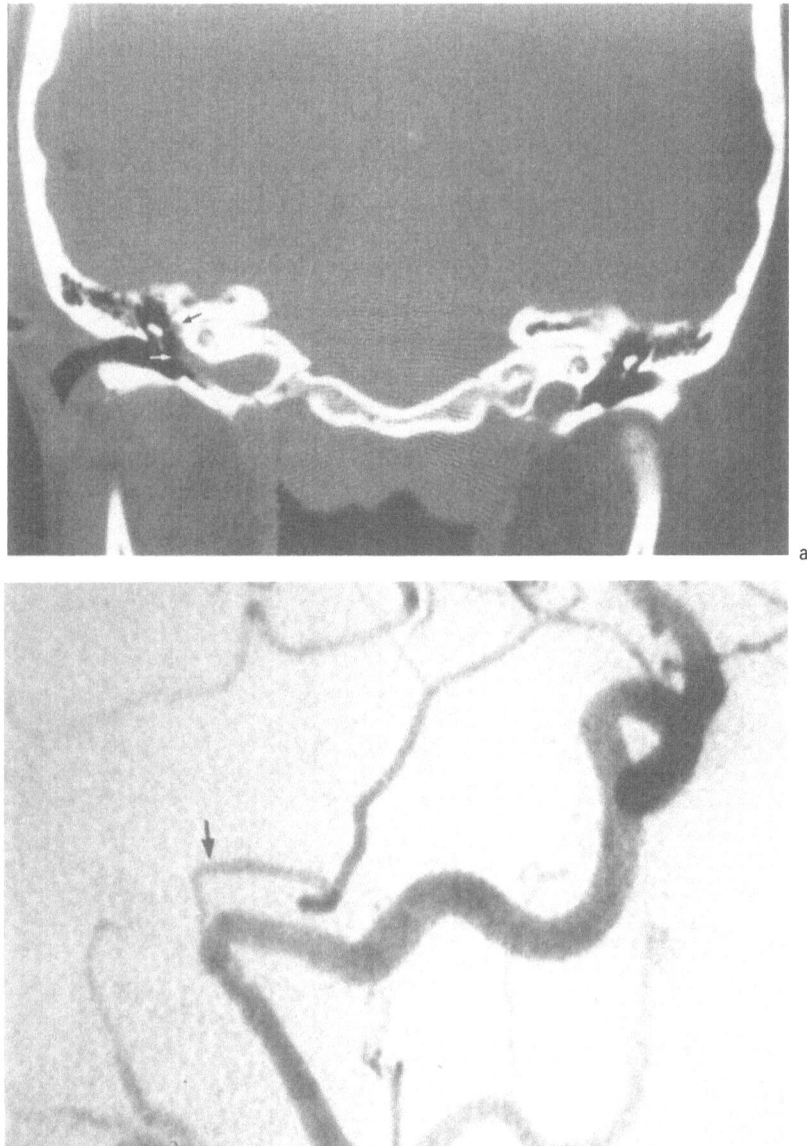

Fig. 2.14 a. Coronal CT section shows a posteriorly placed ascending carotid canal. The canal for the second part of the facial nerve (*black arrow*) appears larger on the affected side but the presence of a persistent stapedial artery in association with this aberrant carotid (*white arrow*), was only shown convincingly by angiography. **b.** Lateral view of internal carotid angiogram showing the stapedial artery (*arrow*).

bone and were usually associated with sparse perilabyrinthine pneumatisation. In some cases, the high jugular fossa encroached upon surrounding structures such as the vestibular and cochlear aqueducts, posterior semicircular canal, cochlea, vestibule, internal acoustic meatus and the mastoid segment of the facial canal.

A diverticulum-like protrusion from the top of a high fossa was found in 17 of 58 temporal bones. The diverticulum was usually directed medio-vertically into the space between the internal auditory meatus, the vestibular aqueduct and the posterior cranial fossa. Few diverticula were directed dorsally or laterally and some high fossae exhibited double

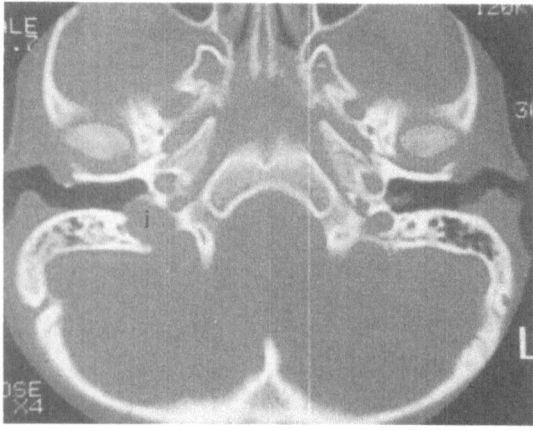

Fig. 2.15. Axial CT scan showing a large jugular fossa (j) bulging into the lower middle ear cavity but with an intact bony covering.

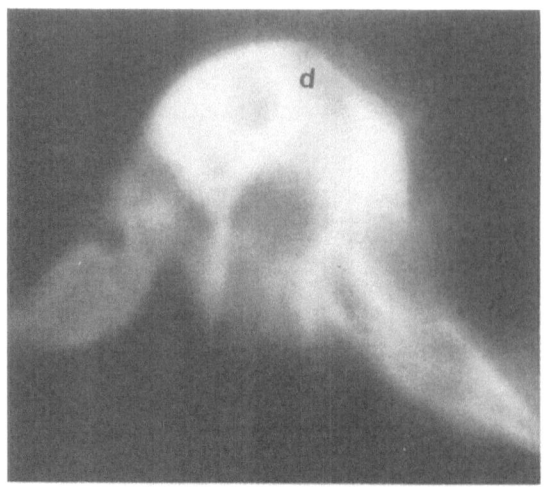

a

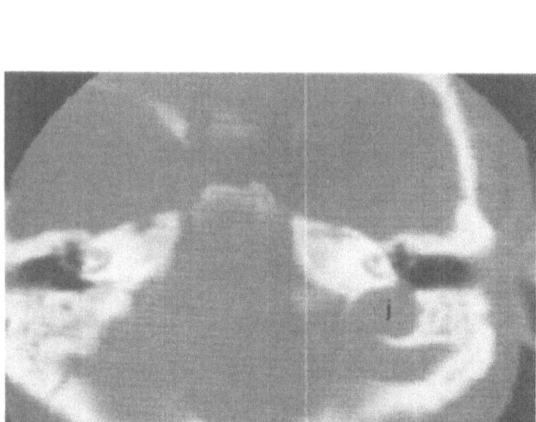

a

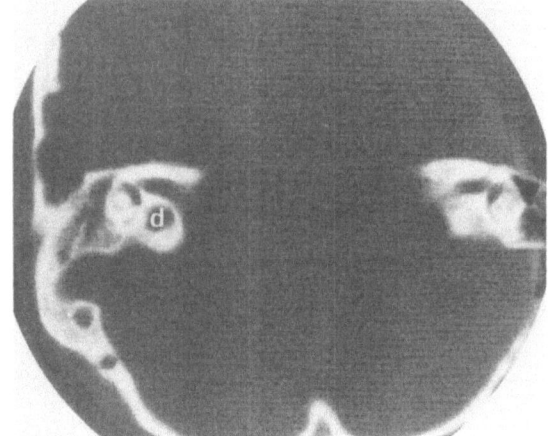

b

Fig. 2.17 a, b. A high jugular bulb with diverticulum (d) reaching to the superior surface of the petrous pyramid; a lateral tomography; b base CT.

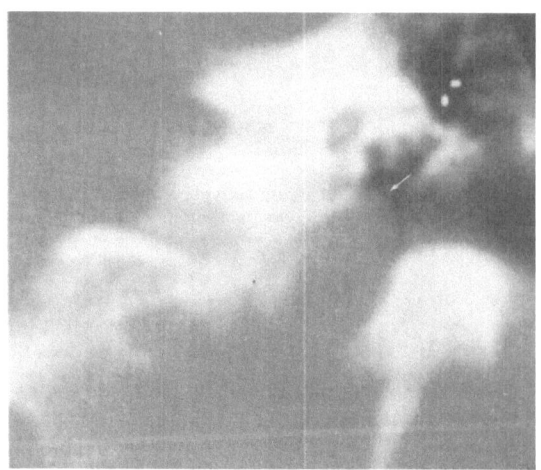

b

Fig. 2.16 a, b. Dehiscent jugular bulb. a Base CT at the level of the cochlea b Coronal CT shows the bare jugular bulb (*arrow*) extending up to the level of the round window.

diverticula. In a clinical material with 112 high jugular fossae, 43 diverticula were found, as diagnosed by multidirectional or computerised tomography (CT). Encroachment of the fossa or diverticulum on surrounding inner ear structures was considered in relation to the clinical symptoms and in some cases no other cause of the symptoms was found. Among 34 patients with Ménière's disease with a high jugular fossa, 35% showed a dehiscence of the vestibular aqueduct, compared with 15% in an unselected material.

We have seen several cases with episodic rotating vertigo, mild sensorineural hearing loss and a giant jugular bulb with diverticulum on the affected side. One of these patients was found to have a purple mass behind an intact eardrum and a jugular venogram showed that the posterior semicircular canal was exposed (Fig. 2.18).

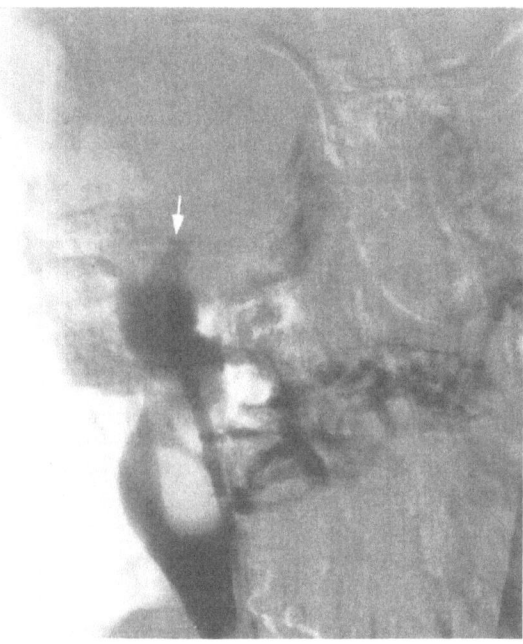

Fig. 2.18. Jugular venogram showing a high jugular bulb with diverticulum (*arrow*) reaching up behind the IAM. More laterally, the bulb can be seen extending into the middle ear cavity.

It is obviously important to define accurately a large jugular bulb either with extension into the middle ear cavity or a diverticulum behind the labyrinth, especially as deafness, tinnitus and vertigo may occur. These can also be presenting features of glomus tumours. Thus, it would seem that a high jugular bulb may cause not only middle ear problems, which can be assessed otoscopically, but also problems from encroachment on inner ear structures which can only be assessed by radiological methods. We still find lateral conventional pluridirectional tomography useful for assessing aberrations of the vascular anatomy in relation to middle ear structures (Fig. 2.19).

Facial Nerve

The facial nerve traverses the petrous bone from the porus of the IAM to the stylomastoid foramen. At the lateral end of the IAM it enters the facial canal, the first part of which runs laterally and forwards above the cochlea to the geniculate ganglion. The second part of the nerve passes backwards and horizontally beneath the lateral semicircular canal. Finally, the third part descends

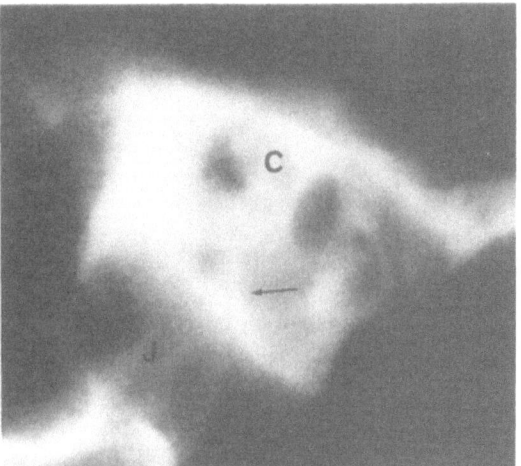

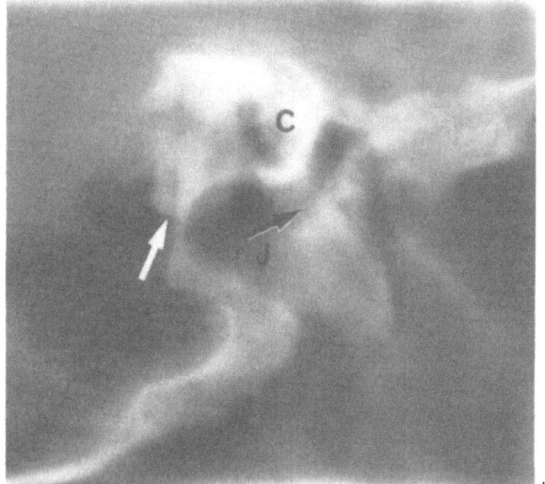

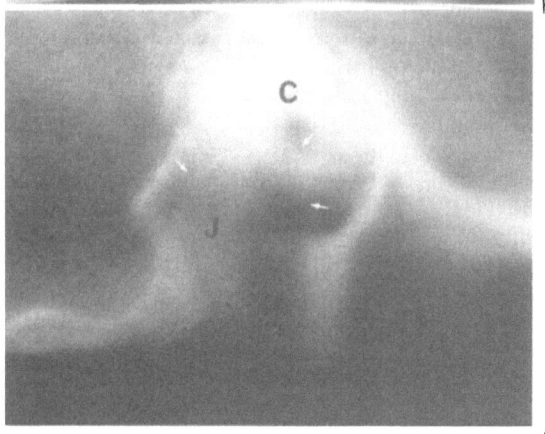

Fig. 2.19 a–c. Lateral tomography showing **a** crest of bone between jugular bulb and carotid artery displaced posteriorly by an aberrant carotid; c = cochlea. **b** large jugular fossa (J) with crest displaced anteriorly. Note the close relation to the vestibular aqueduct (*white arrow*); **c** Large jugular fossa with thin bony covering (*arrows*). This was hit but fortunately not penetrated by a myringotomy knife.

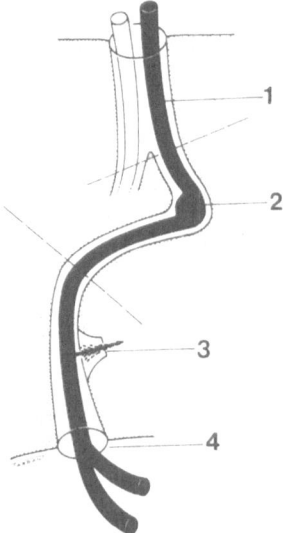

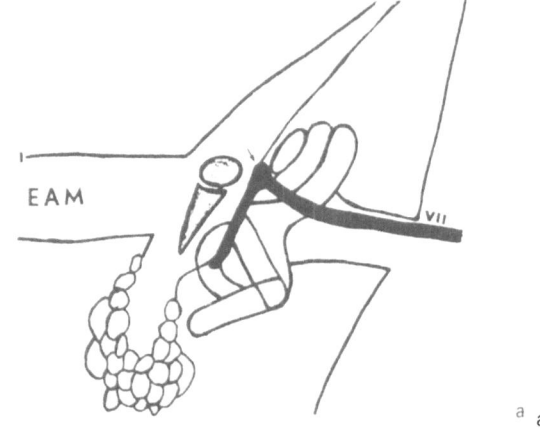

Fig. 2.20. Course of the facial nerve from the porus of the IAM (*top*) to the stylomastoid foramen (4). The nerve runs in the antero-superior part of the meatus (1) turns forwards in the first part of the facial nerve canal to the genicular ganglion (2) then backwards and downwards in the second and third parts of the facial canal. The stapedius muscle and pyramidal eminence (3) are closely related to the third part of the facial nerve.

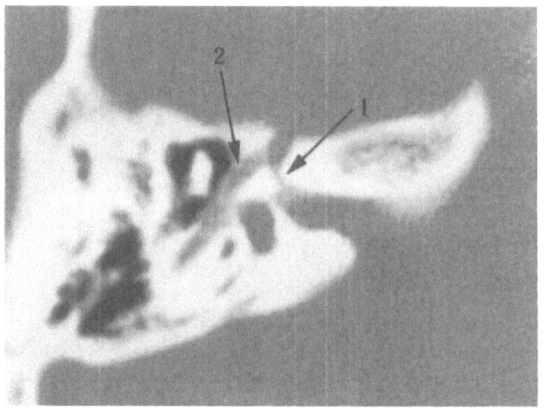

vertically, posterior to the middle ear and external auditory meatus (Fig. 2.20).

Fig. 2.21 a. Diagram to show the course of the first and second parts of the facial nerve and their relations to inner ear structures in the base projection; **b** equivalent base CT section showing first (1) and second (2) parts of the facial nerve canal.

Labyrinthine Part

Starting at the anterosuperior aspect of the lateral end of the internal auditory meatus, this short segment swings anteriorly above the cochlea to the pit for the geniculate ganglion, where the nerve turns sharply backwards to become the second part. This short length of canal may be shown by base CT (Fig. 2.21) but the sulcus for the geniculate ganglion is well demonstrated in coronal sections (see Figs. 1.15 and 1.25). The labyrinthine segment is the narrowest part of the canal, especially where it leaves the IAM and is closely related to the apex of the cochlea.

Tympanic Part

From the geniculate ganglion to the second bend, the nerve runs backwards above the oval window and below the lateral semicircular canal which overhangs it. It is surrounded by a thin bony sheath which may be dehiscent. Its course is somewhat

oblique (Fig. 2.21) and the bony canal is therefore best seen in cross section on the semi-axial projection (Fig. 2.22), although thin base section CT (1 mm) will show its whole length.

Mastoid or Descending Part

The third part of the nerve runs downwards from the second bend to the stylomastoid foramen lying lateral to the jugular fossa and separated from it by a variable distance. Occasionally, a very large jugular fossa, especially with diverticulum, may mean that the jugular bulb is in direct contact with the descending facial nerve (Wadin and Wilbrand 1986). The pyramidal eminence lies just below the second bend. The length of the descending segment,

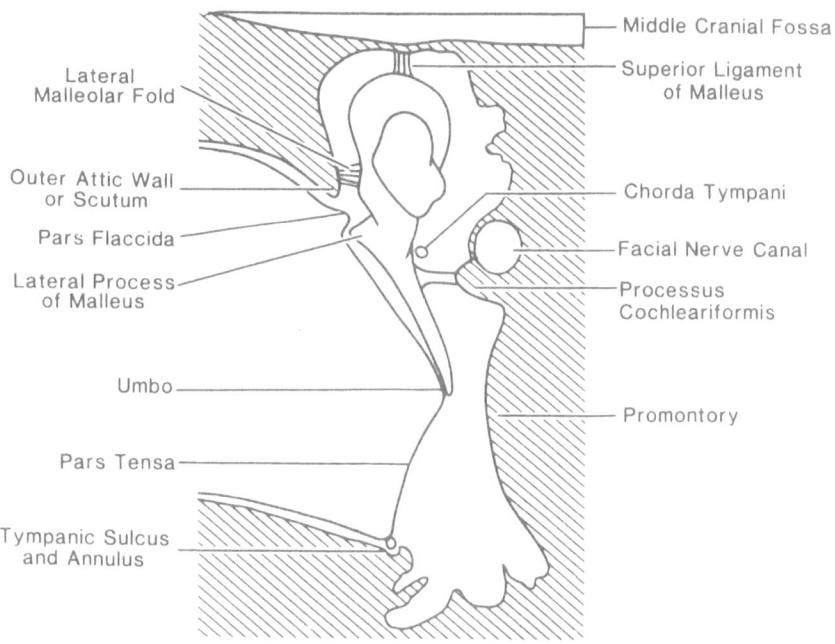

Fig. 2.22. Coronal section of the middle ear at the level of the malleus. Compare with CT section in Chap. 1. Courtesy of Mr. Anthony Wright and Scott Brown's Otolaryngology.

usually about 13 mm, is partly dependent on the shape of the temporal bone and partly on the extent of pneumatisation of the mastoid. Its width varies considerably. The bony canal is best demonstrated by coronal and sagittal sections, and is seen less easily in cross section on base CT.

Recognition is easy where the nerve passes through solid bone, but may be difficult where there is much pneumatisation. In children with congenital ear lesions, it is important not to confuse the facial nerve canal with other dehiscences such as the tympanomastoid fissure.

The Auditory Ossicles

Despite their small size, the three ossicles can be demonstrated in the middle ear cavity by high resolution thin section imaging. The malleus has a head, neck, anterior and lateral processes and a handle. The head is situated in the attic; the handle pointing downwards and backwards is firmly attached to the eardrum (Fig. 2.22). The incus has a body articulating with the head of malleus and a short process, all of which are in the attic (Fig. 2.23). The long process descends behind the handle of malleus and ends in the lenticular process which

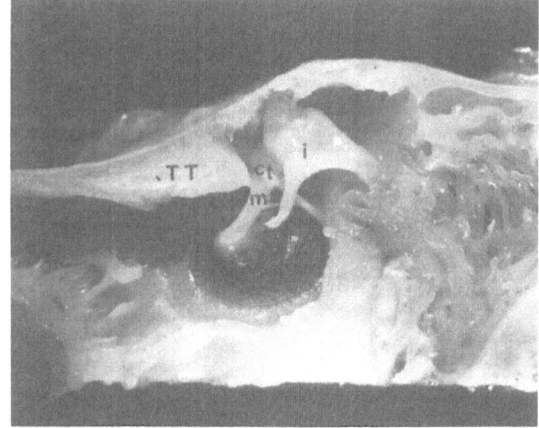

Fig. 2.23. The eardrum viewed from the middle ear showing malleus (m); incus (i); tensor tympani (TT) and chorda tympani (ct).

articulates with the head of stapes. The stapes has a head, neck, anterior and posterior crura and a footplate, which is held in the oval window by the annular ligament. The stapedius muscle arises from the posterior wall of the middle ear cavity in the pyramidal eminence, and it is attached to the neck of the stapes by a thin tendon (Fig. 2.8).

References

Dubois PJ, Roub LW (1978) Giant air cells of the petrous apex. Radiology 129:103–109

Friedman I (1974) Pathology of the ear. Blackwell Scientific Productions, Oxford, p 24

Glasscock ME, Dickens JRE, Jackson CG, Wiet FJ (1980) Vascular anomalies of the middle ear. Laryngoscope 90:77–88

Graham MD (1975) The jugular bulb: its anatomic and clinical considerations in contemporary otology. Arch Otolaryngol 101:560–564

Guinto FC Jr, Garrabrant EC, Radcliffe WH (1972) Radiology of the persistent stapedial artery. Radiology 105:365–369

Jahrsdoerfer RA, Cail WS, Cantrell RW (1981) Endolymphatic duct obstruction from a jugular bulb diverticulum. Ann Otol 90:619–623

Mawson SR and Ludman H (1979) Diseases of the ear: a textbook of otology (4th Edition) Edward Arnold, London.

Michaels, L (1987) Ear, nose and throat histopathology, Springer Verlag, London, Heidelberg.

Muren C, Wilbrand H (1986) Anatomic variations of the cochlear aqueduct: a radioanatomic investigation. Acta Radiol (Diagn) 27:22–28

Myerson MD, Ruben H, Gilbert SG (1934) Anatomic studies of the petrous portion of the temporal bone. Arch Otolaryngol 20:195–210

Wadin K, Wilbrand H (1986) The topographic relations of the high jugular fossa to the inner ear: a radioanatomic investigation. Acta Radiol (Diagn) 27:315–324

Wilbrand HF, Rask-Anderson H, Gilstring D (1974) The vestibular aqueduct and para-vestibular canal: an anatomic and roentgenologic investigation. Acta Radiol (Diagn) 15:337–355

3 Imaging Investigation of Congenital Deafness

The causes of congenital deafness are many and various. Any part of the hearing organ may be affected. The cochlear hair cells and central connections can be damaged in utero by the *Rubella* virus or aberrations in the development of the tympanic bone may result in simple atresia of the external auditory canal. Between these two very different examples of lesions causing congenital impairment of hearing, there is a wide spectrum of abnormalities due to arrested or abnormal development, the aetiology and pathogenesis of which is completely or partially understood in only a few cases. Medical aims consist of prevention and treatment. Prevention by genetic counselling and avoidance of noxious agents is sometimes possible. Surgery may occasionally improve hearing where there is a conduction abnormality but education and provision of a suitable hearing aid are the most important factors in management. If the anatomical deformities are carefully outlined, cases can be judiciously selected for surgical correction involving a minimum of risk to normal structures. Recognition of congenital hearing loss at the earliest possible age is essential, as is recognition of the type and degree of deafness.

Radiology can play a significant role in the management of the child with congenital deafness but, while objective evaluation of bony structures in the ear can be made with accuracy, assessment of the state of soft tissue structures can only be inferred from experience and reports of similar cases. Nevertheless, such indirect information regarding the probable state of the hearing organ is often valuable. Structural deformities of inner and middle ears frequently co-exist to give both a conductive and sensorineural component to the deafness. It is con-

venient to consider the inner and outer ears separately for radiological assessment, the aims of which may be summarised as:

Inner ear
    Probable cochlear function
    Better hearing side
    Risk of CSF fistula

Outer ear
    Feasibility of surgery for better sound conduction
    Most favourable ear for exploration
    Surgical hazards – misplaced facial nerve, carotid artery, jugular bulb

Many abnormalities of the hearing organ do not involve bony structures and so no lesion would be demonstrated by tomography. Moreover, as deafness is usually discovered in 1 or 2-year-old children, for whom imaging is virtually impossible without sedation or general anaesthesia, this technique should only be used for those cases in which useful information may be obtained. Ideally electrocochleography and the tomographic examination should be performed under the same sedation but this is not possible in most hospitals. Suggested guidelines for selection of patients for imaging are:

1. Any syndrome known to be associated with structural deformity of the ear (See Chap. 4)
2. Certain spinal abnormalities including the Klippel–Feil syndrome
3. Abnormalities of the external ears including auricular appendages and pits
4. After attacks of meningitis and CSF rhinorrhoea (see below)

Until recently, tomography provided almost the only objective means of proving the presence of severe hearing impairment in a non-vocalising infant, where the differential diagnosis of profound deafness, mental deficiency, visual problems or autism is difficult. Evoked response audiometry is now of great value in the assessment of these problem infants, and in selected cases can be usefully combined with tomographic studies under the same anaesthetic.

Historical Review of Congenital Deafness due to Malformations of the Temporal Bone and Their Investigations

The earliest accounts were of macroscopic dissections of temporal bones from deaf children. The first and most famous of these was by Carlo Mondini of Bologna in 1791 and was published in Latin in the Bolognese quarterly medical journal with nine drawings of the dissection. Mondini dissected the temporal bones of an 8-year-old boy, who was born deaf. The boy was otherwise healthy but died of gangrene after being knocked down by a horse and cart. Several labelled macroscopic drawings accompanied the account. The oval and round windows and all the semicircular canals and their openings into the vestibule were described as normal in size and position. The vestibule was larger than normal, and the cochlea, described as having one and a half instead of two and a half turns of the spiral, ended in an apical cavity. Neither the cochlear aqueduct nor the IAM were mentioned in the text but the latter is well shown in the diagrams and appears normal in size and shape. The vestibular aqueduct was very large and lacked a medial bony covering (Fig. 3.1).

From 1824 to 1837, the so-called Ibsen–Mackeprang collection of temporal bones was created. It comprises 110 temporal bones from deaf children, all specimens being admirably prepared. This remarkable collection, kept in the University Hospital in Copenhagen, has been the subject of various studies, the most recent and comprehensive account being that of Jensen (1969) who tomographed the specimens and discussed the labyrinthine abnormalities present in 32 of the temporal bones. In England, Cock (1838) described his dissections of the temporal bones of ten patients from the Asylum for Deaf and Dumb. The abnor-

malities seem mostly to be due to inflammatory destruction, but he does describe dilated and absent vestibular aqueducts, and in one case a narrow internal auditory meatus opening directly into a dilated vestibule and communicating via a wide opening with an amorphous cochlear sac. This may have been the type of dysplasia associated with a risk of CSF fistula (vide infra).

Atresia of the external auditory meatus, usually associated with deformity of the pinna, has been recognised since earliest times. The association of facial abnormalities with meatal atresia, and the fact that these deficiencies arise in derivatives of the first and second branchial arches, seems to have been first described by Thomson (1847), who reported three cases of bilateral atresia. Two of these cases are recorded as having deficiences of mandible, malar bones and zygoma, although it is not clear from the description whether these now would be classified as mandibulo-facial dysostosis or as cranio-facial microsomia. All three patients had had surgical exploration attempted. Not surprisingly these operations were unsuccessful, both with regard to evaluation of middle ear structures or to improvement of hearing. However, Thomson did test the hearing of his patients carefully and, correlating the results with the patholgical material available at the time, correctly deduced that in these cases the hearing loss is predominantly conductive due both to the meatal atresia and to deformities within the middle ear cavity. In his paper he describes a temporal bone in the anatomical museum of Edinburgh University which shows "entire obliteration of the meatus externus" and a fused ossicular mass "assuming very much the form and appearance of the columella of birds". In the same journal Toynbee (1847) also describes his personal dissection of a similar case with absence of the meatus and tympanic ring. The middle ear cavity was small and very narrow with two abnormal ossicles only – a globular malleus and a single strut stapes fixed in the oval window. Moreover there was deficiency of the zygoma, malar bone and lateral part of the orbit, so that this must have been one of the first dissections of a case of hemifacial microsomia. The inner ear was normal.

In 1863 Michel described a case of bilateral aplasia of the entire labyrinth with almost normal outer and middle ears. Michel is quoted by all authors as being the first to report on this, the most complete type of malformation of the inner ear, and this rare malformation has been named after him. In fact this lesion had been described in 1819 in a French medical dictionary. In his paper Michel (1863) quotes lesser deformities of the middle ear found in dissections by other authors. In particular

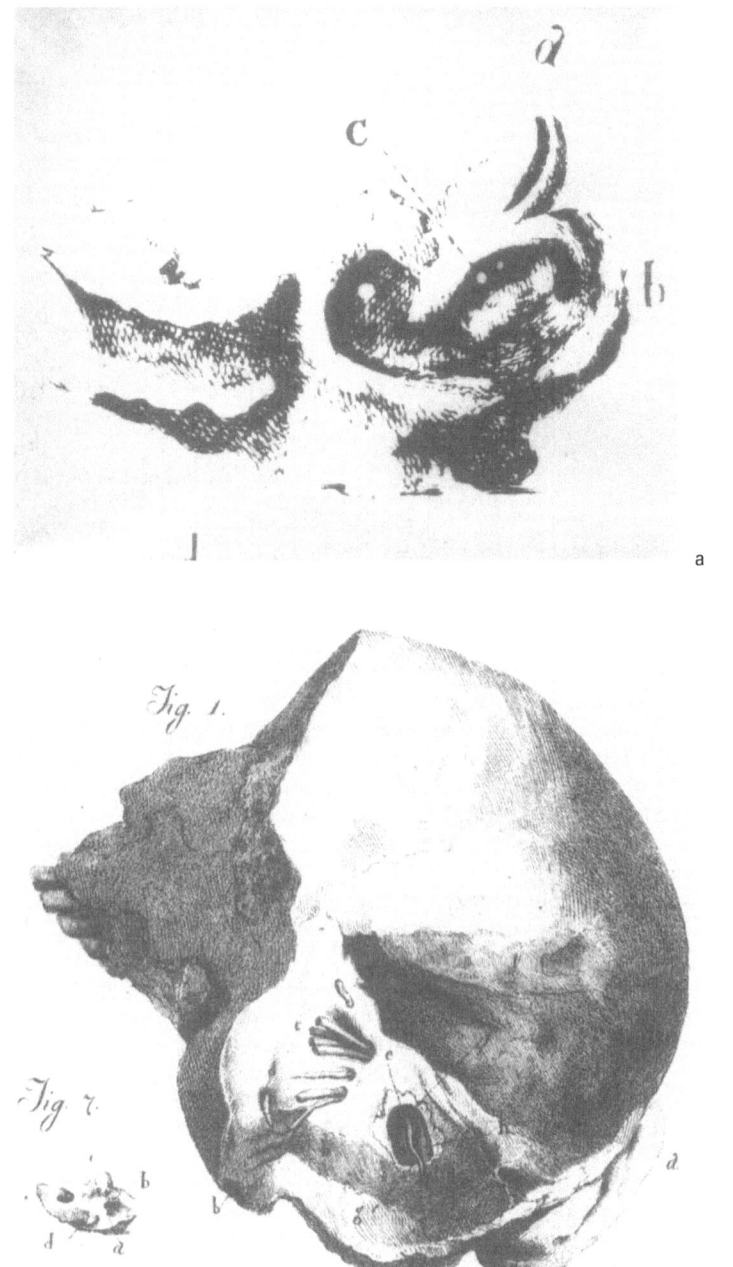

Fig. 3.1 a, b. Two line drawings from Mondini's original paper of 1791 showing, **a**, vestibule and cochlea with a basal turn and distal sac. Note the normally shaped IAM; **b** dilated vestibular aqueduct 15-mm (.7. lines) wide. In the middle is the labyrinthine vein of Cotunnius (from Soc 1996 d. 210, vol 7, 1791 Acata Acad Bononiensis courtesy of the Bodleian Library, Oxford).

there is a description of grossly underdeveloped labyrinths represented by a curved tube on one side and a simple sac on the other. In fact this type of primitive otocyst is commoner than the true "Michel" type (vide infra). Also described is a cochlea reduced to a unilocular bony cyst, and another case in which the lateral semicircular canal on each side was replaced by an evagination from the vestibule. This is the commonest labyrinthine anomaly shown by imaging (vide infra).

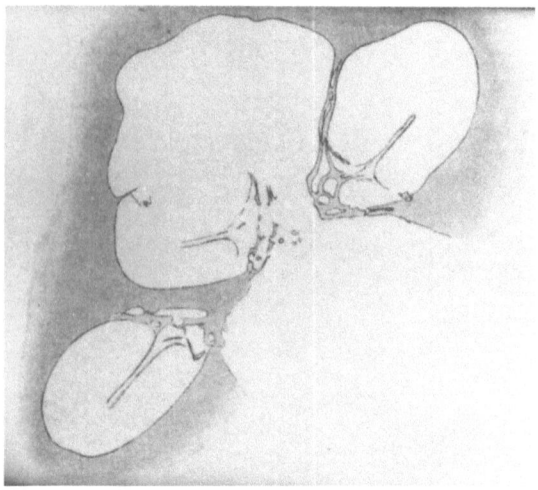

Fig. 3.2. The first histological section of a Mondini defect by Alexander in 1904.

Mygind (1890) published an extensive survey of those cases of pathological changes of the temporal bones from deaf persons, which had been described up to that date. In 32 of the 118 cases described, the deafness was considered to be congenital.

Alexander (1904) was the first to describe histologically a case of the Mondini malformation. Mondini's name, however, is not mentioned, but the findings correspond closely to earlier (macroscopic) findings and to later histological studies (Fig. 3.2).

No attempt at classifying the pathological changes found in the temporal bones from deaf subjects had been made so far, but with the introduction of modern histological technique it became possible to establish a detailed differentiation. Siebenmann's book on the pathology of deafness was published in 1904. In his very limited classification, two types of structural (i.e., bony) abnormality of the labyrinth were recognised: namely, those of Michel and Mondini. The lesions in the other types were confined to the membranous labyrinth.

Ormerod (1960), in a more recent review, presented a similar classification system, and this limited account is still being quoted. Many of these early descriptions stress the difficulty of distinguishing congenital from acquired abnormalities of the petrous temporal bone, in particular labyrinthitis obliterans due to previous meningitis.

Isolated descriptions of histological dissections of abnormal temporal bones continued to appear in the literature, but it was the chance coincidence of the development of pluridirectional tomography in the early 1960s with a spate of ear malformations brought about by the thalidomide disaster, which led to accounts of large series of congenital ear deformities demonstrated by radiological methods. There had been previous descriptions from the 1930s using conventional radiography, but these were mostly concerned with the extent of pneumatisation as only gross abnormalities of the middle ear can be shown by plain films.

The first tomographic study of congenital ear malformations seems to have been by Camp and Allen (1940), who examined four patients using a simple attachment to the Potter–Bucky couch. These patients all had microtia and atresia of the external auditory meatus on one side, and were examined by sections in the coronal and sagittal planes. The linear tomograms published are of good quality and not surprisingly give more information than was appreciated by the authors.

Ombredanne and Francois (1961) published a paper on inner ear malformations. The Polytome was used but nothing else is mentioned about the technique. More than 100 cases with aplasia of the ear were examined. The labyrinth was involved in less than a quarter, but the frequency of solitary abnormalities of the lateral semicircular canal is stressed. There are 16 tomographic reproductions, seemingly in the Stenvers projection, accompanied by line drawings and descriptions, although they do not always seem to agree. From this time most accounts of the radiology of congenital ear malformations were by use of pluridirectional tomography.

Frey (1965) collected 144 ears with malformations during an 8-year period; among these 16 ears (from ten patients) with inner ear malformations. The cause of the malformations was known to be thalidomide in three of the patients. Terrahe (1965) examined 37 children (73 ears) with malformations due to thalidomide. In all, he found 55 ears with malformations of the inner ear, and described his own classification.

A comprehensive account of 34 cases of congenital deformity of the inner, middle and external ears was made by Du Boulay and Bostick (1969), but no attempt was made to classify the great variety of abnormalities found. These included many abnormalities of the semicircular canals and an unusually high incidence of "double" internal auditory meatus. Thalidomide was probably causative in only a few cases.

Correlation of tomographic features with clinical and histological findings was first made by Valvassori et al. (1969) and Jensen (1969), who also gave a detailed account of his tomographic technique. Perhaps the most comprehensive report of investigations for these patients with ear malformations was made by Terrahe in 1972.

Inner Ear

When assessing the initial series of tomograms the state of the inner ears should be considered first, for the following reasons:

1. The level of any tomographic section is best assessed from the part of the labyrinth shown on that section
2. A severe degree of cochlea deformity is obviously incompatible with auditory function, whatever other tests may suggest. This is important in bilateral cases because, although such a melancholy diagnosis is hard to accept, the child will have to be educated by methods not involving sound
3. With the solitary exception of a dysplastic semicircular canal, any deformity of the bony labyrinth indicates a severe degree of sensorineural deafness and is therefore a relative contraindication to surgical attempts to improve the sound conduction mechanism
4. It is possible in some cases of inner ear deformity to assess the likely degree of deafness. For instance, the most common inner ear anomaly shown by tomography, namely shortening and dilatation of the lateral semicircular canal, is usually associated with normal cochlear function. However, if other canals are abnormal and especially if they are absent rather than dilated, there will almost certainly be a severe degree of sensorineural deafness, even if the cochlea appears normal (Phelps 1974). Similarly, there is a range of deformities with underdevelopment of the bony spiral of the cochlea, the best known being that of Mondini, the presence of a basal turn meaning that some degree of cochlear function is possible (Phelps et al. 1978)
5. There is a risk of a CSF fistula developing through the oval window in some types of labyrinthine abnormality, either spontaneously or as the result of stapes surgery

The lesions are so varied both in type and severity that systems of classification are unsatisfactory and incomplete. Anencephalic fetuses provide a fascinating study of a wide range of anatomical abnormalities of the temporal bone. These are similar to, although more severe than, lesions which occur spontaneously.

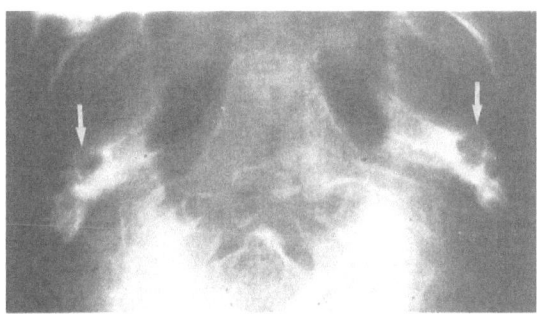

Fig. 3.3. Normal cochlea and hearing but no IAM. Base view showing that no bony sleeve has formed around the VIIIth and VIIth nerves. The arrows point to the cochleae.

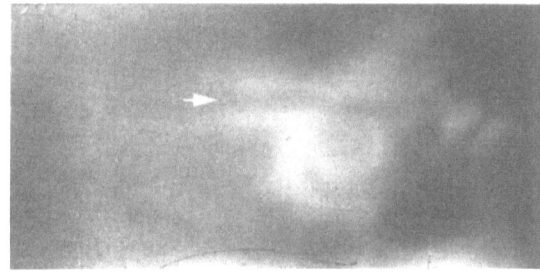

Fig. 3.4. A very narrow IAM of the same calibre as the first part of the facial nerve canal.

Internal Auditory Meatus (IAM)

The IAM is a bony sleeve surrounding four components of two cranial nerves and the vascular supply to the inner ear. It gradually assumes its definitive shape and position during fetal life, with development of the labyrinth, growth of the skull base and ossification of the petrous temporal bone. The IAM is very rarely absent except in Thalidomide deformities and even then a tract for the facial nerve can usually be recognised. Another very rare congenital aberration is failure to form a bony canal around the nerves (Fig. 3.3). If a narrow IAM continues laterally to the labyrinthine portion of the facial nerve canal with no change of calibre (Fig. 3.4), obviously no other neural components can be present, but in the authors' experience any unilateral narrowing of the IAM suggests a severe congenital sensorineural deafness.

Controversy surrounds the association of narrow IAMs with disabling dizziness. We have seen a 14-year-old child with a sclerosing bone dysplasia and an internal auditory meatus narrowed to 1–2-mm diameter who as yet has normal hearing (Fig. 3.5).

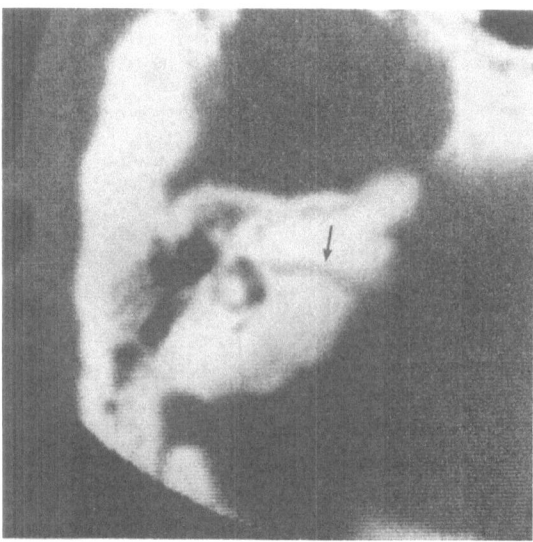

Fig. 3.5. Narrowing of the IAM in van Buchem's sclerosing bone dysplasia.

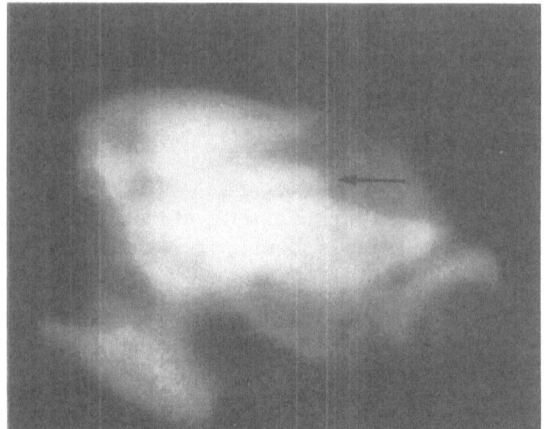

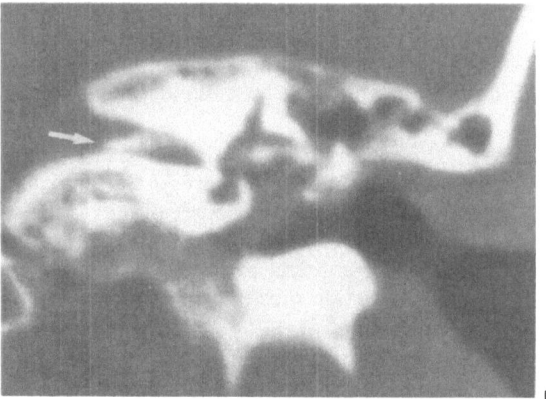

Fig. 3.6 a, b. A bar of bone divides the IAM in two. **a** Coronal tomogram also showing absent semicircular canals; **b** coronal CT of another case with no hearing.

Very wide IAMs, and particularly the ballooned type with widening at the lateral end, are usually of no significance unless there is other evidence to suggest neurofibromatosis. The ballooned meatus may be associated with congenital deafness or with the risk of a cerebrospinal fluid fistula but is unlikely to be due to an acoustic neuroma if the outlines are smooth and uniform. Hypertrophy of the crista falciformis to give a "double meatus" is an important sign indicating severe deafness. In the authors' own six cases, as well as in all cases reported so far, deafness has been complete (Fig. 3.6). Two cases reported by Clemens and Sandstrom (1975) had no hearing in the affected ears but one showed normal caloric responses. No bilateral cases have been reported and, as far as we are aware, no histological sections of this deformity have been published. It does not occur in anencephalics.

A tapered IAM with narrowing of its lateral end (Fig. 3.7) is only seen in combination with severe dysplasias of the labyrinth (Phelps and Lloyd 1978). The risk of development of a cerebrospinal fluid fistula makes its recognition of great importance. Curved IAMs and those that point upwards and backwards are merely the result of base of skull aberration or deformity such as that occurring in the cranio-facial dysostoses or in cranio-facial microsomia (see Chap. 4). This aberration of position is most severe in anencephalics. Fig. 3.8 represents in diagrammatic form some of these anomalies of the IAM.

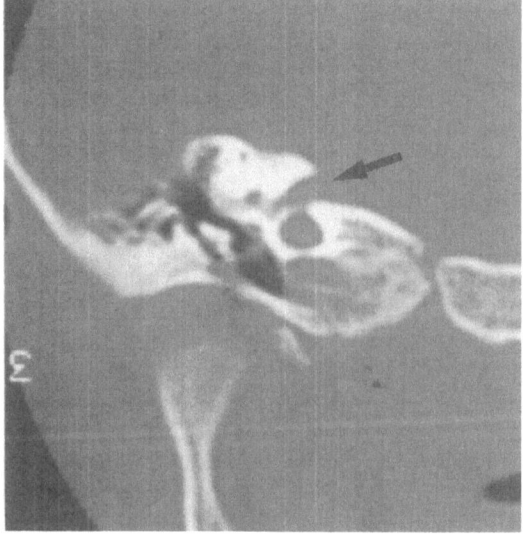

Fig. 3.7. Tapering IAM with severe labyrinthine dysplasia.

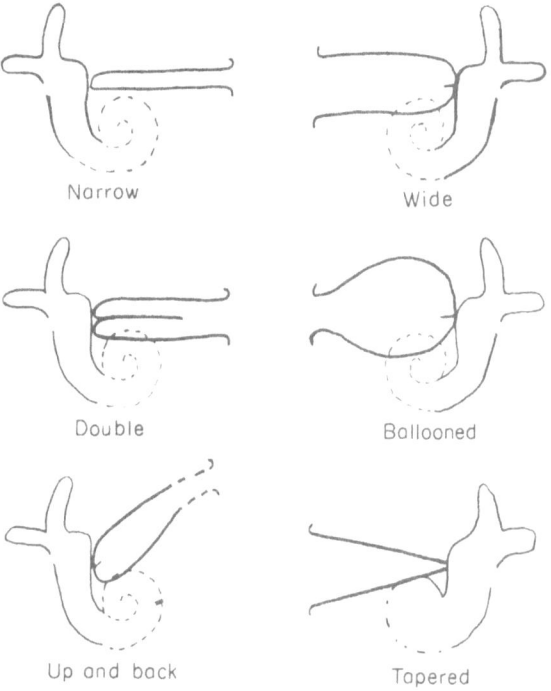

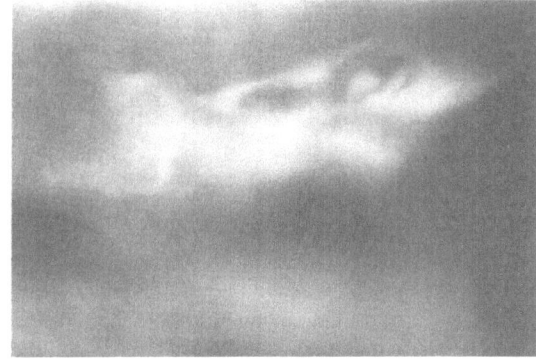

Fig. 3.9. Michel deformity with complete aplasia of the labyrinth. An external auditory meatus and middle ear cavity with ossicle can be seen.

◀ Fig. 3.8. Congenital deformities of the IAM.

Major Deformities of the Labyrinth

Hypoplasia of the petrous pyramid with no vestige of a labyrinth (Fig. 3.9), first described by Michel in 1863, is very rare. Some form of primitive otocyst or curved tube is a more frequent finding (Fig. 3.10). These severe labyrinthine malformations are obviously incompatible with any cochlear or vestibular function and are therefore of little interest, except for the fourth type which carries the risk of a cerebrospinal fluid fistula.

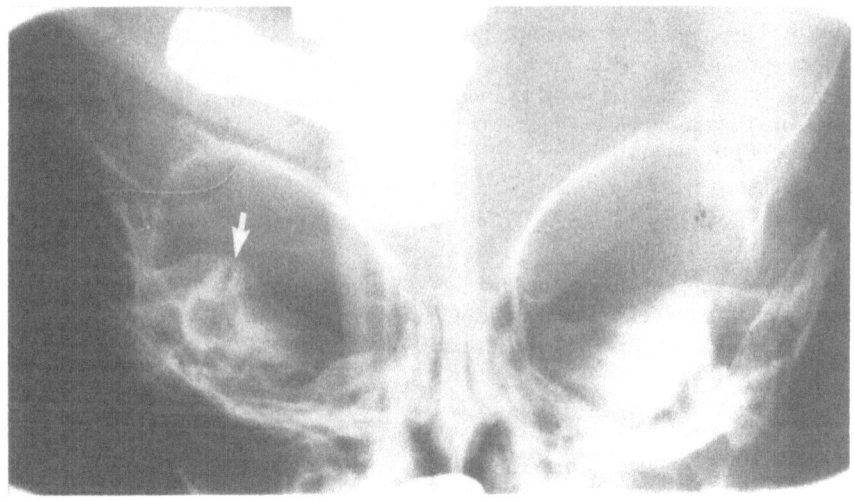

Fig. 3.10. Perorbital view showing a primitive otocyst with endolymphatic appendage on one side (*arrow*).

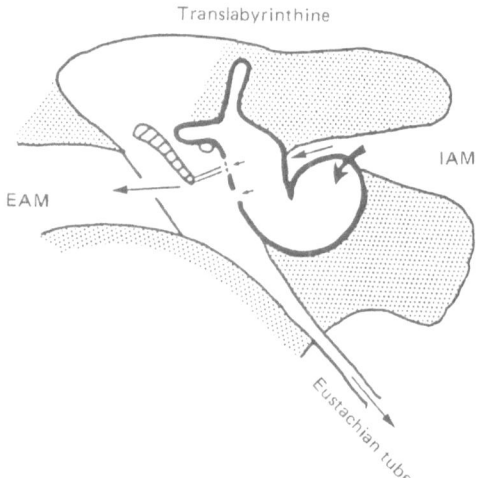

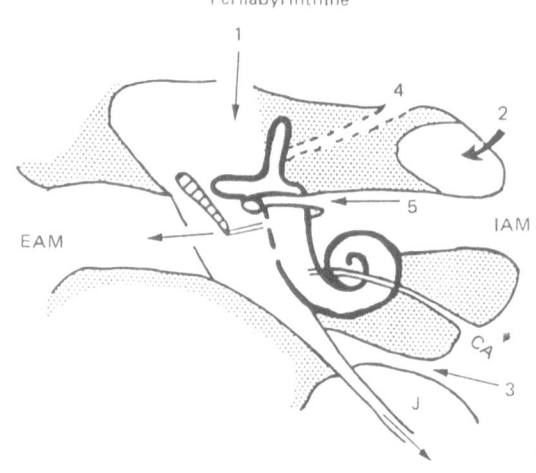

Fig. 3.11 a. Diagram to show the commonest inner ear anomaly associated with cerebrospinal fluid fistula. Note the wide communication between vestibule and cochlear sac. This diagram is based on coronal section tomograms. **b** Diagram based on coronal section tomograms to show the various routes of perilabyrinthine fistulae around a labyrinth of normal configuration: 1 through the tegmen tympani; 2 through large apical air cells; 3 via Hyrtl's fissure; 4 via petromastoid canal (not a proven route); 5 via the facial nerve canal. EAM, external auditory meatus; IAM, internal auditory meatus; ET, Eustachian tube; CA, cochlear aqueduct; J, jugular fossa. (From Phelps (1986), with permission.)

Congenital Deformities of the Labyrinth associated with Cerebrospinal Fluid (CSF) Fistula

Congenital cerebrospinal fluid fistula into the middle ear cavity is a rare but potentially fatal condition which is frequently misdiagnosed. When the fistula occurs spontaneously it usually presents in the first 5 or 10 years of life as:

1. CSF rhinorrhoea. If the eardrum is intact, CSF passes down the Eustachian tube causing a nasal discharge
2. CSF otorrhoea. If there is a perforation in the eardrum, or if myringotomy has been performed for presumed serious otitis media
3. Attacks of meningitis which are usually recurrent. At times meningitis is the sole presenting manifestation of a CSF fistula

Deafness is usually severe or complete but it is difficult to diagnose and assess, especially in a young child. It is frequently unrecognised if unilateral. The conductive and sensorineural components of the deafness are also hard to define.

It is well recognised that congenital fixation of the stapes footplate is likely to be associated with a profuse perilymph or CSF leak following stapedectomy. The surgical results of stapedectomy for congenital stapedial fixation are not very sat-

isfactory (von Haacke 1985) and often lead to a profuse leak of perilymph. It is assumed that the "stapes gusher" is associated with a wide cochlear aqueduct, although this has not yet been convincingly proven.

The following account is concerned with spontaneous fistulae which may be associated with:

1. A normal bony labyrinth and normal hearing, at least initially; (Fig. 3.11a)
2. Deformity of the bony labyrinth with anacusis (Fig. 3.11b)

The first category is extremely rare if one excludes stapes gushers. Fistulae via the following pathways have been shown by us, or have been reported by others (Phelps 1986).

Perilabyrinthine Fistulae

Via the Tegmen (Fig. 3.12)

Kaufman et al. (1977) have described four cases of cerebrospinal fluid rhinorrhoea involving defects in the antero-medial portion of the middle cranial fossa. Gavilan et al. (1984) report an apparently unique case of congenital encephalocoele in the middle ear (Fig. 3.12).

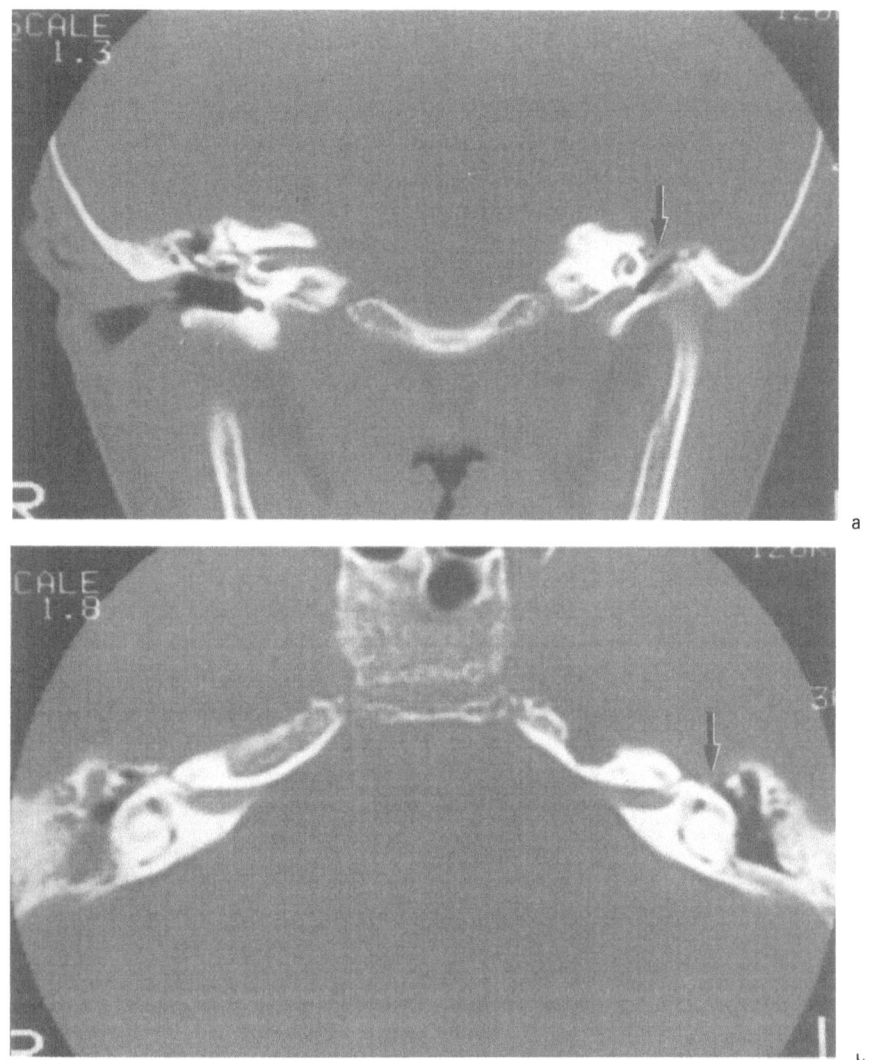

Fig. 3.12 a, b. Coronal (a) and base (b) CT sections showing intracranial structures bulging through the tegmen (*arrow*).

Via a Giant Apical Air Cell

Kraus and McCabe (1982) describe a dehiscence in the medial wall of the middle ear anterior to the cochlea. The defect contained ruptured pulsating arachnoid, and there was a copious leak of cerebrospinal fluid down the Eustachian tube.

Via Hyrtl's Fissure

Gacek and Leipzig (1979) describe a large meningocoele of the middle ear which extended through Hyrtl's fissure. The patient presented with CSF otorrhoea following a myringotomy for serous otitis media. A meningocoele was found to extend through a cleft which appeared to represent a fissure between the bony labyrinth and the jugular bulb. We have seen two similar cases; in one there was an overall deficiency of the medial part of the petrous pyramid. An air CT cisternogram showed air, filling not only the very large internal auditory meatus, but also the large jugular fossa on the affected side. The close association with the introduced air and the air in the middle ear cavity below the cochlea, and only separated by a thin membrane (Fig. 3.13), suggested that this was the site of the CSF leak. This was confirmed at surgery and a muscle pack in the hypotympanum cured the leak. In another case a

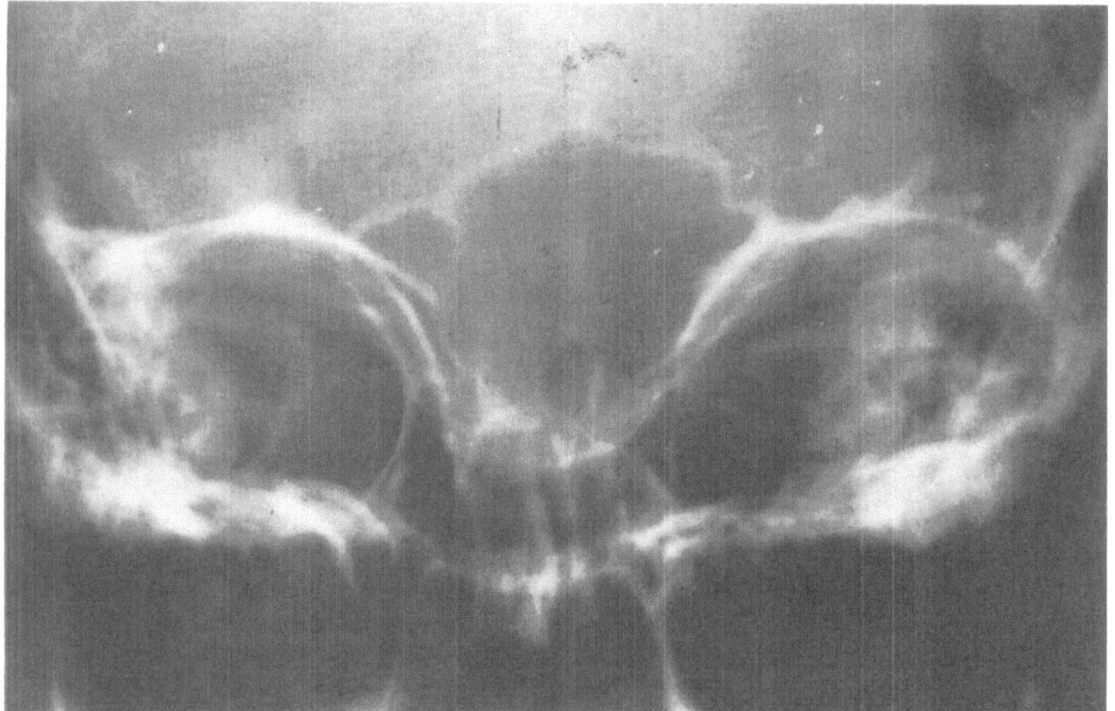

a

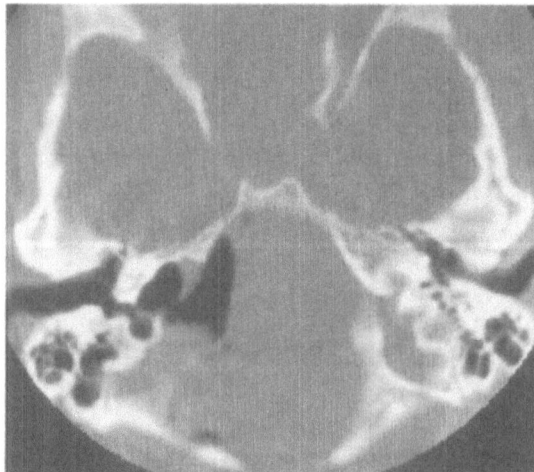

b

Fig. 3.13 a. Perorbital view showing the labyrinth and hypoplasia of both petrous pyramids. b Hypoplastic petrous pyramids with a bone defect in the region of Hyrtl's fissure. The axial CT air cisternogram shows air in the jugular fossa on the affected side, and extending to close apposition with air in the hypotympanum of the middle ear cavity, with only a thin membrane separating. At tympanotomy, a leak of CSF was demonstrated below the cochlea.

large tract extending to the middle ear below the cochlea was shown by base CT sections.

Via the Petromastoid Canal

A small bony canal carrying the subarcuate vessels passes under the arch of the superior semicircular canal before terminating in cells around the mastoid antrum. It can sometimes be demonstrated on tomograms or CT, and has been proposed as a route for a fistula or meningitis (Schuknecht 1974). This evidence, however, is not convincing at least for the passage of cerebrospinal fluid into the middle ear cavity.

Via the First Part of the Facial Nerve Canal

A wide first part of the facial nerve canal may, rarely, occur with a normal labyrinth as shown by the following two cases. Gacek and Leipzig (1979) describe a 2-year-old child who presented with meningitis and was shown, by an iophendylate study and at surgery, to have a lateral extension of the subarachnoid space through the initial segment of

Fig. 3.14 a. A lateral tomogram showing an expanded first part of the facial nerve canal eroding into the top of the cochlea. At surgery, an arachnoid cyst around the facial nerve was found extending into the antrum. **b** Base CT section showing the "soft tissue mass" (*asterisk*) in the attic and the wide first part of the facial canal (*arrow*).

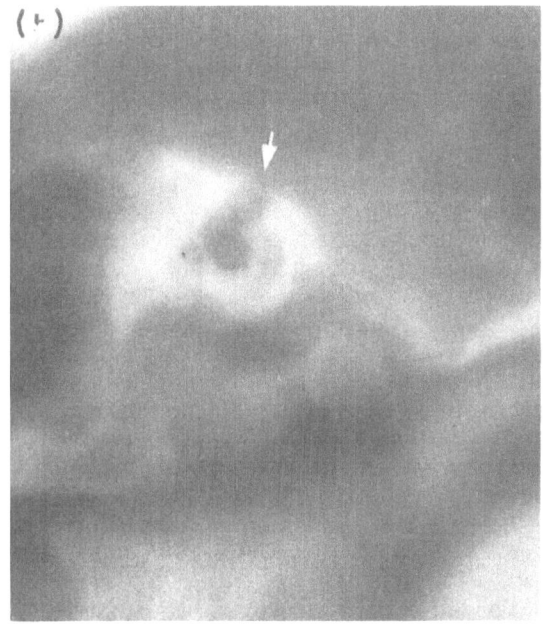

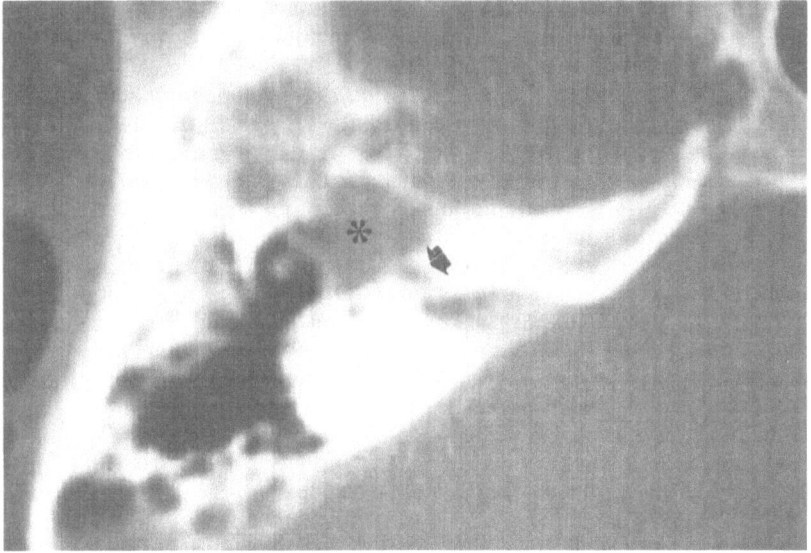

b

the facial canal. This produced a fistulous tract but tomography of the temporal bone was considered unremarkable. We have seen a similar case in a 10–year–old girl who presented with progressive sensorineural deafness followed by a facial palsy. Tomograms and high resolution CT showed widening of the first part of the facial nerve canal with erosion of the top of the cochlea and a soft tissue mass in the attic (Fig. 3.14). This was thought to be a facial nerve neuroma, but an iophendylate study showed contrast filling the "tumour". Sur-

gical exploration revealed an arachnoid sac extending into the attic with the facial nerve lying in its floor. A fistulous track via the facial nerve canal may occur in the second group with deformed labyrinth (vide infra).

Translabyrinthine Fistulae

Before considering the types of labyrinthine deformity which are associated with cerebrospinal fluid fistulae, a brief consideration of normal development would seem pertinent. At an early stage the major compartment of the auditory vesicle (otocyst) differentiates into semicircular canals and cochlea. From the dorsal part of the chamber 3 disc-like evaginations appear and, with further absorption of their centres, by 9 weeks become semicircular canals. From the ventral part of the chamber, a single evagination pushes medially as the cochlear duct, and by 12 weeks it becomes fully coiled. From 8 weeks the mesoderm investing the differentiating auditory vesicle becomes converted to cartilage and then to bone. In the cartilage the scala tympani and scala vestibuli gradually extend along each side of the cochlear duct until they come together and fuse at the helicotrema. The utricle, saccule, endolymphatic sac, and the ducts between them, differentiate.

Arrest of this normal process of development at various stages, collectively or in parts of the labyrinth, seems to be the most important factor in the congenital malformations of the inner ear under consideration. Radiological studies can only show the abnormality of the bony capsule, and this may not necessarily faithfully reflect the abnormalities of the membranous labyrinth (Johnsson 1971). Nevertheless, experience shows that useful assessment of likely hearing status and the route of a fistula, or the risk of one, can be demonstrated by radiological methods. Some minor labyrinthine anomalies with large vestibule and cochlea, the latter having a normal number of coils but with hypoplastic partitions, have been described (Jensen 1974). The lateral end of the IAM is also dilated in this type of malformation. The associated mixed type of deafness has prompted stapes surgery, with resultant stapes gushers. In some cases there appears to be an X-linked hereditary factor (Nance et al. 1971; Glasscock 1973; Bento 1985). In the two families described by Glasscock (1973), three patients were fully investigated, and two developed stapes "gushers" following stapes surgery. The cochlea was not shown radiologically or by exploration, but in one case the leak stopped when the IAM was packed with muscle.

Although the type of labyrinthine deformity shown in Fig. 3.15 seems the most common and most important anomaly associated with cerebrospinal fluid fistulae, other types have been described. Jensen (1974) saw three cases with inner ear malformations who were referred with a mixed hearing loss of about 60 dB. The tomograms of the six ears in question were essentially identical. The outer and middle ears were normal. The overall impression of the inner ear structures was that of enlargement. All of the osseous structures were undoubtedly present, but appeared dilated and irregular. The vestibule was enlarged and its long axis, normally vertical, was horizontal. All semicircular canals were present but the lumina were irregularly dilated. The IAM was normal at its medial end with a normal porus. Laterally, it widened and apparently divided into two. One minor part continued its normal course toward the vestibule, whereas the greater part turned downward, pointing toward the basal coil of the cochlea. All of the coils were seen with an irregularly dilated lumen but the number of coils was normal.

Spontaneous CSF fistula through the labyrinth is probably always associated with underdevelopment and deformity, not only of the membranous labyrinth, but of the bony capsule as well. The evidence comes from three sources: 1 post-mortem studies, 2 radiology, 3 observations at surgery to cure the leak. To our knowledge, histological studies, while showing potential fistulous routes, have never indicated a proven fistulous tract that had been present in vivo.

The important considerations are the routes of "entry" and the "exit" of the fistula to and from the labyrinth (Pimontel-Appel and Vignaud 1979). The exit route into the middle ear is usually readily apparent at tympanotomy and better still by a wider surgical exposure. Almost always the leak is through the oval window, through or around a deformed stapes. A hole in the stapes footplate has been described in many of these cases and it is uncertain whether this is the result of the long-term pressure from behind by the CSF, or a developmental anomaly perhaps related to the stapedial artery and its involution. However, a persistent stapedial artery has been described in only one case with a fistula (Pashley and Shapiro 1978). Leaks from the round window or through defects in the promontory are unusual. Surgical observations on the entry route to the labyrinth from the subarachnoid space are made less frequently and less convincingly because of the limited exposure. Nevertheless, defects of the medial wall of the labyrinth have been observed through the oval window (Gundersen and Haye 1970; Bottema 1975; McNab Jones and Fairburn 1977). The defect or defects in the lamina cribrosa seemed to vary in size and position but from the illustrations shown the defect in one case appeared to be anterosuperior, i.e., in the region of the first part of the facial nerve canal (Gundersen and Haye 1970).

This leaves radiology as the most useful means of assessment, and involves the following:

1. Demonstration of the bony labyrinth by multidirectional tomography or high-resolution CT.

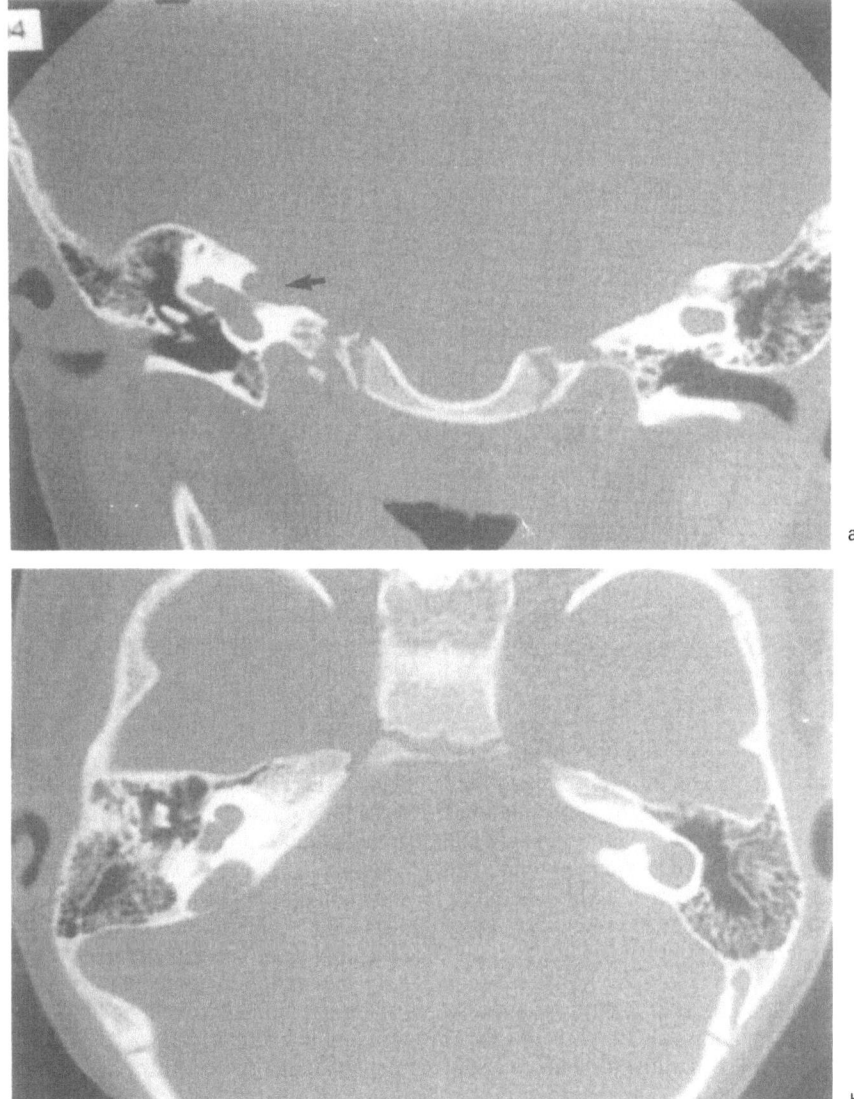

Fig. 3.15 a, b. Coronal CT section showing a combined cochleovestibular sac and tapering IAM (*arrow*). The patient had two attacks of unexplained meningitis. Both ears are affected. **a** Coronal and **b** base CT sections.

Plain films are of little value, although the more severe types of labyrinthine deformity can be recognised

2. Dyes such as fluorescein or indigo carmine, which merely confirm that there is a leak of cerebrospinal fluid without showing anatomical details and are rarely useful

3. Contrast agents such as iophendylate and the more recent water-soluble agents for cisternography which are much more satisfactory when combined with tomography or CT.

Labyrinthine Dysplasia associated with Cerebrospinal Fluid Fistula

Jensen (1974) was the first to draw attention to the more severe type of cochlear dysplasia without a normal basal coil. The best tomographic demonstrations of abnormal labyrinths associated with CSF fistula clearly show that in such cases cochlea and vestibule are abnormal, and there is wide communication between them. Stool et al. (1967) demonstrated iophendylate passing from the IAM into the vestibule and subsequently into the middle ear in two cases. Carter et al. (1975) used tomography with iophendylate to show the contrast material entering the region of the geniculate ganglion and ending in a sac overlying the oval window. Curtin et al. (1982) used metrizamide which extended directly into the abnormal vestibule from the IAM.

We have studied the radiographs of 28 patients whom we consider to have the type of severe labyrinthine deformity under consideration. Ten of these patients developed a spontaneous fistula when the middle ear was explored. Unfortunately, we do not have full clinical documentation and the tomograms were not all done under our supervision. The patients were all in the first decade of life. The lesions were bilateral and virtually symmetrical in two although only one side leaked (Bridger and Phelps 1983), and unilateral in the remaining eight. The hearing in the unaffected ears was normal but there was no evidence of any cochlear function in the affected ears.

The inner ear deformity in these 28 cases consisted of dilatation and dysplasia of the labyrinth. In particular, the cochlea was an amorphous sac which lacked a modiolus or central bony spiral (Fig. 3.15). The cochlea sac may be bigger or smaller than a normal cochlea. No proper basal turn can be recognised as in a true Mondini deformity, and there is a wide communication between the cochlear sac and the vestibule, which is itself abnormal and enlarged, especially in the horizontal plane. The semicircular canals may be dilated in varying degrees, especially the lateral. Characteristically, the internal acoustic meatus tapers, being narrower at its lateral end than at the porus. It is usually narrower than normal overall, but may be wide at the medial end (Fig. 3.16). No contrast investigations were done, being considered unnecessary. The clinical features and the appearance of the bony labyrinth are almost always sufficient to recommend exploratory tympanotomy.

Fistulous communication between the subarachnoid space and the middle ear cavity via an abnormal labyrinth is now a well recognised entity and no longer are these patients subjected to fruitless anterior cranial fossa explorations. The inner ear deformity is readily demonstrable by sectional imaging (either pleuridirectional tomography or CT) in these young patients presenting with CSF otorrhoea, rhinorrhoea, or recurrent attacks of meningitis. The lesion can be identified on plain films, especially in the neonate. Nevertheless, there is often considerable delay in relating the recurrent meningitis to the ear lesion (Hirakawa et al. 1983). Although patients with this deformity have no hearing function in the grossly dysplastic cochlea,

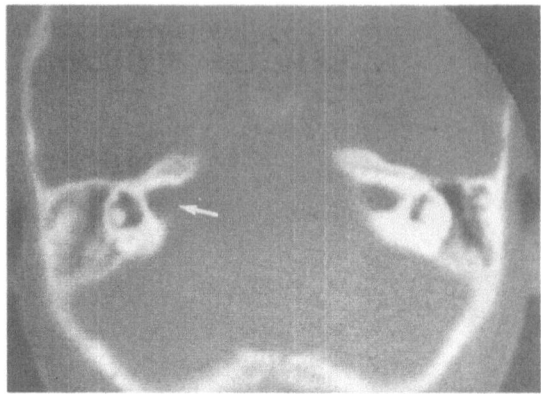

Fig. 3.16. Another case with a fistula presenting with meningitis. There is a wide tapering IAM and dilated vestibule on one side shown on this base CT section.

this may not be recognised if the lesion is unilateral. Meningitis is itself a potent cause of deafness, and on clinical grounds it may not be possible to decide which came first – the meningitis or the deafness. However this distinction can usually be made radiologically. A labyrinth destroyed by meningitis will either appear normal on tomograms, or partially obliterated by labyrinthitis ossificans. The outline of the bony labyrinth can usually be distinguished even if the lumen has been completely obliterated, but good quality pictures and skill in interpretation are necessary.

Serous otitis media is a common problem in children and causes deafness, albeit conductive, and an abnormal eardrum. Often only the volume of fluid aspirated after myringotomy leads the surgeon to suspect that it is cerebrospinal fluid.

The evidence that the usual route of a spontaneous translabyrinthine fistula is from the IAM, through a deformed vestibulo-cochlear sac, and into the middle ear cavity through the oval window, is overwhelming. The stapes is very often deformed and may have a hole in the middle of the footplate (Fig. 3.17). The entry route into the labyrinth from the IAM requires some explanation.

It is readily apparent to anyone doing air CT meatography for the investigation or exclusion of acoustic neuromas that the subarachnoid space extends around the VIIth and VIIIth cranial nerves to the fundus of the IAM (Fig. 1.27). This extension was perhaps even better demonstrated by the now-defunct polytome iophendylate examinations, when contrast could sometimes be seen reaching the pit for the spiral ganglion in the base of the modiolus. In normal cases there are two obstacles to the further extension of the subarachnoid space into the perilymph spaces of the labyrinth. These

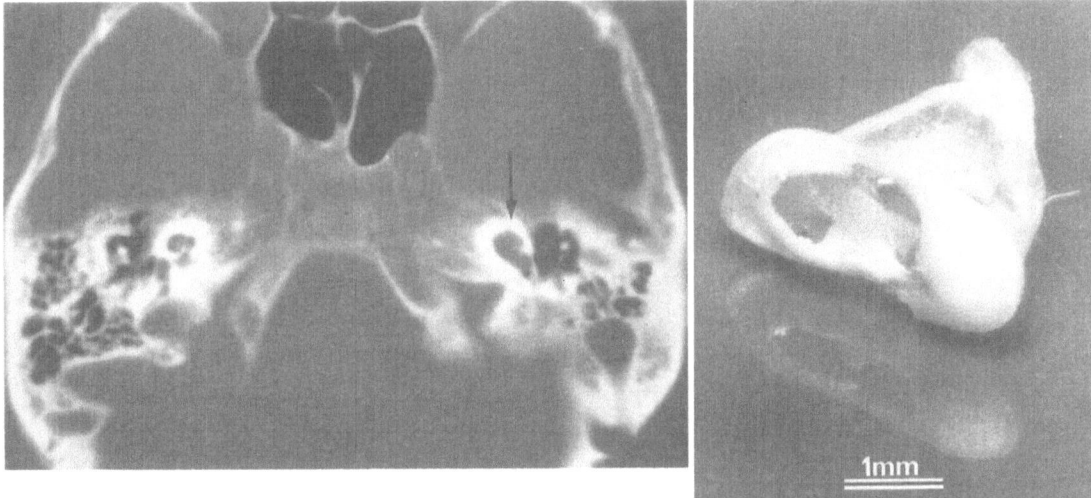

Fig. 3.17 a. Unilateral cochleovestibular dysplasia. Base section at the level of the cochlea coils; compare with the normal side. **b.** The stapes from this patient with a hole in the footplate.

are the bony medial wall of the labyrinth, which consists partly of the base of the modiolus of the cochlea perforated by the branches of the cochlear nerve, and the spiral ganglion itself. When these are deficient, as in severe cochlea dysplasia, there is a ready pathway into the cochlear sac. Although there is no histological evidence of this pathway in cases with a fistula in vivo, nevertheless cases have been shown of severe cochlear dysplasia with thin fragile bony shelves between the IAM and the cochlear sac and a grossly hypoplastic modiolus (Curtin et al 1982). We believe that the narrow lateral end of the IAM often shown by tomography in cases of severe cochlear dysplasia is a "compensatory narrowing to close the gap".

The importance of a normal basal turn and the presence of at least some part of the spiral ganglion now becomes apparent (Fig. 3.2). It seems to us unfortunate, therefore, that the term "Mondini dysplasia" is now used to cover almost every type of abnormality of the bony labyrinth that can be detected by sectional imaging and necessitates some additional qualification of the term "Mondini deformity".

Recognition of severe cochlea dysplasia depends on two types of investigation – audiological and radiological – both difficult in the infant. Ideally, when such a lesion is suspected, imaging and electrocochleography should be carried out under the same anaesthetic, but these can be done as a combined procedure in very few centres. Severe dysplasia of the labyrinth with no cochlear function should necessitate careful follow-up and instant action for any suspected leak or attack of meningitis,

although we do not think that prophylactic packing of the abnormal labyrinth is indicated. Imaging studies should assist the electro-physiological investigations in deciding whether or not a basal turn of the cochlea, as in a "true" Mondini defect, can be identified in a severely deaf infant.

Lesions of the cochlea

In the above section severe deformities of the cochlea incompatible with cochlear function were considered. Minor congenital abnormalities of the bony cochlea, which may be associated with some hearing, will now be described. Assessment of them is difficult and, where they occur on coronal sections, it depends on defining an intact or deficient "curl" of the bony spiral lamina. Further views in the base or axial pyramidal projection, as described in Chapter 1, are necessary for adequate assessment of the coils.

The cochlea may be bigger than normal as in Jensen's three cases (Jensen 1974), or it may be smaller. Most anomalies of the bony cochlea tend to be labelled as Mondini defects so an initial account of Mondini's precise description will be made.

Mondini Deformity

As described by Mondini, the malformation which bears his name consists of a cochlea with a normal

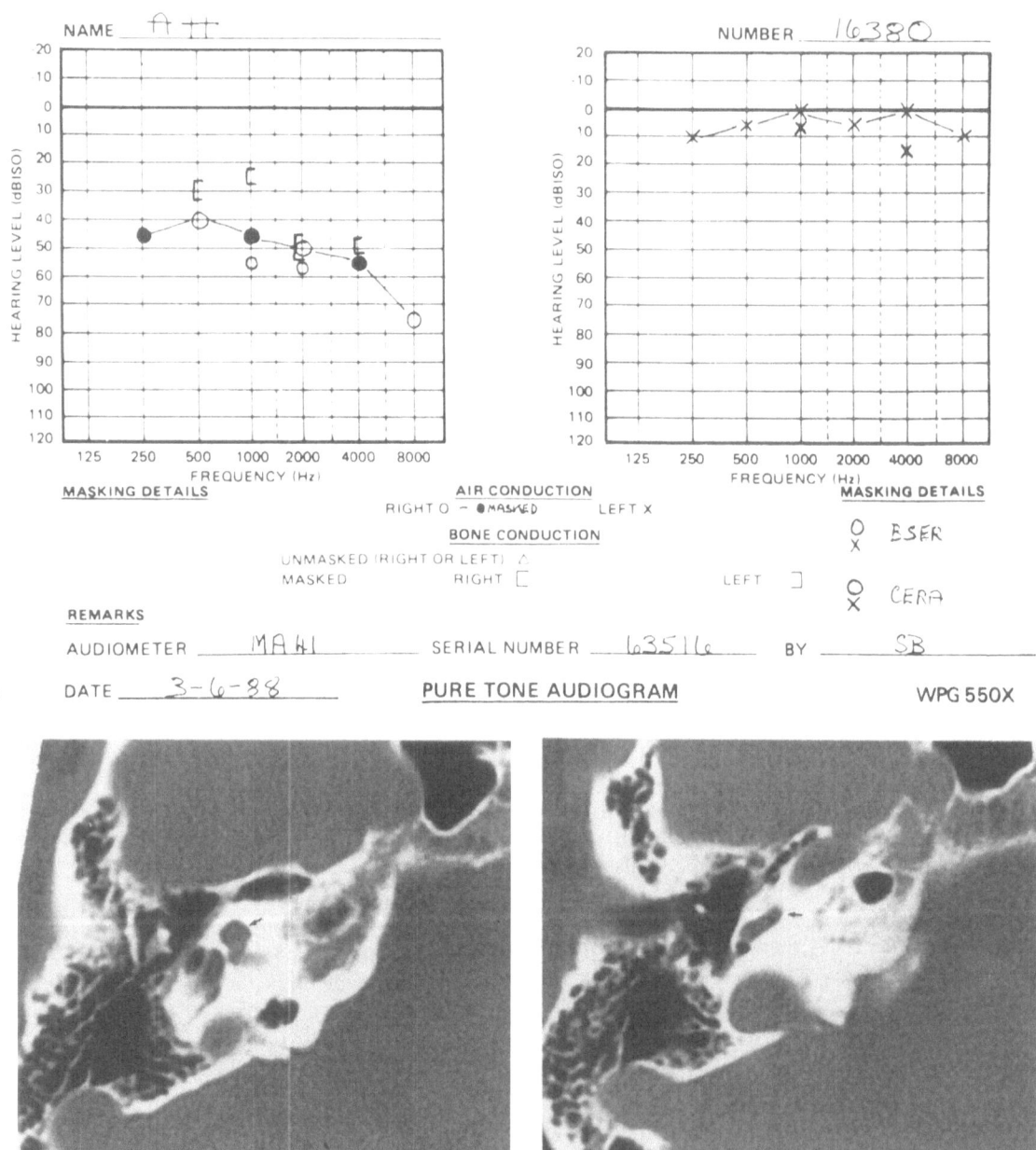

Fig. 3.18 a. Unilateral Mondini deformity with surprisingly good hearing in the affected ear. **b** Base CT sections showing normal basal turn and distal sac.

basal turn but with the distal one and a half turns being replaced by a sac. Some hearing is, therefore, possible in this type of dysplasia and we have seen examples with confirmed cochlear function (Fig. 3.18). Fluctuating and progressive hearing loss with electrocochleography patterns showing multiple acoustic nerve action potential waves similar to Ménière's disease has been observed (Mangabeira-Albernaz et al. 1981). Occasionally the deformity is bilateral (Fig. 3.19).

When the basal turn is dilated, there is no cochlear function. Minor deficiencies of the bony spiral lamina may be detected by tomography. They are usually associated with some degree of sen-

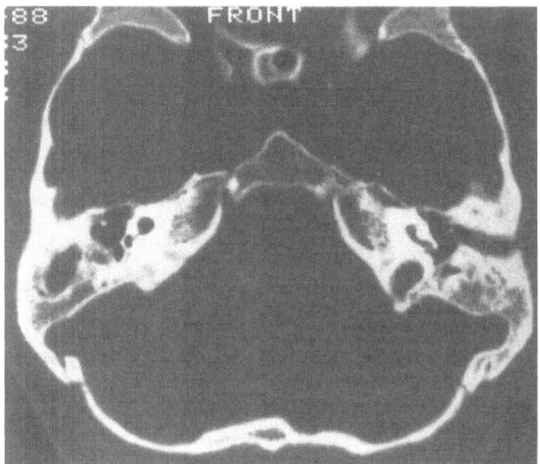

Fig. 3.19. Base CT section showing bilateral Mondini defects.

these are Pendred's syndrome and Ear-pits Deafness syndrome,

To summarise, therefore: some cochlear function is possible if the basal turn of the bony cochlea is shown to be normal, but deficiencies of the apical part of the central bony spiral, resulting in a scala communis of the membranous cochlea, are most likely to be associated with severe sensorineural deafness. Assessment of overall size of the cochlea and normality of the central "curl" is made on coronal section. For full assessment of individual coils, multiple sections in the base projection are required.

Lesions of the Vestibule and Semicircular Canals

sorineural deafness. However, the distinction of normal, abnormal and normal variant for the coils of the cochlea and central bony spiral has not been fully defined (Fig. 3.20). This problem was discussed by Jensen (1969) who considered that two instead of two and a half turns of the cochlea should be considered a normal variant. There is a need for further correlation of radiological, histological and audiometric findings in these cases. A wide range of similar structural cochlear abnormalities occurs in anencephalics. The Mondini deformity may very rarely have a familial tendency and it is also a feature of two syndromes to be described in Chap. 4:

A short dilated lateral semicircular canal incompletely separated from the vestibule (Fig. 3.21) is the most common anomaly of the inner ear shown by tomography. Phelps (1974) reviewed 157 patients with congenital lesions of the external and middle ears studied by tomography. The tomograms showed that 34 of these patients had additional deformities of the inner ear. Eight patients had bilateral dysplasia of the lateral canals in association with bilateral deformities of the external and middle ears. In each of the eight cases cochlear function appeared to be normal, the deafness being of the conductive type.

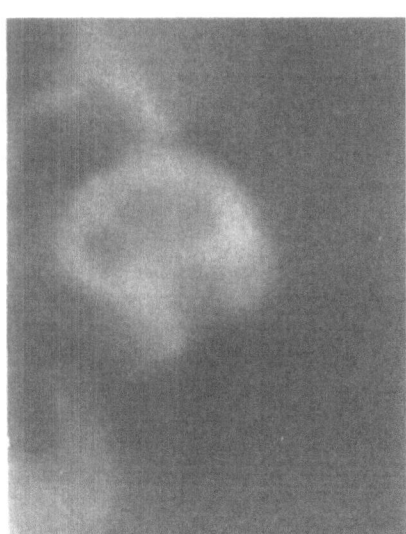
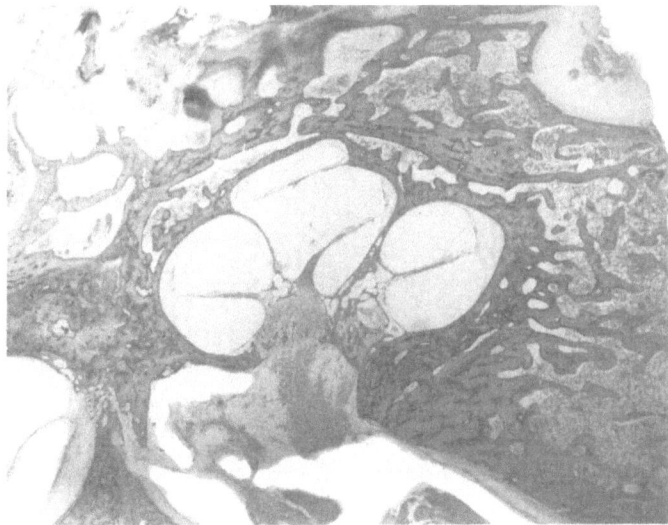

Fig. 3.20. Tomographic and base histological sections showing a reduced number of coils in the cochlea.

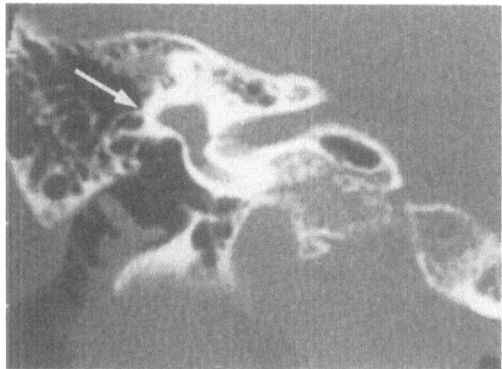 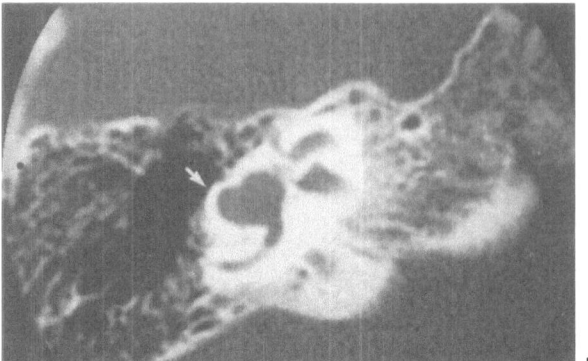

a   b

Fig. 3.21 a, b. Dysplasia of the lateral semicircular canal. **a** Coronal and **b** base views.

The authors have also seen dysplasia of the lateral semicircular canals as an incidental finding, and in one child with unilateral atresia a dilated lateral canal was present in the opposite, otherwise entirely normal ear. Although not of significance as an isolated finding, a dysplastic lateral semicircular canal is very likely to be associated with other abnormalities of labyrinth and IAM. It is common in many syndromes, including cranio-facial dysostosis, cranio-facial microsomia and anencephaly. It is the only inner ear anomaly found in the Treacher Collins Syndrome (See Chap. 4), and one report by Sando et al. (1968) shows histological sections of the ampulla of the lateral canal joined with the utricle into one common large space that contained the crista of the lateral canal and the

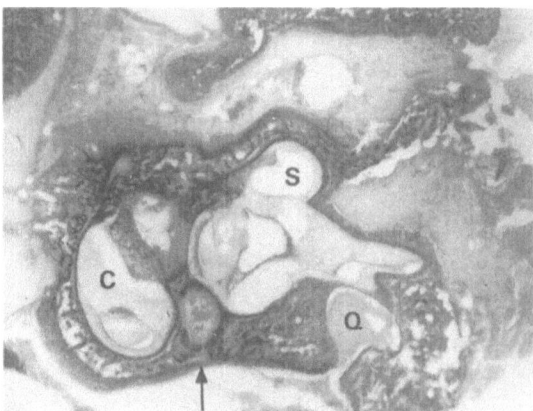

Fig. 3.22. A histological section of the deformed labyrinth in an anencephalic showing a single coil cochlea (c) and a dysplastic lateral semicircular canal, both of which appear to have a virtually normal endorgan. The vestibular aqueduct (Q) is large. The *arrow* points to the IAM.

macula of the utricle. The canal then bulged laterally for a short distance from the vestibule towards the middle ear and ended in a blind pouch. It appears that the canal failed to differentiate fully, although its end organ was present. We have seen similar appearances on a histological section of anencephalic temporal bones (Fig. 3.22) and in one case of cranio-facial microsomia. The caloric response in patients with this anomaly is variable but reduced.

The lateral semicircular canal may, rarely, be entirely absent in whole or in part, or may have an abnormal angulation. Similar anomalies may rarely affect the superior and posterior semicircular canals (Fig. 3.23). Generally speaking, the more severe the anomalies of the semicircular canals, the greater the degree of deafness, whatever the state of the bony cochlea. However, we have seen two cases with absence of the ampullary end of the semicircular canal, as well as a dysplastic lateral canal, where there was normal cochlear function. Dilatation of the vestibule, especially in the horizontal plane, must always be considered to constitute a risk of a stapes gusher.

Of other inner ear structures the cochlear aqueduct has been considered in the section on CSF fistulae and the vestibular aqueduct, which may be dilated in association with congenital ear deformities, will be discussed in the chapter on vertigo (Chap. 10). An attempt to assess the oval and round window should always be made. The oval window appears on coronal sections as a dehiscence in the medial wall of the middle ear. The average size of the normal oval window is approximately 3 mm × 2 mm (Rovsing 1970) and so it can usually be demonstrated adequately by sections at 2-mm intervals. The round window, situated about 2 mm below the oval, is smaller and less often identified. It is best assessed by base CT.

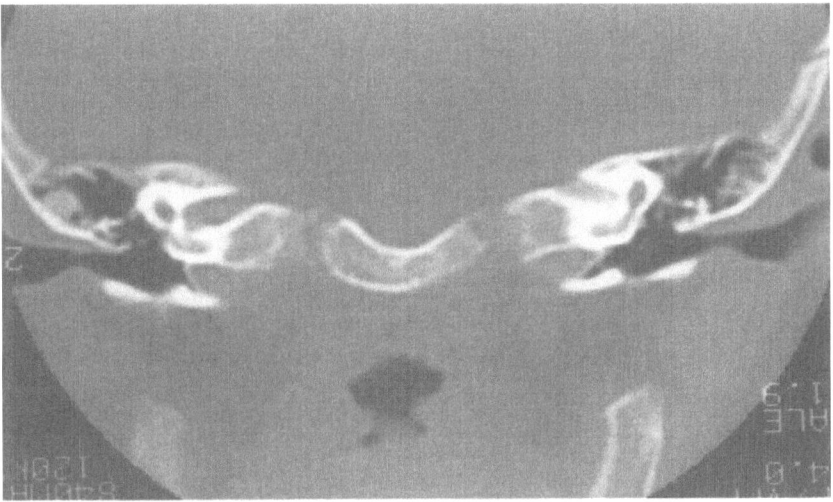

Fig. 3.23. Coronal CT section showing bilateral absence of the semicircular canals in a patient with the CHARGE association.

Abnormality of the Vestibular Aqueduct

Credit for drawing attention to the dilated vestibular aqueduct in cases of congenital deafness must go to Valvassori (1983), although such dilatation represents merely arrested development and is often associated with other severe labyrinthine abnormalities (Fig. 3.22).

Dilatation was defined as a diameter of 1.5 mm or more in the mid portion of the descending limb of the vestibular aqueduct. In 160 cases examined, there was enlargement of the vestibular aqueduct only in 61, enlargement of the vestibular aqueduct with anomalies of vestibule and semicircular canals in 75, and enlargement of the vestibular canal with associated anomalies of the whole labyrinth includ-

ing the cochlea (usually a Mondini-type deformity) in 24. No correlation between audiometry and the tomographic findings was apparent, but fluctuation and progression of the hearing loss were noted. The case illustrated, with a dilated vestibular aqueduct as the only anomaly shown (Fig. 3.24), had some speech in his first 2 years but is now severely deaf, suggesting a progressive hearing loss.

The only work we have been able to find where the radiological appearances have been correlated with full clinical assessment is in a recent paper by Emmett (1985), whose findings were in general agreement with ours. We are presently assessing ten cases (nine children and one adult) with the dilated vestibular aqueduct syndrome. There appears to be a high incidence of depressed vestibular function as shown by rotational and caloric testing but the most striking feature has been the history of head injury, often minor, which preceded the hearing loss; in fact, in the one adult case, the radiological examination was undertaken for a suspected fracture. Thus greater awareness of the vestibular aqueduct syndrome may lead to finding more cases in trauma victims, especially as base CT appears the best method for showing dilated vestibular aqueducts. Those of normal calibre are best shown by lateral tomography (see above).

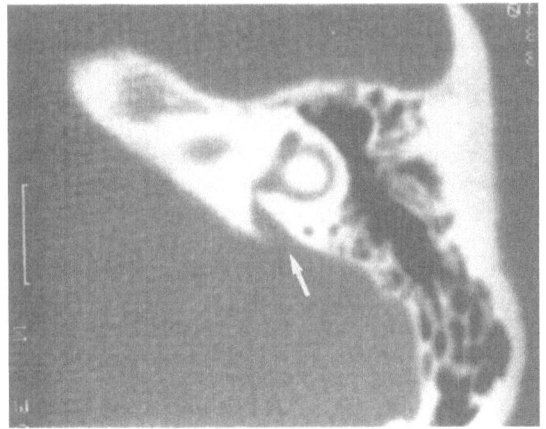

Fig. 3.24. Base CT section showing a dilated vestibular aqueduct.

Middle Ear

Radiology of congenital deformities of the middle and external ear relates almost exclusively to the

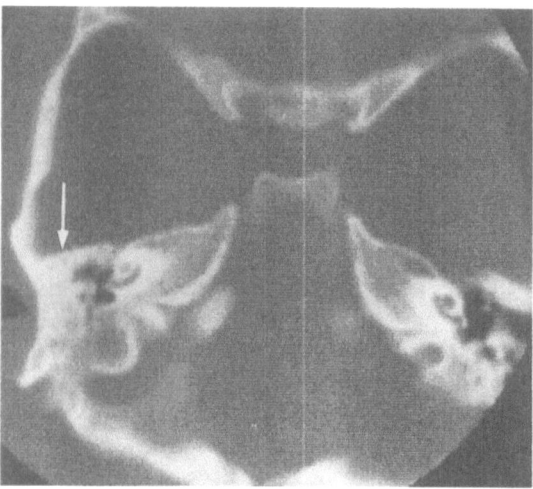

Fig. 3.25. Basal CT at the level of the round windows, showing a thick bony atresia encroaching on the air-containing middle ear (*arrow*). No ossicles can be identified. Compare with the normal side.

prospects of improvement of conductive deafness by surgical intervention. The size and shape of the middle ear cavity is the most important assessment to be made, especially where there is atresia of the external auditory meatus (Fig. 3.25).

In the majority of unilateral atresias with associated deformity of the pinna but no other congenital abnormality, there is a normally formed mastoid with good pneumatisation and the middle ear cavity is of relatively normal shape. Even in the most severe deformities there is rarely complete absence of the middle ear and usually at least a slit-like hypotympanum can be shown lateral to the basal turn of the cochlea. The middle ear cavity may be

reduced in size by encroachment of the atretic plate laterally, by a high jugular bulb inferiorly or by descent of the tegmen superiorly. In cranio-facial microsomia and mandibulo-facial dysostosis, the attic and antrum are typically absent or slit-like, being replaced in varying degree by solid bone or by descent of the tegmen.

If the middle ear is air-containing, its shape and contents are relatively easy to assess and prospects for surgery are promising. Frequently, however, the middle ear in congenital abnormalities contains undifferentiated embryological mesenchyme, a thick glue-like substance, which is radiologically indistinguishable from soft tissue, retained mucus or serous otitis media. Because of persistant tubal dysfunction and recurrence of mesenchymatous tissue, surgical results in such cases are usually bad (Marquet 1981). Thin bony septa may divide the middle ear cavity into two or more compartments. These may cause problems of orientation for the surgeon if only one compartment is opened.

Cholesteatoma may occur behind an atretic plate, presumably from squamous epithelium situated between the plate and the malformed eardrum. This type of congenital cholesteatoma is, in fact, surprisingly rare and in a review of the world literature, Peron and Schuknecht (1975) could find only 20 recorded cases. Ombredanne and Porte (1962) found 12 cholesteatomas in 330 operations on major aplasias, but only one in cases with minor abnormalities of the ossicles and middle ear.

We found four cases of cholesteatoma in 300 patients with congenital ear lesions. One case presented with an inflammatory swelling in the neck and a sinus tract leading to the middle ear, which was found to be full of squamous debris with the dura exposed. No ossicles or other normal structures could be recognised and these had presumably been eroded by the cholesteatoma. In two other cases the cholesteatoma was an unsuspected finding at operation and a tympanic membrane could be identified deep to the cholesteatoma sac (Fig. 3.26).

The destructive nature of cholesteatoma makes its recognition important but, unfortunately, we were unable even in retrospect to distinguish any suggestive features such as bone erosion on the tomograms. This may be because the cholesteatoma was situated beyond a soft tissue atresia in all three cases. Computed tomography does not appear to be any more discerning.

The existence of a normal ossicular chain is rarely found where there is atresia of the external ear but complete absence of the ossicles is also unusual. In most cases, at least some vestige of the ossicular chain is evident. The ossicles are often thicker and heavier than normal or, less frequently, thin and

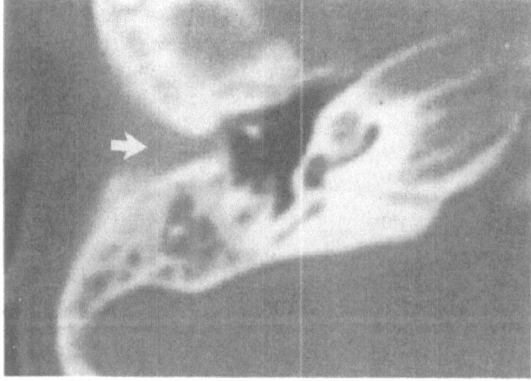

Fig. 3.26. Base CT at the level of the round window. Soft tissue opacity in the narrow bony external auditory meatus.

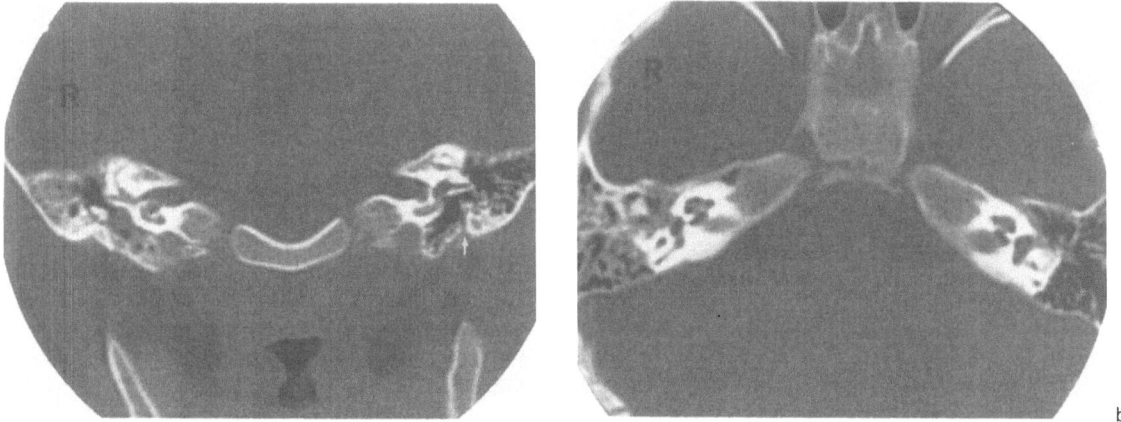

a   b

Fig. 3.27 a, b. Coronal (**a**) and base (**b**) CT sections showing bilateral bony atresia and well pneumatised mastoids. The ossicles, although deformed and fused, are of normal size on the right but hypoplastic on the left. The descending facial nerve canal is anteriorly placed (*arrow*). These findings were surgically confirmed.

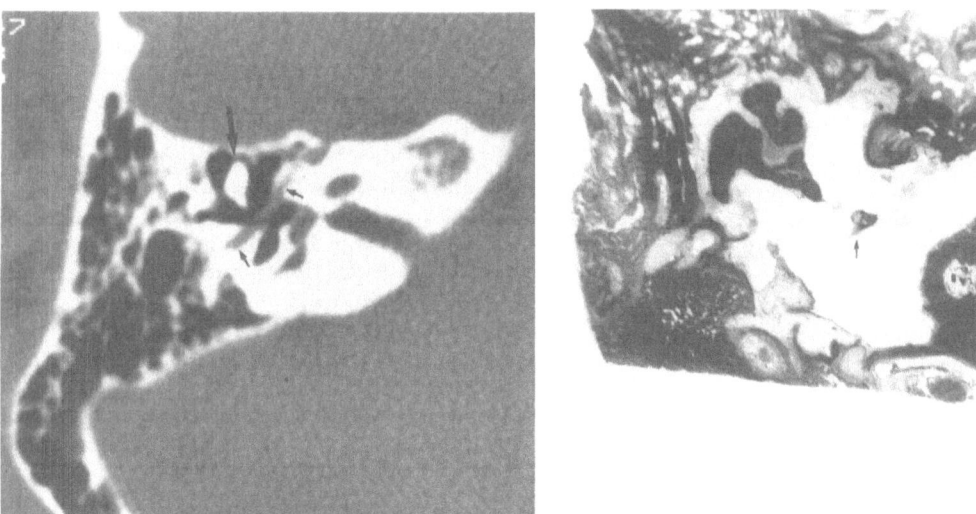

a   b

Fig. 3.28 a. Ossicular mass (*large arrow*). Note the dehiscent second part of the facial nerve canal on the base CT section (*small arrows*). **b.** A histological section from an anecephalic showing a similar ossicular mass which fails to articulate with the head of the stapes (*arrow*).

spidery (Fig. 3.27). They may be fixed to the walls of the middle ear cavity but the more usual deformity discovered at surgery is a fusion of the bodies of the malleus and incus. The ankylosis varies in degree and may be bony or fibrous. The radiological recognition of this ossicular union is difficult but is, in any case, not of great practical importance, and an irregular lump of bone in the middle ear cavity usually represents an ossicular mass (Fig. 3.28).

Because of the partial or complete replacement of the tympanic membrane by a bony plate, the handle of the malleus is not surprisingly that part of the chain which is most often abnormal and most easily recognised on the tomograms. If the handle is absent the "molar tooth" appearance of the ossicles will no longer be evident in the lateral projection and a triangular appearance of the ossicular mass will be seen (Fig. 3.29). Often, the handle of the malleus is bent towards the atretic plate to which it may be fixed and this gives the typical L-shaped appearance to the ossicular mass. A slit-like attic so typical of mandibulo-facial dysostosis or an over-

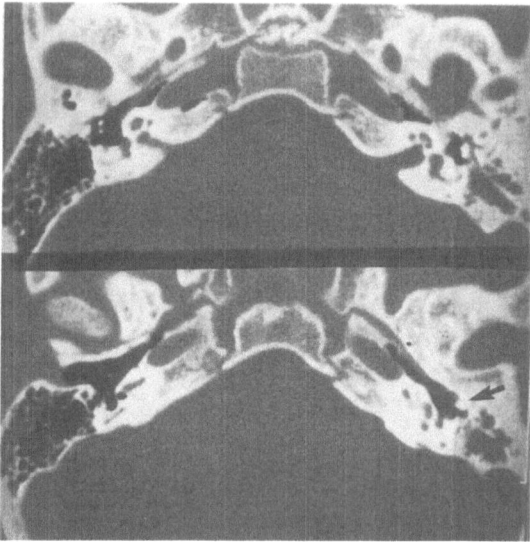

Fig. 3.29. Two base sections showing fusion of the bony processes of malleus and incus to each other and the bony atretic plate (*arrow*). Compare with the normal side.

hanging facial ridge may obstruct the free movement of the ossicular chain.

Deformities of the stapes superstructure cannot usually be recognised and fixation, or absence, of the footplate is best considered in conjunction with the oval window. Sometimes a massive stapes with fixed footplate may be demonstrated. Unfortunately, the common discontinuity at the incudo-stapedial junction is difficult to show. The ossicles are not usually found far from their normal site, although

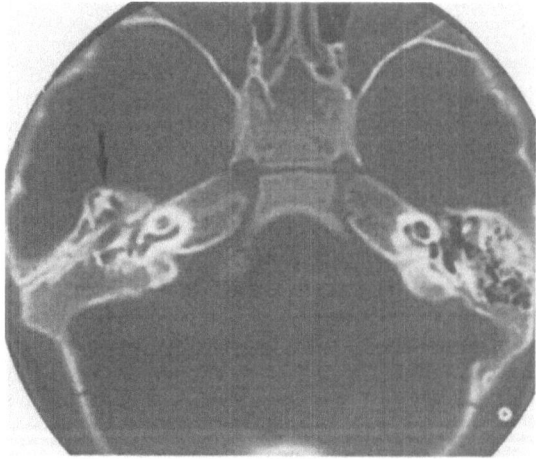

Fig. 3.30. Bilateral bony atresia. The ossicles on the right are deformed and situated anteriorly and laterally. Base CT at round window level.

sometimes they are a little more anterior than normal. Ossicles situated in a lateral position (Fig. 3.30) are a feature of hemifacial microsomia (see Chap. 4).

External Auditory Meatus (EAM)

In congenital deformities of the external ear, the external auditory meatus may be narrow, short, completely or partially atretic or it may run in an abnormal direction. It often slopes up towards the middle ear and in such cases it may be curved in two planes, becoming more horizontal at its medial end. The obstruction in atresia may be due to soft tissue or bone, but usually both are involved. The tympanic ring may be deformed, hyperplastic or absent. Complete aplasia of the tympanic ring occurred in one third of Terrahe's cases but is in fact only common in thalidomide malformations (Terrahe 1972). In these patients, the temporo-mandibular joint is situated more posteriorly than usual and is in direct contact with the mastoid process, which may itself be hypoplastic.

A rudimentary, incomplete or grossly misshapen tympanic bone can often be recognised and is best demonstrated by lateral tomograms. The external auditory meatus will appear to lack a floor if the ring is incomplete. Hyperplasia of the ring is not common, accounting for only 6% of Terrahe's cases. In these patients a cylindrical uncannulated bone which is separate from the squamous temporal may appear to protrude from the side of the head (Fig. 3.31). It is uncertain to what extent the atretic plate is due to a deformed tympanic bone or to extension of the squamous temporal bone downwards to meet the floor of the middle ear but, sometimes, there seems to be a solid bony wall continuous with the side of the skull. The atretic plate may be pneumatised, presumably by extension of the mastoid air cells.

It is not difficult to estimate the thickness of the atretic plate from coronal section imaging, but the position of an abnormal auditory meatus should be carefully assessed in relation to surrounding structures such as the middle ear and the temporo-mandibular joint. This is important if surgery is contemplated, as the pinna is often low in relation to the middle ear cavity and the surgeon will want to know whether to approach the cavity via the existing meatus or to create a new opening.

A diagrammatic representation of some of the congenital structural abnormalities of the middle and external ears as shown by tomography is given in Fig. 3.32.

Facial Nerve

The demonstration of the three parts of the facial nerve canal in the temporal bone is described in Chap. 2. The canal is 24–30 mm in length and extends from the fundus of the IAM to the stylomastoid foramen. It is about 1 mm in diameter in its first part but usually widens considerably as the stylomastoid foramen is reached.

Abnormal Development

In early embryonic life the developing VIIth cranial nerve lies anterior to the otocyst so, if development is arrested at this stage, a tract for the facial nerve is found anterior to the otic sac. If development is arrested at a later stage, when the cochlea has formed to some extent, then the first part of the facial nerve is found in its usual situation above and lateral to the cochlea. The facial nerve is, therefore, relatively unaffected by developmental abnormalities of the labyrinth, and aberrations of the first part of the facial nerve canal are most unusual.

The course of the second and third parts is, however, dependent on normal development of the branchial arches, the facial nerve being the nerve of the second arch. During its development and migration, the facial nerve curves behind the branchial cartilage to reach the anterior aspect of the same cartilage. At the same time, part of the cartilage adheres to the otic capsule to form the Fallopian canal. Should the branchial cartilage not develop as usual and be hampered in facial canal closure, defects may occur and, consequently, the facial nerve may extend in a more frontal direction (Rohrt and Loretzen 1976). Dehiscences in the Fallopian canal of the second part of the facial nerve were common in the cases reported by Marquet (1981); in 7% the geniculate part was covered only by the middle fossa dura, while in the posterior part the nerve was exposed in 12%. Terrahe (1972), in his comprehensive treatise on the radiology of congenital ear lesions, states that, with severe deformities, the facial canal is shortened and anteriorly placed or the nerve may cross the middle ear from the genicular ganglion. If the mastoid is hypoplastic, the nerve tends to pass out laterally with no descending portion. Steep descent of the facial nerve, associated with shortening of the middle ear cavity and stapedial abnormalities, was found in 50% of cases with severe narrowing or absence of the oval window. Variations in width, either widening or apparent narrowing, are probably not of significance. Bifurcation of the descend-

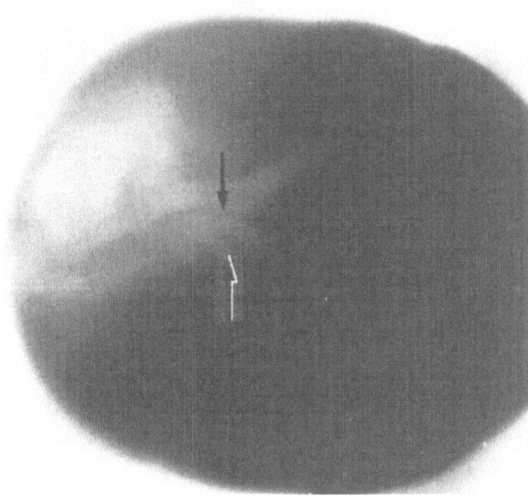

Fig. 3.31. A cigar-shaped uncannulated tympanic bone.

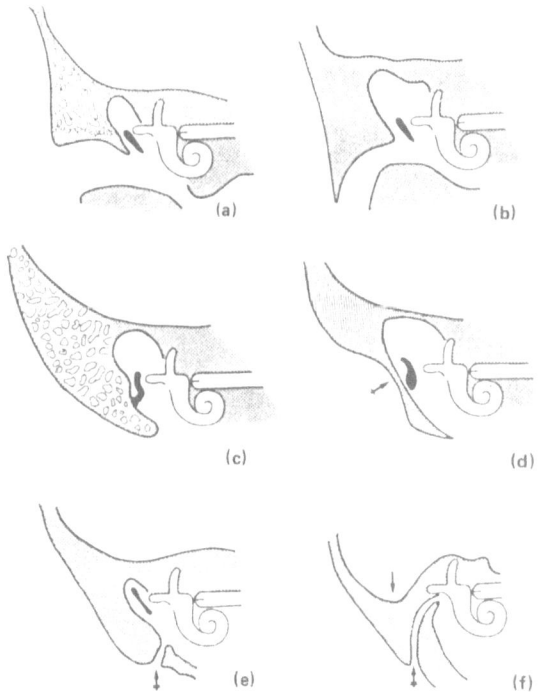

Fig. 3.32 a–f. A diagrammatic representation of congenital deformities of middle and external ears based on coronal section tomograms. **a** Normal appearances; **b–f**, various types of atretic plate, reduced middle ear cavity, ossicular deformity and anterior facial nerve ↑, → = thin atretic plate, ↓ = depression of the tegmen. (From Phelps et al. (1977), with permission.)

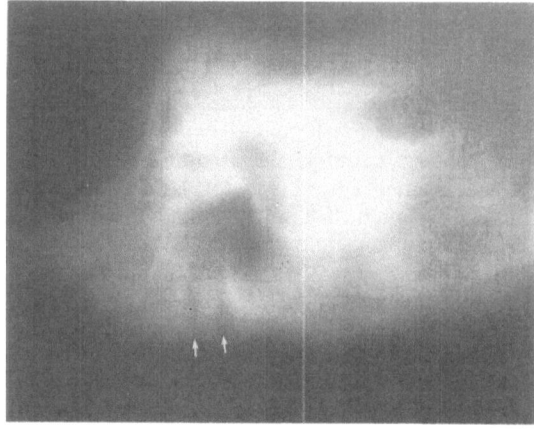

Fig. 3.33. Coronal tomogram showing the descending facial canal dividing into two parts.

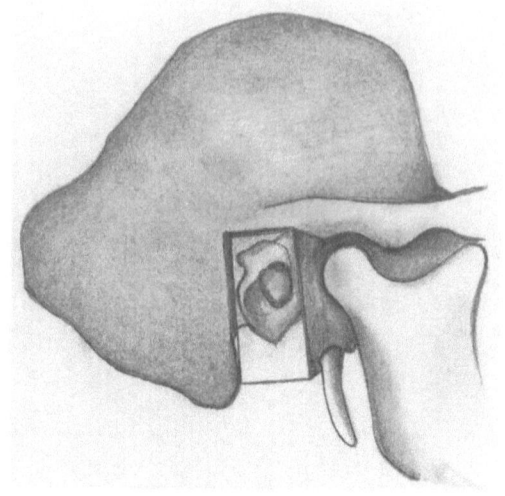

a

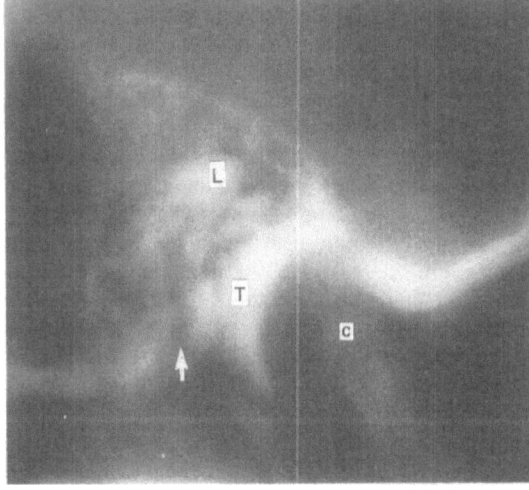

Fig. 3.34. Lateral tomogram of congenital atresia with well-pneumatised mastoid. T, the uncannulated tympanic bone; L, lateral semicircular canal; c, condyle of the mandible. The *arrow* points to the descending facial canal, which is in normal position.

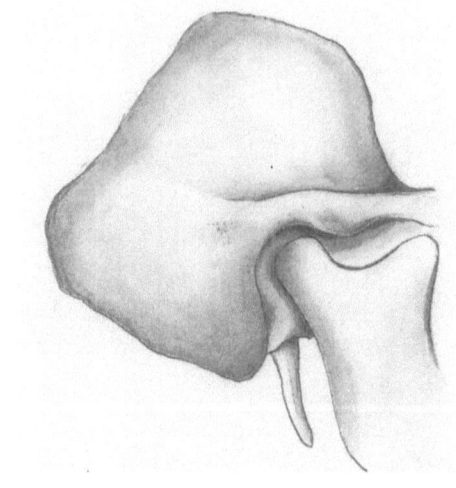

b

Fig. 3.35 a, b. External auditory meatal atresia. **a** When the pharyngeal groove was active embryologically; **b** absence of induction of the tympanic bone. Courtesy of Professor J Marquet, Antwerp.

ing portion is far more common with congenital malformations than in normal ears (Fig. 3.33).

It is believed that if the external pharyngeal groove of the first branchial arch is active during development and atresia is due only to maldevelopment of the tympanic ring, the Fallopian canal follows its normal course (Fig. 3.34). In major atresias, when the external pharyngeal groove is not active, development of malformations is much worse. The temporomandibular joint may abut directly on to the mastoid process and the topography of the Fallopian canal is always disturbed

and abnormal (Fig. 3.35). Several operative descriptions of aberrant facial nerves, found during exploration of congenital ear deformities, have been recorded. Two thirds of the facial nerves in the cases reported by Scheer (1967) had marked variations in their course and appearance, while Crabtree (1974) found 22 abnormal facial nerves out of 50, of which four were exposed and partly over the oval window, and two completely covered it. The greater the deformity, the more marked the tendency to a shortening of the third vertical segment. When the mastoid is small and sclerotic, the nerve often takes an almost straight line outwards from the horizontal portion to the surface. In such cases, it may lie below the skin and fascia in front of the pinna.

Phelps and Lloyd (1981) found that exposed facial nerves in the middle ear cavity were the most common abnormalities reported at surgery – usually dehiscences of the Fallopian canal but with the descending segment often affected. In several cases, severe and important abnormalities were found – usually a marked overhang of the facial ridge with absence of the second genu (Fig. 3.36). In only three cases did the nerve cover the oval window. In two other cases, the nerve crossed the eardrum, turning forwards in the floor of the external auditory meatus. Although CT will demonstrate soft tissue structures in an air-containing middle ear, nevertheless recognition of the exposed facial nerve is difficult. Two useful signs of aberrant pathways through the middle ear cavity may help.

1. An exit foramen through the floor of the middle ear cavity or lateral atretic plate may be identified (Fig. 3.32)
2. Absence, at the back of the middle ear cavity, of the pyramidal eminence which normally contains the stapedius muscle and tendon

The pyramid was identified in only two of the cases noted at operation to have marked anomalies of the facial canal in the middle ear and, in these, the dehiscence was in the second part. Absence of the pyramid is, therefore, good presumptive evidence of an exposed facial nerve.

When there are deformities of the external and middle ear, the descending facial canal is often more anteriorly situated than normal (Fig. 3.37). This anterior displacement may be observed on lateral tomograms but it appears to be best assessed on coronal sections by relating the position of the descending canal to labyrinthine structures. The two sections which best demonstrate the descending facial canal and the oval window, respectively, are noted as well as the distance between these sections. If the oval window is absent, this method can still be used, as the site of the oval window can be assessed from the configuration of the labyrinth.

The patients with mandibulo-facial dysostosis (Treacher Collins syndrome) and ear malformations had a very high incidence of facial nerve anomalies, even when the eardrums were normal. In three cases the facial nerve was completely exposed in the middle ear cavity: one nerve passing below the oval window, one adherent to the stapes and one fixed to the head of the malleus in the attic. In the nine other ears that were explored, there was an overhanging facial ridge, and in several the second part of the facial nerve canal was partially

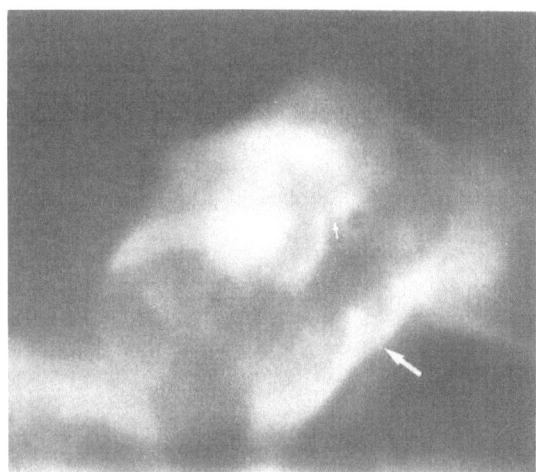

Fig. 3.36. The Fallopian canal for the second part of the facial nerve overhangs the oval window (*arrow*). The large arrow shows the atretic plate. This feature would make it difficult or impossible to insert any form of strut during attempts at reconstructive surgery.

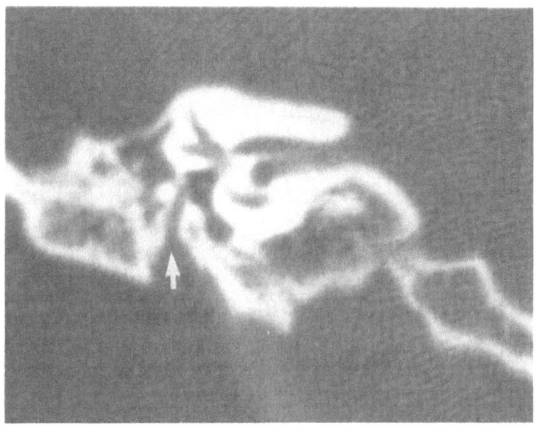

Fig. 3.37. Coronal CT section showing the descending facial canal at the level of the oval window.

dehiscent. Tomograms showed the descending facial nerve to be anteriorly situated in most cases and in five ears it was at the level of the oval window. In two cases, the descending portion of the nerve ran out more laterally than normal, but in all, the facial nerve seemed to follow a more direct path out of the temporal bone with the bends opened to some degree (Fig. 3.38). In the whole of the series there was no indication of any facial nerve misplaced in its first part, and the pit for the genicular ganglion was nearly always demonstrated above and lateral to a normal cochlea. Even with quite severe labyrinthine deformities, the

FACIAL NERVE

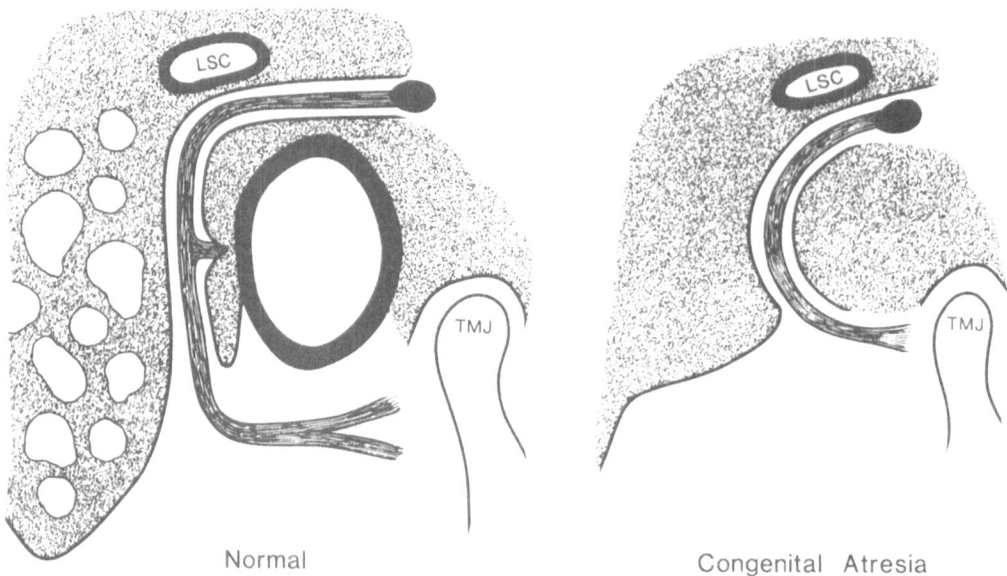

Normal   Congenital Atresia

Fig. 3.38. Diagram based on sagittal section imaging of the course of the facial nerve in congenital deformities.

nerve followed a normal course, provided that the middle and external ears were normal. A very narrow IAM may contain nothing but the facial nerve, even when there is a relatively normal-looking labyrinth. This is confirmed by tomography when the IAM is continuous with the first part of the facial nerve canal, there being no change in calibre. When the labyrinth is grossly abnormal with no recognisible cochlea, a tract for the facial nerve can usually be identified anterior to the primitive otic sac.

In the most common type of congenital atresia occurring as an isolated anomaly, normal mastoid pneumatisation is present and a recognisible, although often grossly deformed, tympanic bone between mastoid and temporo-mandibular joint. In these patients the course of the facial nerve is likely to be normal.

Regime for Investigation

A limited amount of information can be obtained from plain films. The extent of mastoid pneumatisation and some details of labyrinth and ossicles may be assessed, especially in the neonate. The base view gives most information. To this end, any previous relevant films including skull views should be studied before beginning the definitive investigation of the temporal bones, which is by base and, if possible, coronal section CT at 2-mm intervals.

The question of the optimum age for the examination is a difficult one, particularly as the hearing deficit is often discovered at the age of 2–3 years, when some form of sedation and often a general anaesthetic is necessary. The authors believe that a child born with a deformed pinna, with or without external meatal atresia or with manifestations of a syndrome, such as mandibulo-facial dysostosis (in which deafness is a known feature) should have imaging in the neonatal period, preferably before mother and baby are discharged from the maternity unit. Examination at this stage has the following advantages:

1. Usually no more sedation than a large feed is required
2. A few sections should give a full assessment of the state of the middle and inner ears
3. The information obtained, provided that it is not lost in the meantime, can be usefully correlated with the hearing assessments undertaken from 1–2 years of age. Severe labyrinthine deformities preclude any auditory function. When the external ears are normal but a severe degree of deafness is suspected, imaging may be useful as an

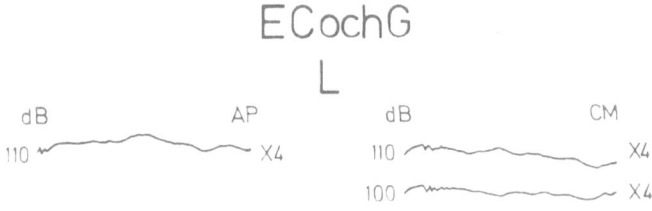

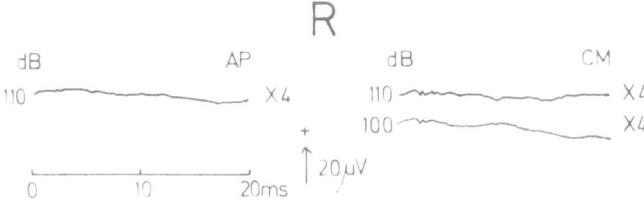

a   ♀ 2 yr Bilateral Cochlear and Vestibular dysphasia

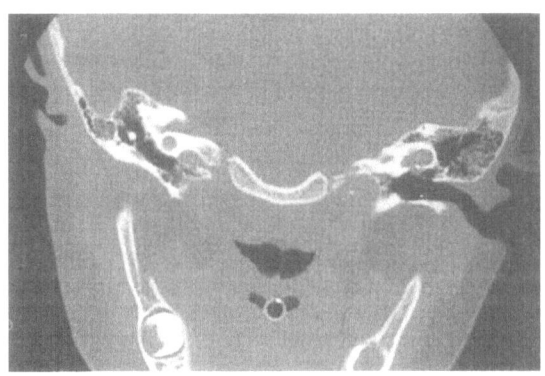

b

Fig. 3.39 a, b. Electrophysiology (a) and imaging (b): complementary procedures in severe deafness.

adjunct to electrocochleography for assessment (Fig. 3.39). Any unexplained attacks of meningitis or suspected CSF rhinorrhoea, associated with deafness, also necessitate imaging of the temporal bones

Surgical attempts to improve the sound conduction mechanism in unilateral malformations are now rarely undertaken, if the hearing in the other ear is normal. Opinions differ as to the best age to operate on bilateral cases. Above the age of 5 years the child will often co-operate sufficiently, but below this age a general anaesthetic is usually necessary for the examination.

References

Alexander G (1904) Zur Pathologie und pathologischen Anatomie der kongenitalen Taubheit. Arch Klin Exp Ohren Nasen Kehlkopfheilkd 61: 183–219

Bento RF (1985) X-linked mixed hearing loss – four case studies. Laryngoscope 95: 462–468

Bottema T. (1975) Spontaneous cerebrospinal fluid otorrhea. Arch Otolaryngol 101: 693–694

Bridger WMN, Phelps PD (1983) Recurrent meningitis due to congenital malformation of the inner ear. Br Med J 286: 626–627

Camp JD, Allen EP (1940) Microtia and congenital atresia of the external auditory canal. Roentgenol 43: 201–203

Carter BL, Wolpert SM, Karmody CS (1975) Recurrent meningitis associated with an anomaly of the inner ear. Neuroradiology 9: 55–61

Clemens F, Sandstrom J (1975) Double barrelled hypoplastic internal auditory canal in unilateral deafness. Acta Radiol (Diagn) 16: 342–346

Cock E (1838) The pathology of congenital deafness. Guys Hospital report 7: 289–307

Crabtree JA (1974) The facial nerve in congenital ear surgery. Otolaryngol Clin North Am 7: 505–510

Curtin HD, Gignaud J, Bar D (1982) Anomaly of the facial canal in a Mondini malformation with recurrent meningitis. Radiology 144: 335–341

Du Boulay G, Bostick T (1969) Linear tomography in congenital abnormalities of the ear. Br J Radiol 42: 161–183

Emmett JR (1985) The large vestibular aqueduct syndrome. Am J Otol 6: 387–403

Frey KW (1965) Die Tomographie der Labyrinth-Missbildungen, Fortschr Geb Roentgenstr Nuklearmed 102: 1–3

Gacek RR, Leipzig B (1979) Congenital cerebrospinal otorrhea. Ann Otol 88: 358–363

Gavilan J, Trujillo M and Gavilan C (1984) Spontaneous encephalocele of the middle ear. Arch. Otolaryngol 110: 206–207

Glasscock ME (1973) The stapes gusher. Arch Otolaryngol 98: 82–97

Gundersen T, Haye R (1970) Cerebrospinal otorrhea. Arch Otolaryngol 91: 19–23

Hirakawa K, Kurokawa M, Yajin K, Harada Y (1983) Recurrent meningitis due to a congenital fistula in the stapedial footplate. Arch Otolaryngol 109: 697–700

Jensen J (1969) Malformations of the inner ear in deaf children. Acta Radiol Supp 286: 11–90

Jensen J (1974) Congenital anomalies of the inner ear. Radiologic Clin North Am 3: 473–482

Johnsson LG (1971) Degenerative changes and anomalies of the vestibular system in man. Laryngoscope 10: 1682–1694

Kaufman B, Jordan VM, Pratt LL (1969) Positive contrast demonstration of a cerebrospinal fluid fistula through the fundus of the internal auditory meatus. Acta Radiol (Diag) 9:83–90

Kaufman B., Nulsen FE, Weiss MH, Brodkey JS, White RJ and Sykora CF (1977) Acquired spontaneous, nontraumatic normal-pressure cerebrospinal fluid fistulas originating from the middle fossa. Radiology 122: 379–387

Kraus EM, McCabe RF (1982) The giant apical air cell: a new entity. Ann Otol Rhinol Laryngol 110: 237–239

McNab Jones RF, Fairburn B (1977) Spontaneous cerebrospinal fluid otorrhea. J Laryngol Otol 91: 897–902

Mangabeira-Albernaz PL, Fukuka Y, Chammas F, Cananca MM (1981) The Mondini dysplasia – a clinical study. Oto-Rhino-Laryngol 43:131–152

Marquet J (1981) Congenital malformations and middle ear surgery. Proc R Soc Med 74: 119–128

Michel (1863). Mémoire sur les anomalies congenitales de l'oreille interne. Gazette Medicale de Strasbourg 4:55–58

Mondini C (1791) Anatomica surdi nati sectio, Bononiensi scientarium et artium instituto atque academia commentarii, Bonaniae VII: 419–428

Mygind H (1890) Übersicht über die pathologisch-anatomischen Veränderungen der Gehörorgane Taubstummer. Arch Ohrenheilk. 30: 76–118

Nance WE, Setleff F, McLeod A, Sweeney A, Cooper C, McConnell T (1971) X-linked mixed deafness with congenital fixation of the stapedial footplate and the perilymphatic gusher. Birth Defects 7: 64–69

Ombredanne M, Francois J (1961) Malformations radiologiques de l'oreille interne dans les aplasies de l'oreille. Ann Otolaryngol (Paris) 78: 557–566

Ombredanne M, Porte L (1962) Cholesteatome primitif de la caisse et aplasie mineure. Ann Otolaryngol 79: 427–430

Ormerod FC (1960) The pathology of congenital deafness. J Laryngol Otol 74: 919–950

Pashley NRT and Shapiro R (1978) Spontaneous perilymphatic fistula. J Otolaryngol 7: 110–117

Peron DP, Schuknecht HF (1975) Congenital cholesteatoma and other anomalies. Arch Otolaryngol 101: 498–505

Phelps PD (1974) Congenital lesions of the inner ear demonstrated by tomography. Arch Otolaryngol 100: 11–18

Phelps PD (1986) Congenital cerebrospinal fluid fistulae of the petrous temporal bone. Clin Otolaryngol 11: 79–82

Phelps PD, Lloyd GAS, Sheldon PWE (1977) Br J Radiol 50: 714

Phelps PD, Lloyd GAS (1978) Congenital deformity of the internal auditory meatus and labyrinth associated with cerebrospinal fluid fistula. Adv Oto-Rhinol-Laryngol 24:51–57

Phelps PD, Lloyd GAS (1981) Course of the facial nerve in congenital ear deformities. Acta Radiol (Diag) 22: 475–483

Pimontel-Appel B, Vignaud J (1979) Cerebrospinal fluid otorrhoea due to a congenital defect of the petrous bone. J Neuroradiol 6: 15–31

Rohrt T, Lorentzen P (1976) Facial nerve displacement within the middle ear. J Laryngol Otol 90: 1093–1094

Rovsing H (1970) Otosclerosis. Acta Radiol Supp 296:54

Sando I, Hemenway WG, Morgan WR (1968) Histopathology of the temporal bone in mandibulofacial dysostosis (Treacher Collins Syndrome). Trans Acad Ophthalmol Otolaryngol 72: 913–924

Scheer AA (1967) Correction of congenital middle ear deformities. Arch Otolaryngol 85:55–63

Schuknecht HF (1974) Pathology of the ear. Harvard Univ Press, Cambridge, Mass.

Siebenmann F (1904) Grundzüge der Anatomie und Pathogenese der Taubstummheit, Wiesbaden, quoted by Jensen (1969).

Stool S, Leeds NE, Shulman K (1967) The syndrome of congenital deafness and otic meningitis. Diagnosis and management. J Pediat 71: 547–552

Terrahe K (1965) Missbildungen des Innen und Mittelohre als Folge der Thalidomid-embryopathie. Fortschr Geg Roentgenstr Nuklearned 102: 14–29

Terrahe K (1972) Diagnostik der Missbildungen des Ohres und des Ohrschadels. Arch der klinischen experimentellen Ohr, Nasen und Kehlkopp Heilkunde 202: 85–151

Thomson A (1847) Notice of several cases of malformation of the external ear, together with experiments on the state of hearing in such persons. Edinburgh J Med Sci 76: 730–740

Toynbee J (1847) Description of a congenital malformation in the ears of a child. Edinburgh J Med Sci 76: 738–740

Valvassori GE, Naunton RF, Lindsay JR (1969) Inner ear anomalies: clinical and histopathological considerations. Ann Otol 78: 929–941

Valvassori GE (1983) The vestibular aqueduct and associated anomalies of the inner ear. Otolaryngol Clin North Am 16: 95–101

Von Haacke NP (1985) Juvenile stapedectomy. Clin Otolaryngol 10: 9–13

4 Syndromes with Congenital Hearing Loss

Many syndromes are associated with deafness and an even greater number with abnormalities of the pinna – usually a real or apparent low position on the side of the head. These combinations of deformities are well described in various reference books (Gorlin et al. 1976; Konigsmark and Gorlin 1976). However, while there are some specific clusters of anomalies many, or perhaps most, of these children do not fit the description of any particular syndrome. There may be associated congenital heart disease and also abnormalities of the genito-urinary system. Potentially serious renal anomalies may go undetected in early life and it has been suggested that all children with malformed ears should have an intravenous pyelogram (Rapin and Ruben 1976).

Sensorineural deafness in these children is most likely to have been caused by deformed development or degeneration of the cochlear end organ. Conductive deafness may be the result of an increased liability to suppurative or secretory otitis media, as with cleft palate for instance. In such cases, the bony architecture of the ear is normal and tomography unrewarding.

The present inadequate understanding of the pathogenesis for all of these syndromes makes any system of classification less than satisfactory. The most recent and comprehensive classification for anomalies of the inner ear is by Suehiro and Sando (1979). In a review of 108 articles they made a special effort to find and classify inner ear anomalies and associated diseases. The study showed that most of the diseases associated with inner ear anomalies are also associated with anomalies in other parts of the body. Hereditary characteristics comprise the most common aetiological factor among the diseases associated with inner ear anomalies. Of anomalies observed in the cochlea, the vestibule and the semicircular canals, those in the cochlea were found to be most frequently associated with various diseases and were observed in 30 of 43. Anomalies in both the osseous and the membranous cochlea were observed in 18 diseases. Among them the most common were anomalies of the modiolus and interscalar septum. Anomalies of the vestibule were observed in 25 diseases and those of the semicircular canals in 18. Anomalies in both the osseous and membranous labyrinth were most frequently associated with the diseases studied.

Tomography, surgical exploration or post-mortem histological sections have shown structural abnormalities of the ear in the syndromes shown in Table 4.1. This chapter is intended as a guide to the likely abnormalities that may be demonstrated by imaging and also to suggest in which of these children it may be rewarding.

The otocranio-facial group of syndromes are amongst the most common and most important of those with malformations of the middle and external ears. The lesions of the face, palate and jaws are the most obvious and receive early attention from plastic and oral surgeons, but the ear abnormalities tend to be less fully investigated. Because these cranio-facial anomalies involve several cephalic organ systems, comprehensive management of the patients reaches beyond the traditional confines of any single subspeciality. Few centres have as yet acquired the full multidisciplinary team approach that is needed. Perhaps the best example of how this comprehensive management can be achieved is the centre for cranio-facial anomalies in Illinois, USA (Calderelli 1981). The role of radiology in the management of these patients is described by Calderelli.

Table 4.1. Syndromes with structural abnormality of the ear

Otocranio-facial (ear, face, skull)			
Cranio-facial microsomia (Goldenhar Syndrome)			C
Mandibulo-facial dysostosis (Treacher Collins Syndrome)		D	C
Cranio-facial dysostosis		D	C
Apert Syndrome			
Pfeiffer Syndrome			
Saethre-Chotzen Syndrome			
Crouzon Syndrome			
Cryptophthalmos Syndrome		R	C
Waardenberg Syndrome		D	SN
Ear malformations, cervical fistulae, and mixed hearing loss (Earpits Deafness Syndrome)		D	M
Anencephaly			
Otocervical (ear, face, shoulder)			
Klippel-Feil Syndrome (Wildervanck Syndrome)			SN
Cleidocranial dysostosis		D	C
Otofacial Cervical Syndrome		D	C
Sprengel shoulder			C
Otoskeletal (bone dysplasias)			
Osteogenesis imperfecta (Van der Hoeve Syndrome)		D	M
Dysplasias with increased bone density		D&R	M
Kniest disease		D	M
Otofacial Digital Syndrome type II (Mohr)		R	C
Otopalato-digital Syndrome		XR	C
Chromosome abnormalities			
Chromosome deletion	4p-(Wolf-Hirschhorn)		C
Autosomal trisomy			
with chromosome pairs	13–15		SN
	18		M
	21 (Down's Syndrome)		C
	22		C
Sex trisomy	XO (Turner Syndrome)		C
Miscellaneous			
With endocrine disorders			
Pendred Syndrome			SN
Drug-induced			
Thalidomide embryopathy			M
Neurocutaneo-skeletal disorders			
Neurofibromatosis			M
CHARGE Association			M

Those syndromes in which there is clear hereditary transmission are labelled D for dominant, R for recessive, C for predominantly conductive deafness, SN for sensorineural, and M for mixed.

The authors believe that imaging has an important part to play in assessment of the ear deformities in many of these syndromes.

Otocranio-facial Syndromes

Cranio-facial Microsomia

Hemifacial microsomia was a term introduced by Gorlin and Pindborg (1964) to encompass those closely related syndromes that comprise anomalies of the first and second branchial arch derivatives. It is the commonest of the otocranio-facial syndromes. The distinguishing feature is the underdevelopment of one half of the face (Fig. 4.1). Mandibular and maxillary hypoplasia, macrostromia, microtia, external auditory canal atresia or stenosis, and various middle ear malformations may be present. Abnormalities of the mandibular condyle may be the hallmark of the condition, but abnormalities of the pinna and descent of the tegmen are almost constant features. As the condition is not exclusively unilateral, and often involves the bones of the skull vault and base, the term "cranio-facial microsomia" seems preferable. The malformations are bilateral in about 20% of patients, but there is always considerable dissymmetry between the two sides. The pathogenesis of the syndrome has been investigated by Poswillo (1973) using animal models. Phenocopies of cranio-facial microsomia followed the administration of various teratogens, and the causal mechanism appeared to be one of embryonic haematoma formation.

Patients with cranio-facial microsomia are not infrequently found to have additional malformations of the eye and vertebral column, and Gorlin

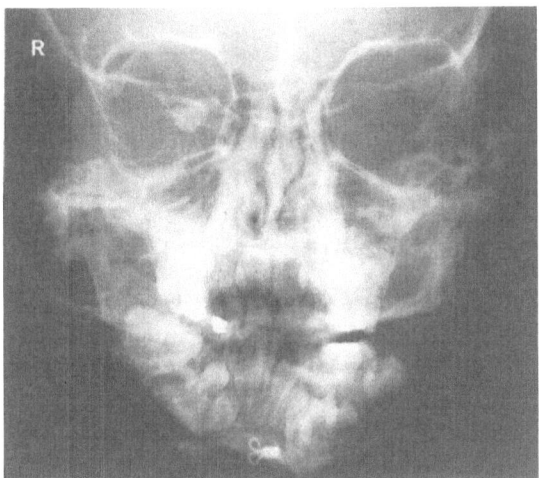

Fig. 4.1. Hemifacial microsomia. The right side of the face is underdeveloped with small orbit and short mandibular ramus.

and Pindborg recommend the term oculo-auriculo-vertebral dysplasia, although the eponym "Goldenhar's syndrome" is still used for this combination of deformities. It is considered to be a variant of cranio-facial microsomia. Goldenhar's original description (1952) was of a solitary case of epibulbar dermoids and auricular pits and appendages. There were apparently no deformities of the petrous temporal bone. Although the majority of cases of oculo-auriculo-vertebral dysplasia are sporadic without evidence of any genetic basis, nevertheless there have been reports of both autosomal dominant and recessive transmissions (Regenbogan et al. 1982).

Comprehensive descriptions have been made of the jaw lesions (Converse et al. 1979; Kaban et al. 1981). Facial asymmetry increases progressively during the formative years since the growth disparity between the affected and unaffected sides causes the mandible to deviate laterally and upwards towards the affected side. Alteration in pull of the rudimentary muscles contributes to further deformity of the developing skeleton.

There have been few comprehensive accounts of the temporal bone malformation in hemifacial microsomia, and even fewer descriptions in the radiological literature (Mafee and Valvassori 1981). Seventy patients (85 ears) were studied radiologically by Calderelli and Valvassori (1979), who found correlations between the severity of the microtia, mandibular deformity and the status of the ossicles. In 1983 we described the petromastoid lesions in 29 affected temporal bones in 22 patients (Phelps et al. 1983). This study was based on tomographic appearances correlated with surgical findings in eight, and histological sections in one case. This case has been more fully reported in another paper (Wells et al. 1983). Since then we have been able to assess a further 29 cases, including 20 from a visit to Ecuador with the Por Cristo Organisation.

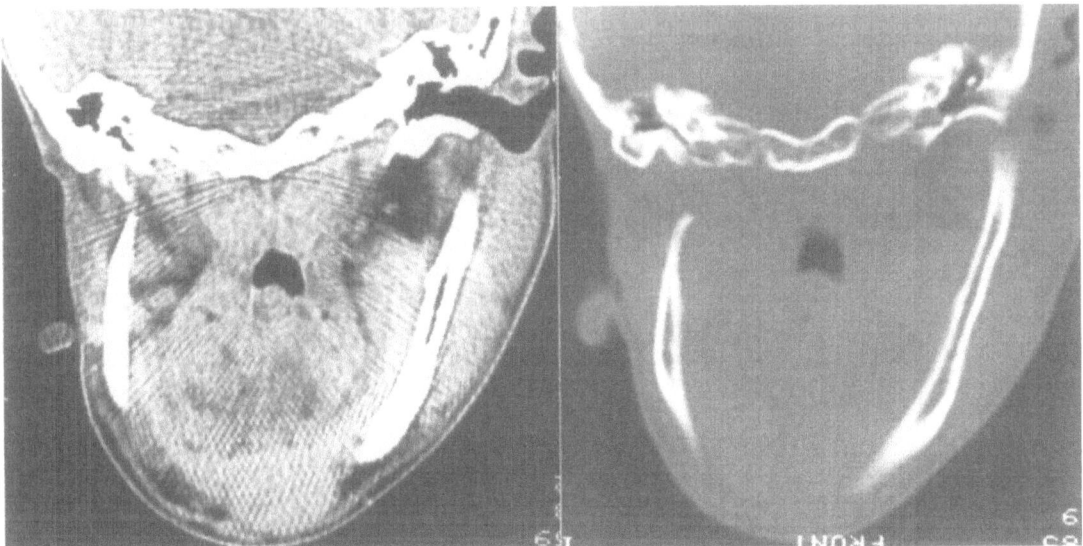

Fig. 4.2. Coronal CT section at the level of the cochleae showing the typical ear and jaw lesions of hemifacial microsomia. There is marked reduction in the right middle ear cavity and the parotid gland, masseter and medial pterygoid muscles in particular on the affected side.

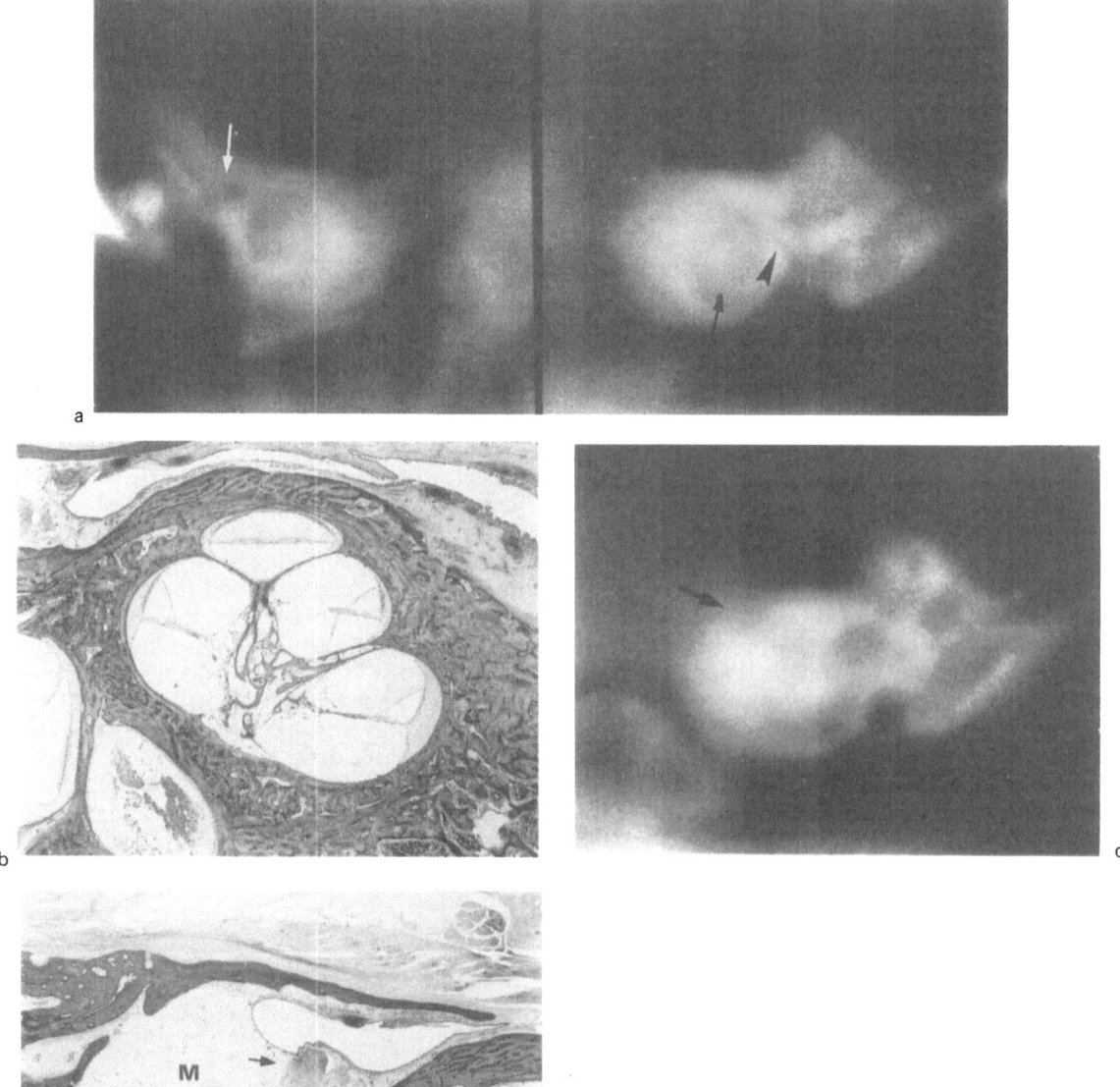

Fig. 4.3 a–d. Coronal tomograms and base section histology. (a,b) at cochlea level. The *black arrow* indicates the deficient central bony spiral. The arrow head indicates the narrow facial nerve canal pointing downwards. Compare with the cochlea and sulcus for the geniculate ganglion (*white arrow*) on the normal side: (c) at vestibule level. Note the small middle ear cavity with absent oval window and ossicles. Also the small IAM (*arrow*). The histology section (d) shows the bare facial nerve running downwards between cochlea (c) and vestibule (v). There is no oval window.

These radiological assessments have included the use of computerised tomography for the otofacial deformities. Although CT has no particular advantage for the study of bony deformities, including the state of the auditory ossicles, it nevertheless gives an excellent demonstration of soft tissue abnormalities, particularly hypoplasia of the muscles of mastication which formerly could not be demonstrated by conventional imaging techniques. CT can be used to assess both ear and jaw, soft tissue and bony abnormalities in one examination (Fig. 4.2). The following account is therefore based on examination of 61 affected temporal bones. Regarding the overall appearances of the petrous temporal bones, the most impressive feature was the tilt in the horizontal axis, so that the lateral part forming the external ear was displaced caudally, the porus of the IAM therefore being situated much higher than the opening of the external meatus in some cases.

Inner Ear

The appearances of the bony labyrinths were normal in most cases, and this correlated with assessment of normal cochlear function. The commonest anomalies found were lateral semicircular canals that were mildly dysplastic and dilated. These anomalies are not considered significant and were usually associated with good cochlear function. Narrow IAM (two ears) and a single tube labyrinth (one ear) were associated with severe or complete deafness. A dilated vestibular aqueduct in one petrous temporal bone was associated with sensorineural deafness. Minor anomalies of the bony cochlea were harder to assess. Our one case with histological verification showed minor deficiencies of the central bony spiral, and a somewhat flattened cochlea (Fig. 4.3). Similar abnormalities of the cochlea were present in the case reported by Chandra Sekhar et al. (1978).

Middle Ear

In only a few ears was there pneumatisation of the mastoid and rarely was the middle ear cavity of normal size and shape. The most characteristic feature was descent of the floor of the middle cranial fossa between the arcuate eminence and the squamous temporal bone. This lowering of the tegmen to form a gutter-shaped depression in the cranial floor varied in degree as shown in Fig. 4.4. The tegmen was at the level of the lateral semicircular canal in 13 cases and below it in nine. In some cases the middle ear cavity was very small, being further constricted by the bony atretic plate and amounting only to a slit-like hypotympanum. In only one case was there a high jugular bulb, but the bony septum forming the floor of the middle ear was intact.

The ossicles were frequently completely absent, and in other cases abnormal in size, shape and situation. Hypoplastic malleus and incus were seen

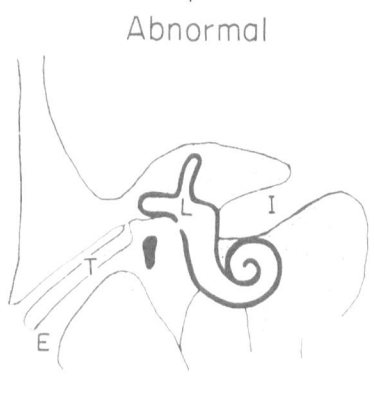

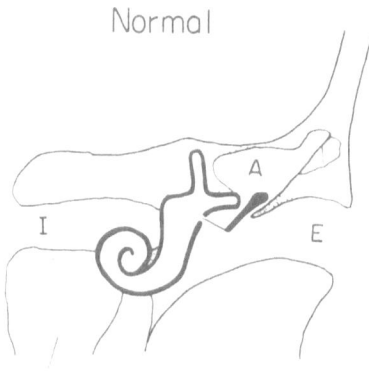

Fig. 4.4. Diagrammatic representation of cranio-facial microsomia based on coronal tomograms. I, internal auditory meatus; L, lateral semicircular canal; T, tympanic bone; E, external auditory meatus.

alongside each other on coronal sections in several cases, and in others there was a half-moon-shaped ossicular mass. One characteristic feature was the lateral position of the ossicles, often far from the oval window (Fig. 4.5). In the seven operated ears, the status of the ossicles was recorded as a fused ossicular mass in two, abnormal malleus and incus in three, one malleus being attached to the tympanic annular ring, and absent in two. There were no ossicles nor an oval window present in the sectioned ear (Fig. 4.3).

Three patients had muscular weakness as well as deformity of one half of the face. These congenital facial palsies were only partial. The facial nerve followed an unpredictable and more direct path in many cases, with opening out of the second bend. Dehiscences of the walls of the facial nerve canal were common findings at surgery. In the sectioned temporal bone the nerve ran straight downwards in the middle ear between cochlea and vestibule with no bony covering.

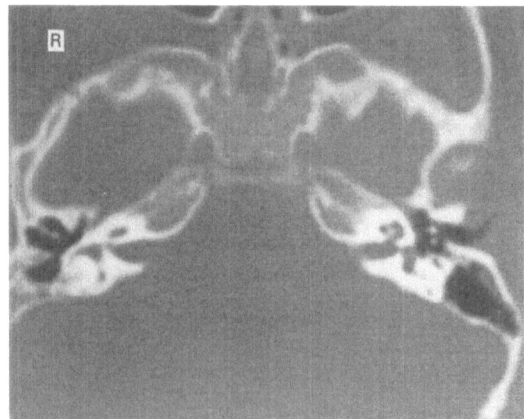
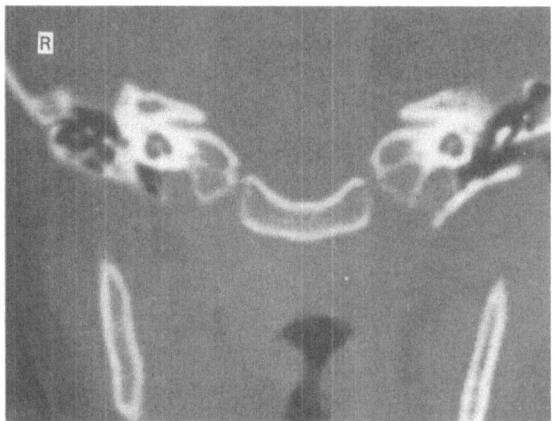

a   b

Fig. 4.5 a,b. Hemifacial microsomia, (a) base, (b) coronal sections. Normal appearances on the left. On the right, there is some depression of the tegmen and thin bony atresia, but there is a large air-containing middle ear cavity. Note, however, that the small hypoplastic ossicles lie medial and lateral instead of anterior and posterior as on the normal side. (From Scott Brown's *Otolaryngology*, Vol 6.)

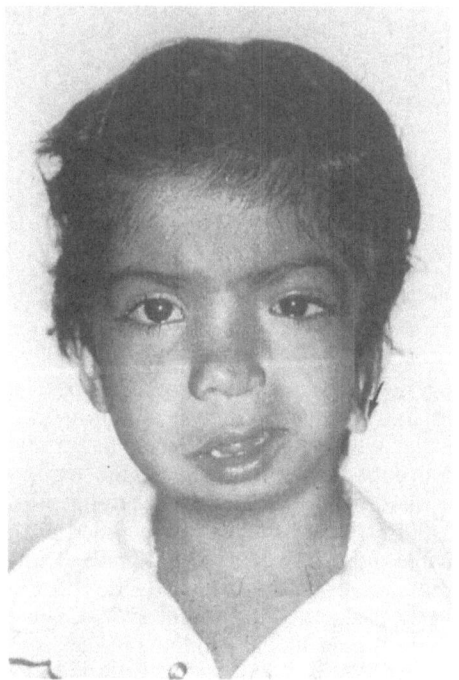
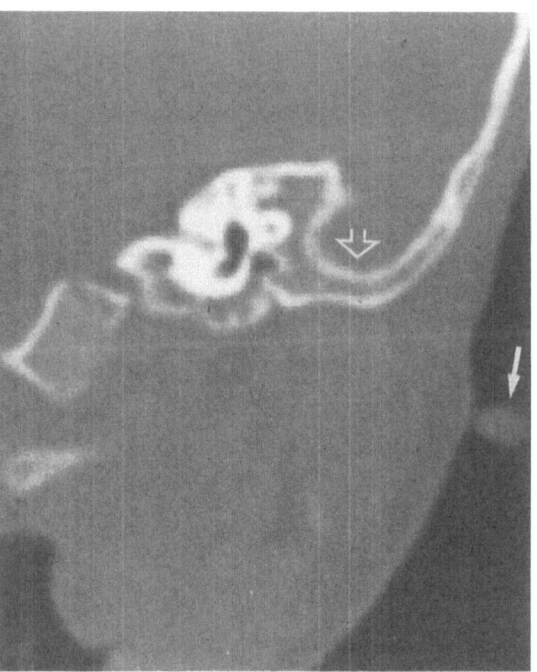

a   b

Fig. 4.6 a,b. Typical hemifacial microsomia. (a) Note the unilateral microsomia, flattened nose and ear lobule (*arrow*). The coronal CT section (b) shows the slit middle ear cavity and severe descent of the floor of the middle cranial fossa.

External Ear

The major structural abnormalities of the petrous bone affected the region of the external auditory meatus and tympanic bone. These were always associated with deformity of the pinna, varying from complete absence to slight microtia. In three cases there was only a lobule present (Fig. 4.6).

There was a normal external auditory meatus (EAM) in some patients, always on the less severely

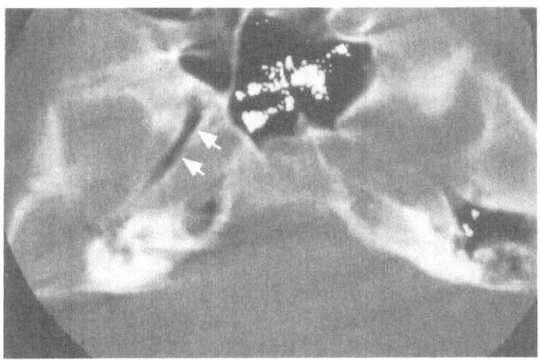

Fig. 4.7. A child with severe hemifacial microsomia. As well as showing the hypoplasia of the muscles of mastication, this base high-resolution CT examination demonstrated a patulous cartilaginous Eustachian tube (*arrow*). There was a typically deformed middle ear cavity but no cleft palate.

Eustachian Tube. A dilated patulous Eustachian tube was present in two cases (Fig. 4.7).

Other Skull Abnormalities. Cleft palate was present in several patients, and deficiencies of the skull base in three. An occipital meningocoele was associated with a large foramen magnum in one patient (Fig. 4.8) and in two others deficiency of the margins of the foramen magnum was shown.

Mandibulo-facial Dysostosis (Treacher Collins Syndrome)

affected side in bilateral cases. There was often complete atresia and in other cases the EAM opened in a low anterior position, running a curving course upwards and making inspection of the eardrum difficult or impossible. In the most extreme examples the course was almost vertical.

Whereas hypoplasia is the dominant feature of the middle ear and ossicles, hyperplasia of the bony structures forming the external ear may occur. This was particularly severe in one case, in which a prominent mastoid process, uncannulated vertical cigar-shaped tympanic bone and large styloid process could be identified.

There is a marked similarity between the abnormalities in the middle and inner ears in both hemifacial microsomia and mandibulo-facial dysostosis. This suggests that, once initiated, the mechanism of malformation is similar. Both appear to be caused by disturbances in the local mesenchyme, craniofacial microsomia caused by a stop-go process of cell death and redifferentiation, and mandibulo-facial dysostosis provoked by fundamental diminution of local mesenchyme ab initio.

Mandibulo-facial dysostosis is an autosomal dominant malformation syndrome of full penetrance but variable expressivity, with the characteristic features of antimongoloid slanting of the palpebral fissures, malar bone hypoplasia, mandibular hypoplasia and, occasionally, cleft palate. In about 75% of cases there is coloboma of the lower eyelid. The

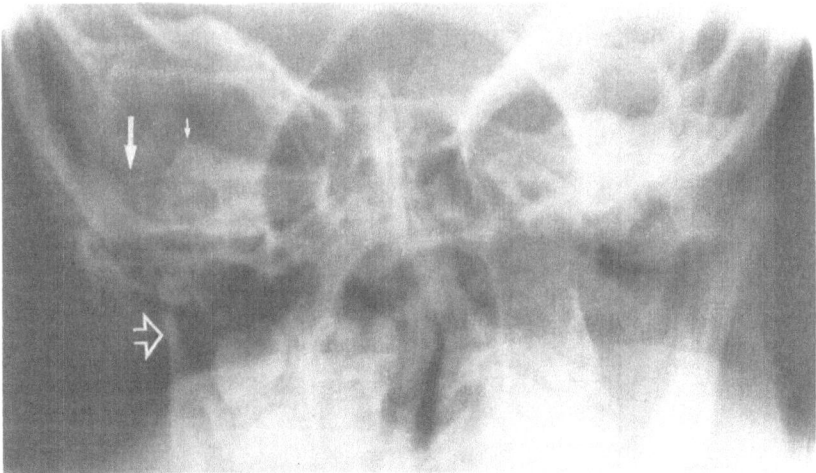

Fig. 4.8. A case of ocular auriculovertebral dysplasia. The Towne's view shows a large foramen magnum which was associated with an occipital meningocoele. The *open arrow* points to the hypoplastic mandibular ramus; the *small arrow* points to the arcuate eminence; the *large arrow* to the depressed tegmen so typical of hemifacial microsomia. (From Scott Brown's *Otolaryngology*, Vol 6.)

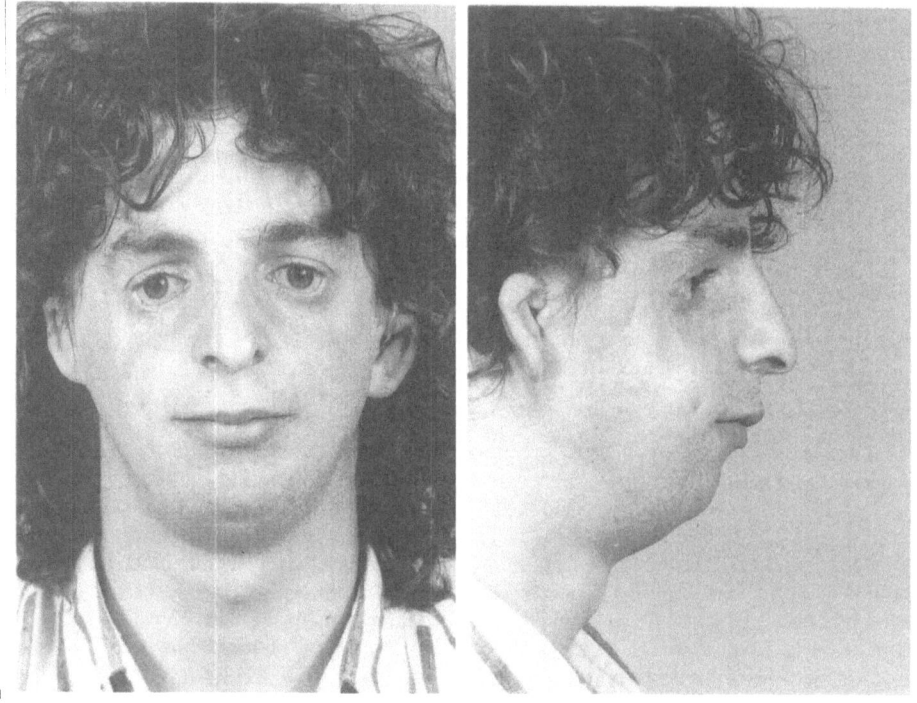

a   b

Fig. 4.9 a,b. Treacher Collins Syndrome.

pinnae are usually malformed and microtia is common. The pinnae may be hypoplastic or cupped and pre-auricular tags or sinuses may be present. The features of the syndrome are characteristically bilateral and surprisingly symmetrical (Fig. 4.9).

Poswillo (1975b) has shown that deficient migration of neural crest cells into the first and second branchial arches is the probable cause of the symmetrical hyoplasia of jaws and face and the characteristic ear deformities (Table 4.2). The ear lesions of the animal model were similar to those occurring in human mandibulo-facial dysostosis.

The authors have described the tomographic and surgical findings in 22 deaf children with true mandibulo-facial dysostosis (Phelps et al. 1981). The patients in this series all had hypoplasia of the middle ear cleft (Table 4.3). The mastoid was always unpneumatised, the antrum and attic were reduced and there was variable descent of the tegmen. This last feature is not a specific finding in mandibulo-

Table 4.2. Features of mandibulo-facial dysostosis and cranio-facial microsomia

Feature	Mandibulo-facial dysostosis	Cranio-facial microsomia
Probable pathogenesis	Deficient neural crest cells in the branchial arches	Focal haemorrhages *in utero*
Family history	Sometimes	Negative
Deformities	Bilateral and symmetrical	Unilateral or asymmetrical
Pinna	Small and shapeless	Often absent except for lobule
Outer-ear anomalies	Deficient and unpneumatised mastoid; may be atresia of EAM, characteristic reduction in attic and antrum – often slit-like	Unpneumatised mastoid; usually atresia of EAM: more bizarre lesions; gross descent of the tegmen
Labyrinth anomalies	Dysplastic lateral canal only; normal cochlea function	Lateral canal commonly dysplastic gross structural abnormalities rarely
Internal auditory meatus	Normal	Often narrow or abnormal direction
Eye anomalies	Typical anomalies of adnexa	Lesions of the globe may be present
Incidence	300 + new cases in USA annually	1:3500 live births

Table 4.3. Narrowing and atresia of the external and middle ears in 22 patients (44 ears) with mandibulofacial dysostosis

External auditory meatus	
Patent	20 (4 narrow)
Soft-tissue atresia	2
Bony atresia	22
Meso and hypotympanum	
Normal size	19
Reduced	10
Slit-like	14
Absent	1
Attic and antrum	
Normal size	nil
Reduced	7
Slit-like	22
Absent	15

Table 4.4. State of the ossicles in 13 operated ears of patients with mandibulo-facial dysostosis

	Normal	Absent	Deformed	Fused mass
Malleus	6	–	4	
Incus	2	3	5	3
Stapes	2 + 2(?)	2	7	

facial dysostosis as even greater tegmen depression is common in hemifacial microsomia. Atresia of the EAM was a less constant feature and in ten patients the meatus was patent, although it tended to be curved, running upwards in its lateral part (Fig. 4.10). Ossicular abnormalities were common (Table 4.4) and, in nearly all the operated ears, the facial nerve followed a more direct path with opening out of the bends. It usually appeared at surgery as an overhanging facial ridge (see Chap. 3). The short descending part can be seen on coronal sections at the level of the oval window in severe cases, with a high stylomastoid foramen (Fig. 4.11). The nerve may less often cross the middle ear cavity and be attached to the ossicles (see Chap. 3).

Cochlear function is nearly always normal in mandibulo-facial dysostosis and the only structural deformity of the inner ear shown by tomography is a short dilated lateral semicircular canal. As previously stated, this is of doubtful significance. Although the radiological appearance of the ears is usually characteristic a thorough assessment is necessary because of the wide range in the severity

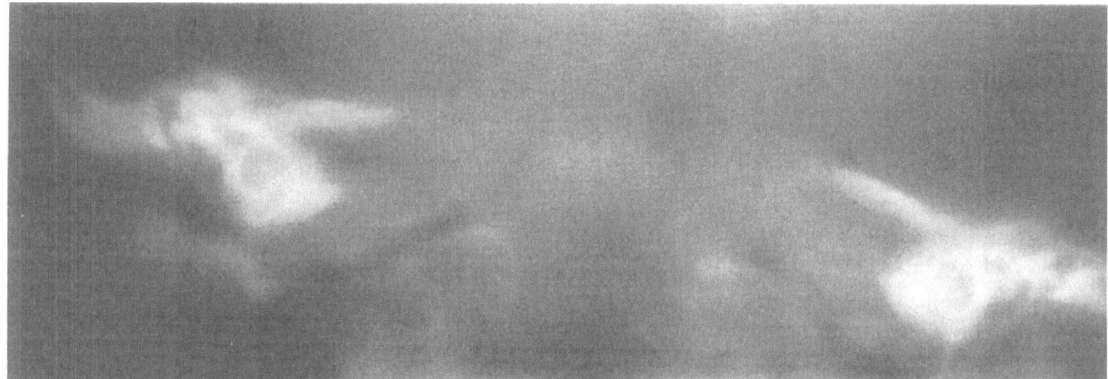
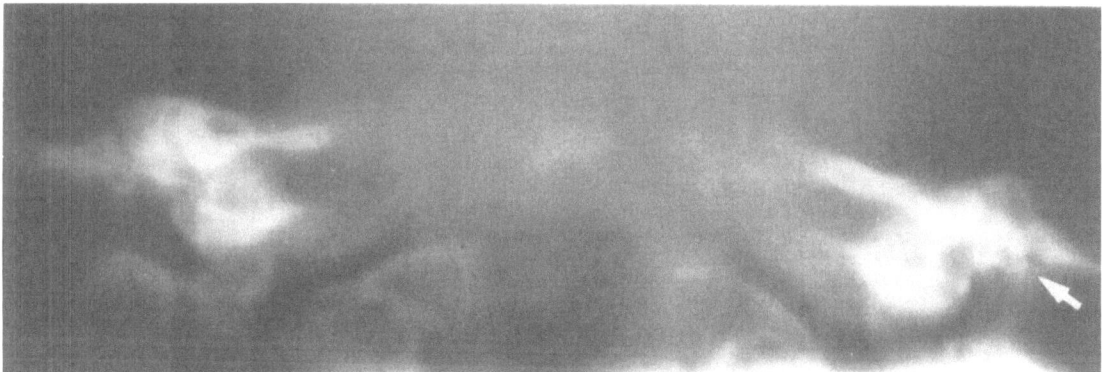

Fig. 4.10. Treacher Collins syndrome with bilateral 60–dB conductive hearing loss and normal ear drums. Coronal tomograms show a normal malleus in a slit attic. Further back at the level of the vestibule and oval window, there is no attic and a hypoplastic incus fused to the medial wall (*arrow*). In this case, the patent EAM makes surgery a reasonable prospect.

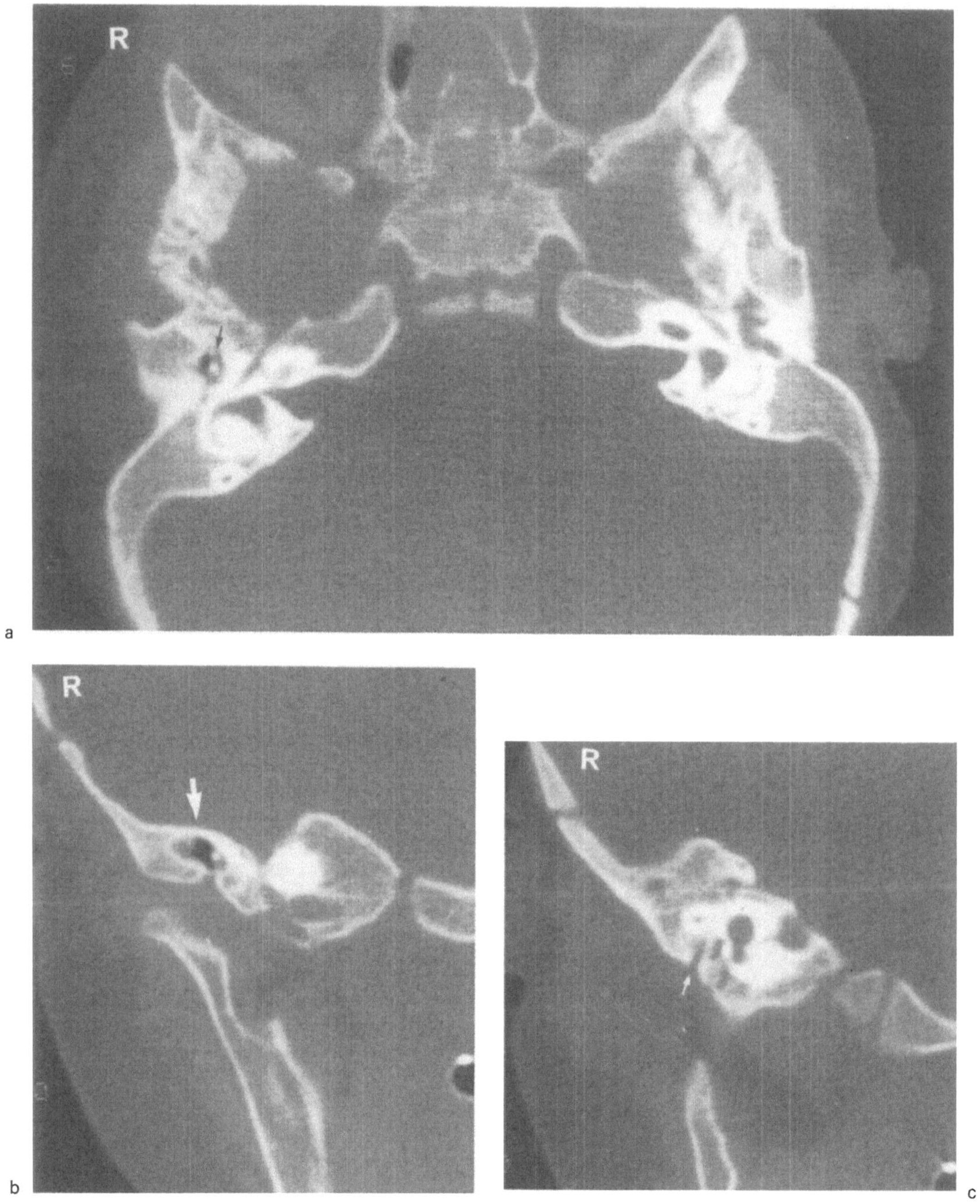

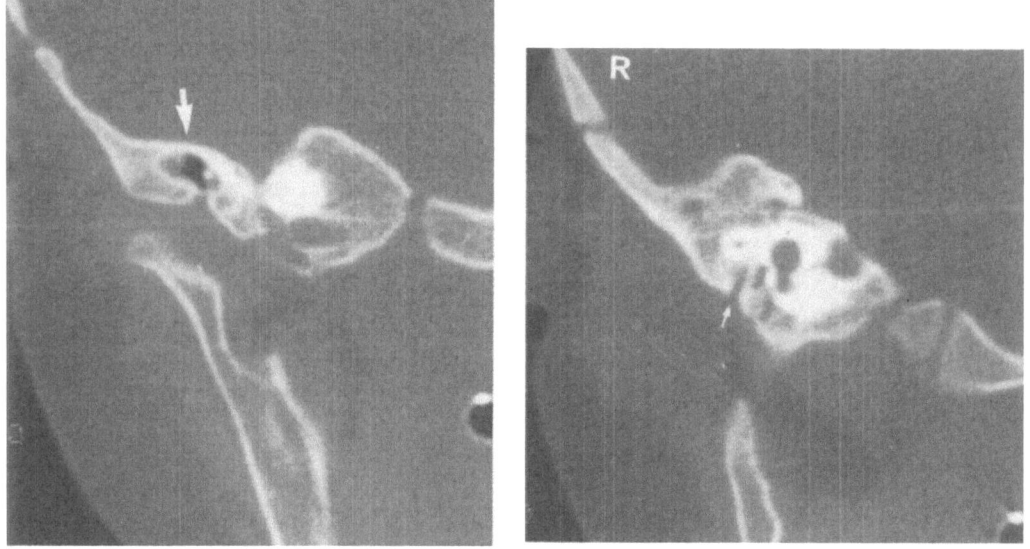

Fig. 4.11 a–c. A poor prospect for surgery. Severe congenital deformity of the middle and external ears in a case of Treacher Collins syndrome. The inner ears are normal. a Base section at the level of the lateral semicircular canals. On both sides the antrum is replaced by solid bone. On the right, a very small air-containing attic encloses a diminutive ossicle (*arrow*). b Coronal section anteriorly shows the small attic. c More posterior coronal section through the vestibule shows the short descending facial canal (from Scott Brown's *Otolaryngology*, Vol 6).

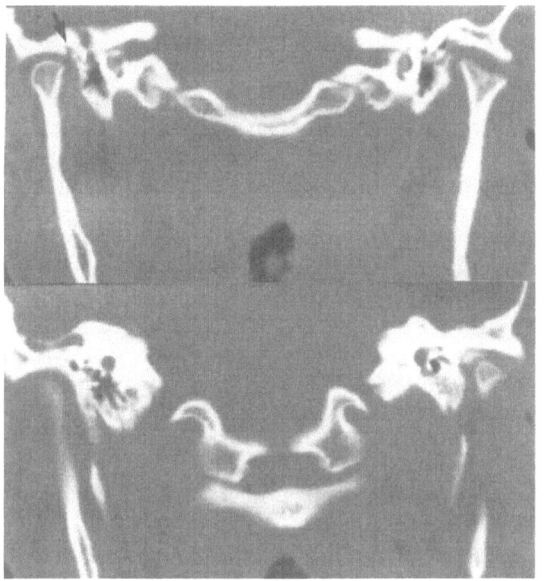

Fig. 4.12. Another case of severe Treacher Collins syndrome. Coronal sections show the slit-like middle ear cavities with mandibular condyles at the level of the cochlea. The *arrow* indicates the solitary ossicle.

of the ear lesions, with or without atresia of the external meatus. Prospects for surgical improvement of the conduction deafness range from good, where there is slight attic atresia and ossicular discontinuity, to poor where only a slit middle ear cavity is present. The general hypoplasia means that the surgeon has very little space between the sigmoid sinus, the middle fossa above and the temporo-mandibular joint (Fig. 4.12).

The Pierre Robin Syndrome

The well recognised combination of micrognathia, glossoptosis and cleft palate is probably the result

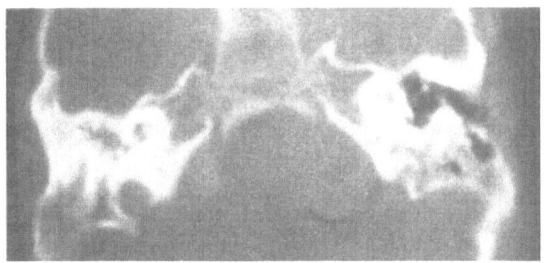

Fig. 4.13. Pierre Robin syndrome with unilateral atresia of the external meatus. Base section at the level of the oval windows.

of arrested development. Temporal bone abnormalities are not a usual feature although the low-slung pinnae may be deformed. However, we have seen ossicular abnormalities and external meatal atresia in this condition (Fig. 4.13).

Cranio-facial Dysostosis

This group of disorders is characterised by craniostenosis from premature closure of skull sutures, which usually results in sagittal shortening of the base of the skull. Abnormalities of the facial bones are often present and other skeletal deformities may occur. Terrahe (1972) believes that deafness with hypoplasia and lack of pneumatisation of the mastoid is, to some extent, the result of this distortion of the skull base and temporal bones. Otopathology is less frequent in cranio-facial dysostosis than in mandibulo-facial dysostosis or hemifacial microsomia (Calderelli 1977). Four cranio-facial dysostosis syndromes with a dominant type of inheritance are associated with deafness.

Acrocephalosyndactyly 1. (Apert Syndrome)

In this condition, irregular craniostenosis with turret skull, facial asymmetry, hypertelorism, dental malocclusion and high arched palate are associated with syndactyly or partial webbing of the fingers.

Perhaps because of frequent mental retardation, the congenital conductive deafness associated with the syndrome has been largely ignored (Konigsmark and Gorlin 1976). Fixation of the stapes is the most consistent abnormality reported and in one case a perilymphatic gusher followed stapedectomy (Bergstrom et al. 1972b).

The authors have also seen a case with severe syndactyly, cleft palate and turret skull, who was found to have ossicular fixation at tympanotomy. Although the eardrums looked normal, compliance testing showed almost no drum movement and at tympanotomy there was gelatinous fluid in the middle ear cavity and the three ossicles were all fixed. The malleus and incus were of normal shape; the stapes was composed of a solid bar but with an apparently normal oval window. There was the usual upward tilt of the petrous pyramids and tomography demonstrated dilatation of the lateral semicircular canal on one side and of the crus commune on the other.

Similar inner ear malformations were noted by Mafee and Valvassori (1981), particularly a short,

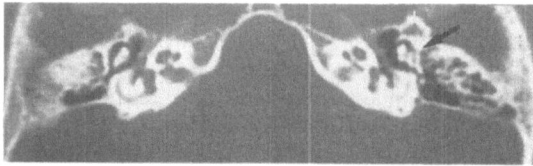

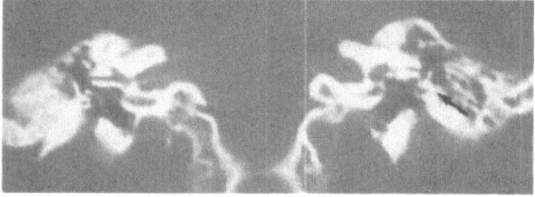

Fig. 4.14. Pfeiffer syndrome. Base and coronal (*below*) sections showing bilateral atresia and on one side an abnormal bulky incus fixed to the outer attic wall (*arrow*).

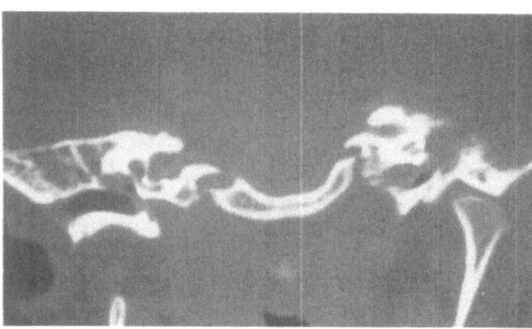

Fig. 4.15. Crouzon syndrome. Bilateral serous otitis media and hypoplastic ossicles.

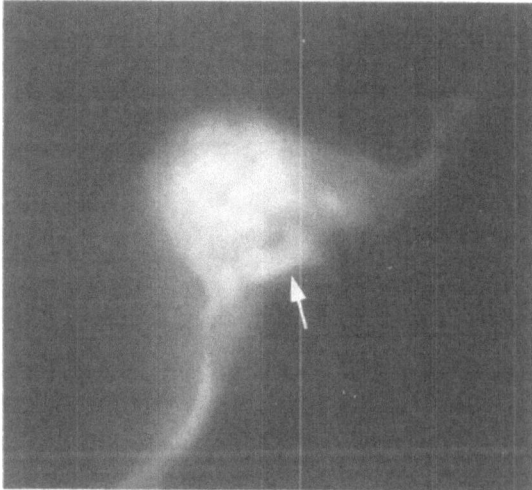

Fig. 4.16. Atresia of the external auditory meatus in Crouzon disease. Lateral tomograms showing deformed tympanic bone (*arrow*).

dilated, lateral semicircular canal. These authors also found deformed and ankylosed ossicles.

Acrocephalosyndactyly 2. (Pfeiffer Syndrome)

This craniostenotic syndrome is very similar to Apert type acrocephalosyndactyly and may be just a less severe form. We have seen one case with bilateral atresia of the external meatus and abnormal ossicles fused to the attic wall on one side (Fig. 4.14).

Acrocephalosyndactyly 3 (Saethre–Chotzen Syndrome). A minor degree of hearing loss is common.

Crouzon Syndrome

This is the commonest of the craniostenosis syndromes. The deformities are confined to the cranium and face. The appearance is distinctive with a beak nose, hypertelorism, hypoplastic maxillae, mandibular prognathism, and proptosis due to shallow orbits. Hearing loss is present in about one third of cases and seems to be due mainly to deformities of the ossicles and, in particular, fixation of the stapes. There is upward tilt of the petrous pyramids and the mastoids are poorly pneumatised. Mafee and Valvassori (1981) consider the prevalence of serous otitis media due to impairment of Eustachian tube function to be the usual cause of the conductive deafness, but atresia of the EAM also occurs (Fig. 4.15). Corey-Grey et al. (1987) made radiographic cephalometric measurements of the nasopharynx and temporal bone in 30 patients with Crouzon's disease. These illustrated growth disturbances of the nasopharyngeal dimensions worsened with age. We have seen cases with bilateral atresia of the EAM and deformed tympanic bones (Fig. 4.16). At operation in one case a fused ossicular mass was found in place of the malleus and incus but the stapes was normal.

Cryptophthalmos Syndrome

The skin of the forehead completely covers one or both eyes giving the distinctive appearance of this syndrome. Sixty cases have been reported with multiple congenital abnormalities, particularly of the urino-genital system. Syndactyly of the fingers occurs and there are abnormalities of the nose in 50%, as well as meningo-encephalocoele in 10% (Konigsmark and Gorlin 1976). The pinnae are small and poorly modelled in 30% and conductive

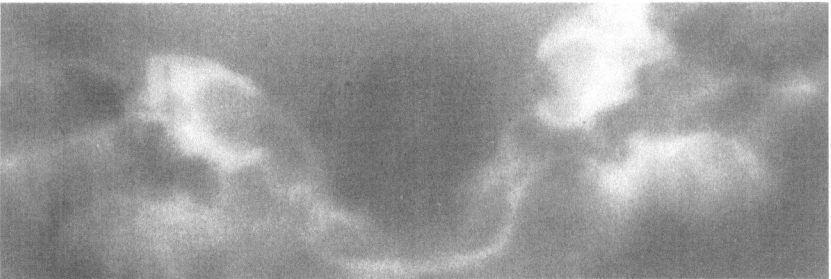

Fig. 4.17. Short wide IAMs with a deep posterior cranial fossa. Other members of this family with the earpits-deafness syndrome showed similar temporal bone anomalies.

deafness due to narrowed atretic auditory meatus has been reported as well as malformed ossicles.

Waardenberg's Syndrome

Hypoplasia of the base of the nose, with lateral displacement of the medial canthi, underdeveloped orbits, heterochromia iridium and a white forelock, are features of this syndrome, which has a dominant inheritance.

Although sensorineural deafness is common, there is usually no structural abnormality of the inner ear and histological section has shown absence of the organ of Corti and atrophy of the spiral ganglion, as occurs in deaf white cats. Anomalies of the vestibular apparatus have been reported. Of 24 patients reported by Nemansky and Hageman (1975), eight had dysplasia of the lateral semi circular canal. Of these, one had malformation of the vestibule and cochlea. Not surprisingly, therefore, abnormal vestibular function is more common than hearing loss in these patients.

Familial Mixed Deafness with Branchial Arch Defects (Earpits Deafness Syndrome)

Pedigrees of families with this distinctive syndrome indicate an autosomal dominant disorder with a high degree of penetrance. Any of the following anomalies may be present: auricular deformities, pre-auricular pits or sinuses, branchial fistulae or clefts, EAM atresia and conductive or mixed hearing loss. Lacrimal duct aplasia occurs rarely, but urinary tract anomalies are common, in which case the syndrome is usually referred to as branchio-oto-renal syndrome. The ear lesions may be unilateral or more usually bilateral in about 75% of all cases.

The most comprehensive recent review was by the Dutch school (Cremers et al. 1981), who noted that 138 cases had been recorded in the world literature, and reported 19 more. Clinical findings were discussed with the results of tomography in 13 cases. Many labyrinthine changes were found, in particular a dysplastic lateral semicircular canal and a cochlear malformation with hypoplasia and reduction in the number of turns. Ossicular abnormalities were noted, both on tomography and at surgical exploration.

We have now seen five families with this syndrome. Four of these have been recorded in a recent paper (Slack and Phelps 1985). A further family of mother and two sons has recently been examined by CT.

The base of the skull and petrous pyramids are somewhat distorted in this syndrome, and it is difficult to be sure on sectional imaging how much the appearances are due to this malrotation, and how much to intrinsic abnormality of the structures. Generally speaking, the petrous pyramids are short and point upwards at their medial end, giving an upwards and backwards slant to the IAM, which appears rather short and bulbous (Fig. 4.17). There is often dysplasia of the lateral semicircular canal, but of more importance is the small cochlea (Fig. 4.18). This seems to have a reduced number of turns, but is not truly a Mondini-type deformity. The middle ear cavities are usually of reasonable size and air-containing, although bony atresia of the EAM may occur. The malleus and incus are usually mobile, though coarse and clumsy in shape. Minor anomalies of these ossicles are frequent, but the stapes is the ossicle usually affected, often with one crus only and fixation in the oval window, which may appear to be absent. The ossicles also appear more anteriorly situated than normal.

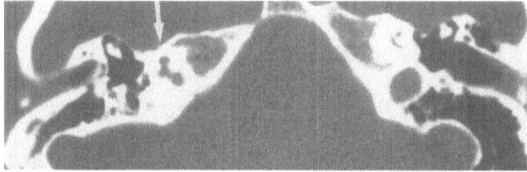

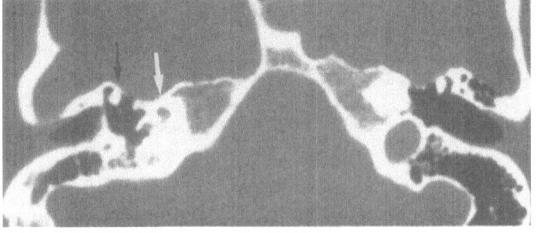

Fig. 4.18. Earpits deafness syndrome. The *white arrow* points to the small Mondini cochlea. The *black arrow* points to the anteriorly placed ossicular mass. Two base sections.

In theory such cases with a conductive hearing loss should be amenable to surgical improvement of the sound conductive mechanism, but unfortunately the results have been disappointing in both our cases, who had exploratory tympanotomy, and in other recorded series. Cremers and Fikkers-Van Noord (1980) have a good discussion on surgery in this condition.

Anencephaly

Anencephaly is a common malformation, characterised by defective development of the skull and brain. The ear structures are present but abnormal, and demonstrate a great range of deformities similar to those occurring as isolated congenital ear malformations. Anencephalics die soon after birth and, consequently, the temporal bone can easily be obtained for histological section. These sections may be compared with the appropriate tomographic sections for research and experimental purposes (Wright et al. 1976).

Several aspects of anencephalic temporal bone pathology are of interest when compared with those of other, non-lethal congenital malformations. The petrous pyramid is shorter and thicker than normal and occupies a more transverse position with its apex higher than its base. Mainly as a result of this, the IAM may run upwards and backwards instead of horizontally and medially (see Chap. 9). Similar, although not so severe, degrees of directional aberration may be seen in other cranial malformations such as hemifacial microsomia, Klippel–Feil syndrome and the cranio-facial dysostoses. The anencephalic cochlea varies from a simple sac to an almost normal structure of $2\frac{1}{2}$ turns, although the bony modiolus is rather squat and spindly (Fig. 4.19). The organ of Corti is essentially normal. The author's experience with cochlear defects, demonstrated by tomography in deaf children, suggests that a similar range of deformities with variable development of the modiolus occurs without neural tube defects.

Otocervical Syndromes

Otopathology occurs less frequently with primary cervical shoulder anomalies than with cranio-facial

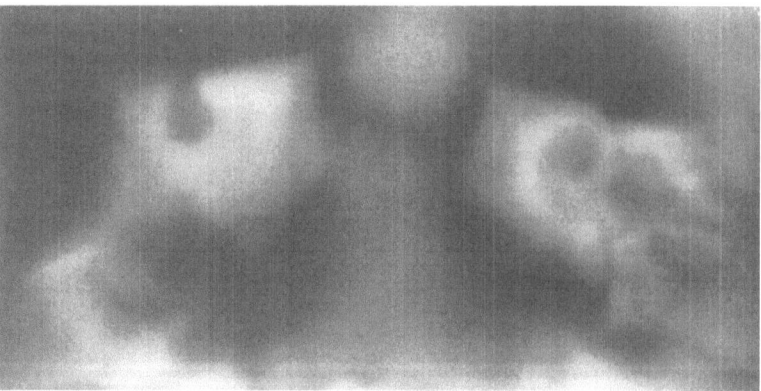

Fig. 4.19. Coronal tomogram of an anencephalic foetus showing the abnormally positioned petrous pyramids. A Mondini type of cochlea is shown on the left and a flask-shaped IAM pointing upwards on the right. This IAM nevertheless contained only scanty nerve elements.

malformations. Sensorineural hearing loss is, however, more common than conductive loss (Calderelli 1977).

Klippel–Feil Syndrome

The characteristic fusion of several cervical vertebrae has long been known to be associated with severe deafness. Although there may be a high-arched or cleft palate, the face is not the main site of deformity. There are not consistent audiometric or otopathological patterns associated with Klippel–Feil syndrome. Sensorineural deafness is more common than conductive and tends to be severe or complete, with gross deformities of the labyrinth shown by tomography. Mondini-type defects are also found and a stapes gusher has been recorded (Daniilidis et al. 1978). There is probably a heterogeneous group of disorders with Wildervanck's syndrome being one entity. We have ten deaf children with Klippel–Feil syndrome (Windle-Taylor et al. 1981). Of the 20 ears examined, 12 showed evidence of severe hearing loss, and of these, 11 had evidence of inner ear dysplasia on tomography. These covered a wide range of severe structural deformities of the labyrinth, often with a narrow IAM. Three of the cases had no proper labyrinths and three had deficiences of the central bony spiral of the cochlea of the Mondini type.

The series also showed a high incidence of both external and middle ear abnormalities (Fig. 4.20). Similar lesions have been reported before but not in such a high percentage of cases (16 out of 20 ears examined). In most of the patients, the sensorineural component predominated, thus reducing the clinical significance of the conduction abnormalities. The problems of the overlap with, and differential diagnosis from, other syndromes with similar features, was also discussed in this paper (Table 4.5). Although we have found more severe structural abnormalities of the inner than of the middle ear, minor anomalies of the ossicles and oval window region have been described, especially of the incudo-stapedial junction (Van Rijn and Cremers 1988). These minor deformities are difficult to show even by the best imaging but are usually amenable to surgical improvement of hearing.

Cervico-oculoacousticus (Wildervanck's) syndrome is an association of Klippel–Feil syndrome with deafness, usually due to severe labyrinthine deformity and Duane's syndrome. Duane's syndrome is a combination of limited abduction and, sometimes adduction of the eyeball with retraction when lateral deviation of the eyes is attempted. This is due to fibrous replacement of the appropriate

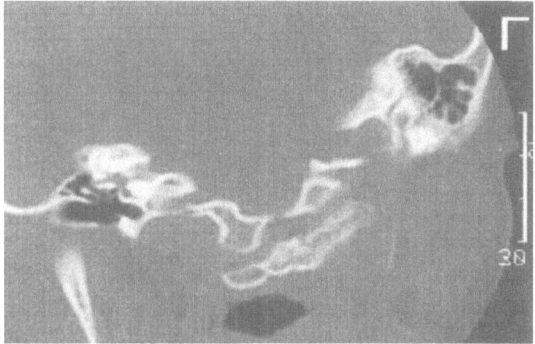
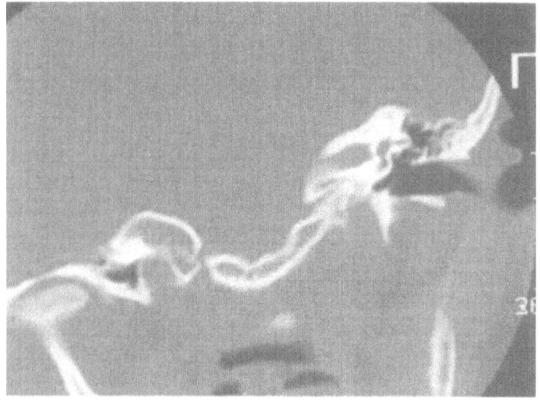

Fig. 4.20. Conductive deafness in a child with Klippel-Feil syndrome. There is considerable skull base deformity and no oval window is apparent on the left. Coronal CT section.

rectus muscles although whether or not it is secondary to a neurological deficit is not clear. If so, it would seem that the condition is related to the Moebius syndrome of VIth and VIIth nerve palsies. Duane's syndrome is inherited as a dominant condition with variable expression and penetrance (Kirkham 1969). This author found the complete triad of Duane's syndrome, sensorineural deafness and Klippel–Feil syndrome in only two patients of 112 with Duane's syndrome. Limitation of lateral movement of the eyes, like facial paralysis, occurs not uncommonly with severe congenital deformities of the temporal bone. These eye lesions were particularly prevalent in the thalidomide era. A particularly severe case of Wildervanck's syndrome is illustrated in Fig. 4.21). The child is totally deaf.

Cleidocranial Dysostosis

Variable deficiency or absence of the clavicles is combined with abnormalities of the skull in cleidocranial dysostosis. There is, usually, a dominant pattern of inheritance. Unlike the Klippel–Feil syndrome, it is middle rather than inner ear which is

Table 4.5. Comparison of the clinical features of five head and neck syndromes. (From Windle-Taylor *et al.* 1981)

	W	G	HM	MFD	GD
Vertebral anomalies	+ + +	+ + +			
Pterygium colli	+				+ + +
Low hairline	+				+
Spina bifida	+	+			
Facial asymmetry	+	+	+ + +		+
Frontal bossing		+			
Microphthalmia		+	+	+	
Epibulbar dermoids	+	+ + +			
Iris and/or choroid coloboma		+	+	+	
Upper lid coloboma		+ + +			
Lower lid coloboma		+		+ + +	
Abducent nerve palsy	+ + +				+
Antimongoloid slant		+		+ + +	
External ear defects	+	+	+ + +	+ + +	+
Ear tags	+	+ + +	+	+	+
Ear pits	+	+	+	+	
Middle ear defects	+	+	+	+ + +	
Sensorineural hearing loss	+ + +		+		+
Malar hypoplasia		+	+	+ + +	
Macrostomia		+ + +	+ + +	+	
Malocclusion		+	+	+ + +	
Aplasia of mandible, ramus & condyle		+	+ + +		
High palate		+	+	+	+
Cleft palate	+	+		+	+
Abnormal karyotype					+ + +
Ovarian agenesis					+ + +
Short stature					+ + +
Digital anomalies					+ + +
Renal anomalies					+

W, Wildervanck's syndrome; G, Goldenhar's syndrome; HM, hemifacial microsomia; MFD, mandibulo-facial dysostosis; GD, gonadal dysgenesis; +, recorded anomaly; + + +, distinctive anomaly.

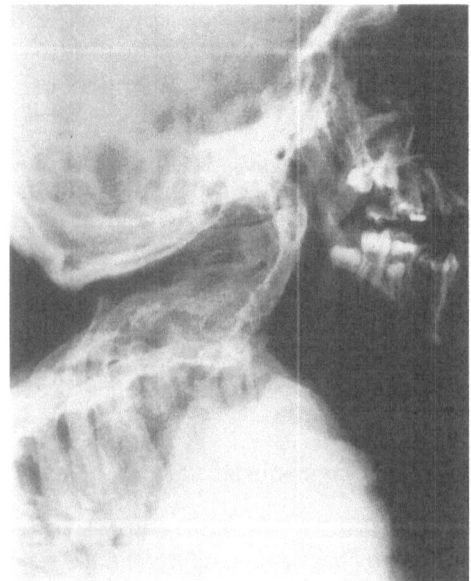
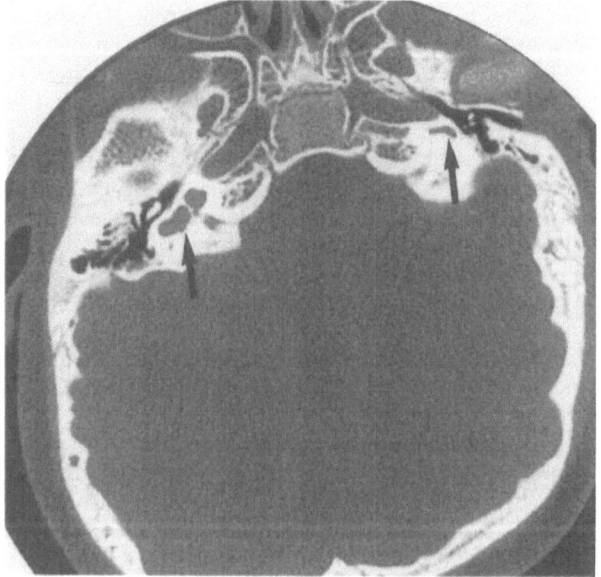

a   b

Fig. 4.21 a,b. Wildervanck Syndrome. As well as cervical fusion and general deformity of the skull (**a**), both labyrinths are severely dysplastic (*arrows*, **b**).

Fig. 4.22 a,b. Cleidocranial dysostosis. Coronal (a) and base (b) CT showing bony encroachment on the upper middle ear cavities with fusion of the left incus to the outer attic wall (*arrow*).

◄────────────────────────────

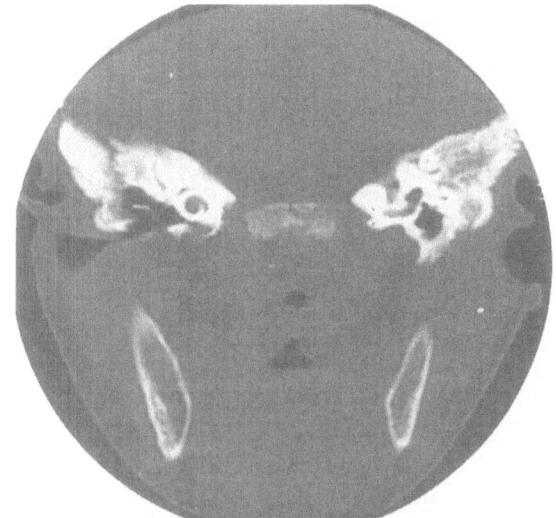

a

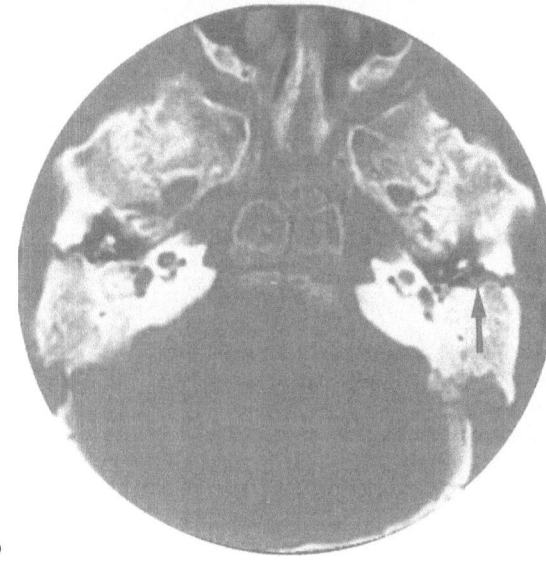

b

the site of deformity. Ossicular chain malformations and atresia of the external auditory meatus have been recorded (Calderelli 1977). We have seen a case in which bony thickening obliterated the attic and antrum on each side (Fig. 4.22). The ossicles appeared normal except that the short process of the incus was fused to the outer attic wall on the left side.

Otofacial-cervical Syndrome

This is a rare condition with dominant inheritance. Narrowing and flattening of the mid-face with cer-

vical and shoulder anomalies are its features. The pinnae are always deformed and conductive hearing loss is a prominent feature.

Sprengel Shoulder

In this condition a high malformed and malrotated scapula is found in combination with other anomalies. Congenital fixation of the stapes may occur but the authors have seen two cases with atresia of the external auditory meatus, narrowed middle ear cleft and absent incus (Fig. 4.23).

Otoskeletal Syndromes (Bone Dysplasias)

Deafness is a common feature of generalised bone dysplasias. Although structural abnormalities of the ear may occasionally be present at birth, acquired deafness is more often due to Eustachian tube obstruction and otitis media. This may result from distortion of the temporal bones tilted upwards at their medial ends. Sensorineural hearing impairment is often severe but it is uncertain how much is due to compression of the inner ear structures and narrowing of foramina by abnormal bone. The main disorders of bone affecting the ears, namely otosclerosis, fibrous dysplasia and Paget's disease are described in Chapter 11. Although these conditions often have a strong hereditary tendency they are mostly diseases of adult or later life, and only the rare congenital dysplasias will be considered here. A good review of bone dysplasias and hearing loss is given by Booth (1982).

Osteogenesis Imperfecta (Van der Hoeve's Syndrome)

The reported incidence of otopathology and hearing loss in osteogenesis imperfecta ranges from 20% to 60% of affected patients (Bergstrom 1977; Quisling et al. 1979). Systemic manifestations include a large skull, bowing of the legs, multiple fractures of the long bones, laxity of ligaments, atrophic skin, blue

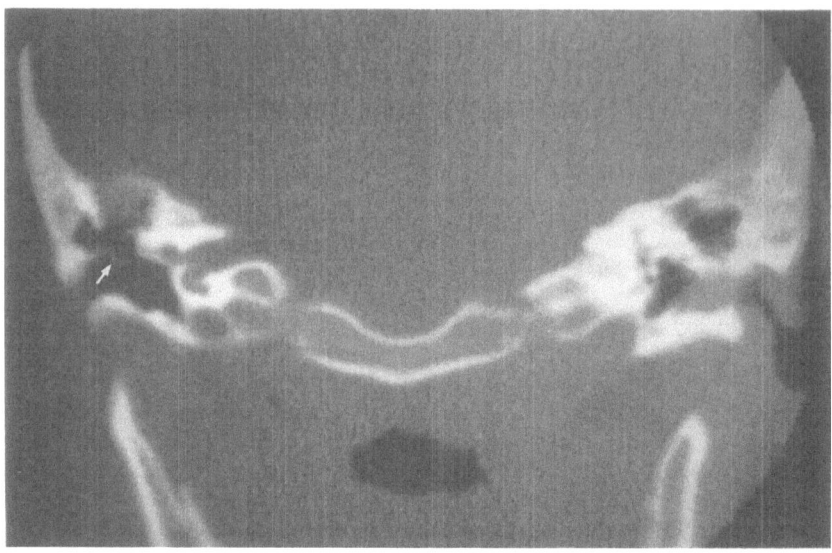

Fig. 4.23. Sprengel shoulder. Coronal CT showing middle ear abnormalities. The *arrow* points to a hypoplastic malleus. There is soft tissue atresia of the opposite external meatus.

sclera, abnormal tooth dentine and various haematological disorders. Only one third of patients present with the complete syndrome. Two forms of the disease are usually recognised: the lethal congenital form, manifestations of which are present at birth (and indeed fractures may occur in utero); and the tarda form, which has a dominant mode of inheritance, developing in the second or third decade. The underlying defect is believed to be an inborn error of osteoblasts or chondroblasts. Blue sclera is considered to be the hallmark of osteogenesis imperfecta and, although not always present, it accompanied conductive deafness in the cases reported by Quisling et al. (1979).

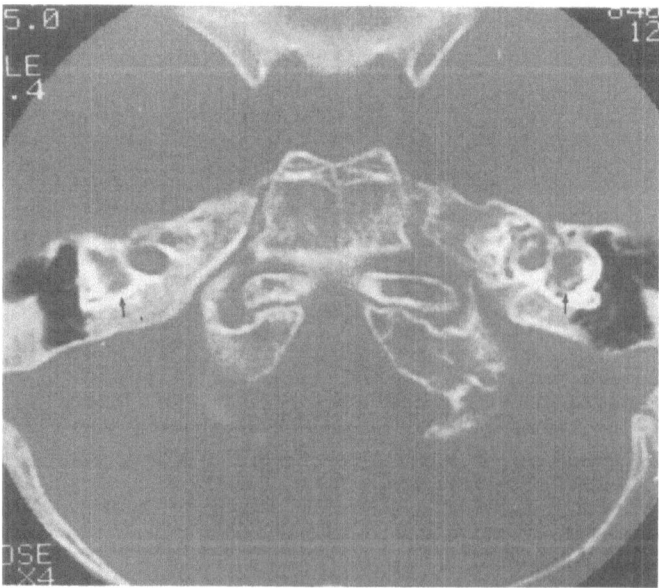

Fig. 4.24. Rarefaction of the bone around the labyrinth by osteogenesis imperfecta. The vestibules (*arrows*) appear larger than normal on this base CT section.

Bergstrom, in an extensive review of the syndrome, concludes that ear abnormalities are present in younger individuals in about the same frequency, although with less severity, as in adults. Conductive deafness usually occurs in the tarda form but mixed or pure sensorineural loss are almost as common. Although there is histopathological confirmation of otosclerosis occurring in the temporal bone of patients with osteogenesis imperfecta, it now seems that the deafness and ear deformities in these patients are not due to otosclerosis. The stapedial crura are often fragile, while the footplate seems heavy. Moreover, although there is often a heavy growth of abnormal bone in the region of the footplate, its margins remain discrete and show only slight fixation (Kosoy and Maddox 1971). Biochemical evidence of distinct differences between the abnormal bone of osteogenesis imperfecta and otosclerosis is accumulating and it appears that there are histological differences

between the affected stapedial footplates in the two diseases. Deficient ossification in multiple sites in the temporal bone has also been found on histological examination in osteogenesis imperfecta (Bergstrom 1977).

The radiographic appearances of the temporal bones of these patients have not been fully described in the literature but the changes in the labyrinthine capsule are virtually indistinguishable from those of labyrinthine otospongiosis. Demineralisation is often extensive and the deposits of abnormal bone may be very thick although the oval window can often be recognised. In one case of the authors', a deposit on the promontory was obstructing the long process of the incus as well as encroaching on the oval window, the margins of which were intact. Thick demineralised bone may replace the labyrinthine capsule, but leave the modiolus of the cochlea: the "cochlea within a cochlea" appearance and excessive rarefaction of bone in the labyrinthine capsule can make the vestibule appear larger than normal (Fig. 4.24). Histological examination of such a case has shown scanty periosteal and endosteal bony trabeculae surrounding the labyrinth (Fig. 4.25).

Dysplasia with Increase in Bone Density

Mixed deafness which is usually progressive occurs in osteopetrosis (Albers–Schonberg disease), in sclerostenosis and hyperostosis corticalis generalisata (Van Buchem's disease), craniometaphyseal dysplasia and frontometaphyseal dysplasia (Gorlin–Hart syndrome), congenital hyperphosphatasia and progressive diaphyseal dysplasia (Engelman's disease).

The osteopetroses are a group of uncommon genetic disorders that are characterised by increased skeletal density and abnormalities of bone modelling. Common to all these disorders is a proclivity for involvement of the calvaria and skull base. An associated constellation of neurological symptoms may result (Miyamoto et al. 1980).

Various cranial palsies occur secondarily to bony encroachment on the cranial foramina. In addition to the facial nerve, the disease process most often involves the optic and vestibulo-cochlear nerves and the mandibular division of the trigeminal nerve containing the motor fibres to the masticatory muscles. In the case of the facial nerve, the characteristic manifestation is that of recurrent, acute, facial palsies identical to Bell's palsy. Conductive hearing impairment has been attributed to narrowing of the EAM, encroachment of the bony walls of the attic on the ossicles or to narrowing of the

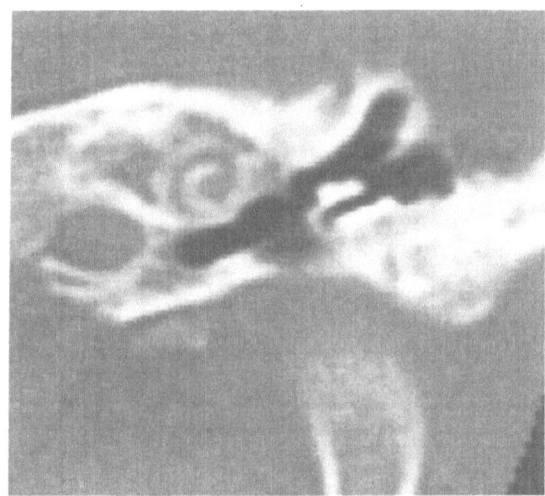

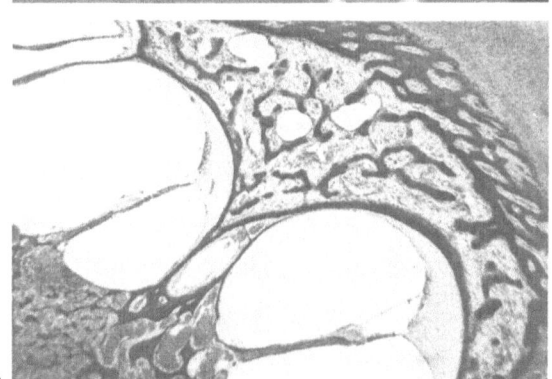

a

b

Fig. 4.25 a,b. Osteogenesis imperfecta. Thin bony trabeculae surround the cochlea. (a) coronal CT; (b) histology section. From Michaels L, *Ear, Nose and Throat Histopathology.*

oval and round windows. Sensorineural hearing loss may be associated with bony constriction of the IAM, although we have recently reported a 14-year-old patient who had sclerosis of the whole of the skull base and other classical features of Van Buchem's disease; yet in spite of gross narrowing of

the IAMs demonstrated by imaging in three planes, the girl has a normal pure tone audiogram.

Imaging of the petrous temporal bones in the osteopetroses shows generalised sclerosis and expansion of the petrous pyramid (Fig. 4.26). Narrowing of the IAM and encroachment by bosses of sclerotic

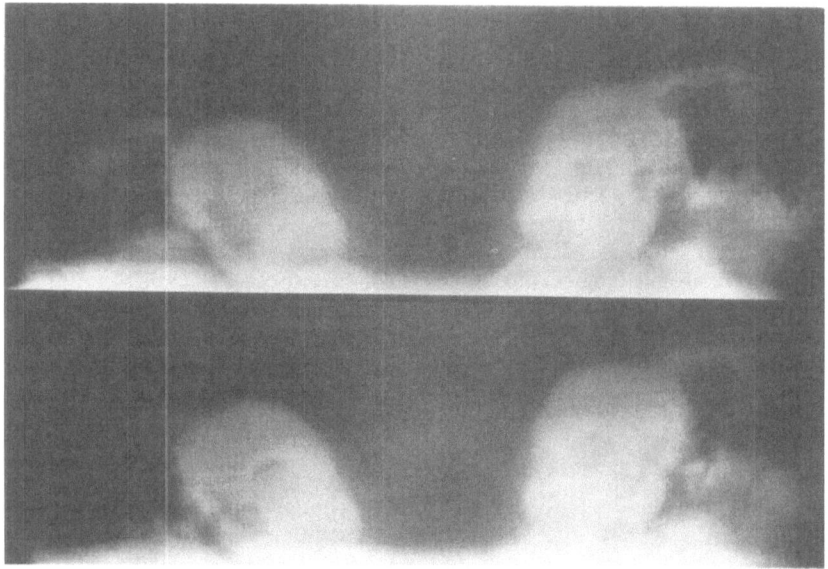

Fig. 4.26. Hypophosphataemic rickets. Sclerosis and expansion of the petrous pyramids.

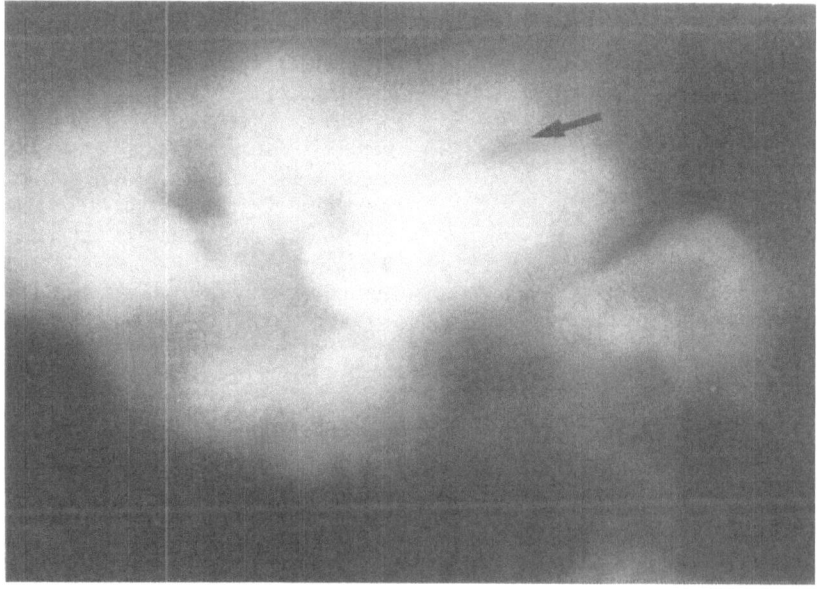

Fig. 4.27. Englemann disease. Sclerotic bone encroaches upon the attic and the incus. The *arrow* shows the IAM.

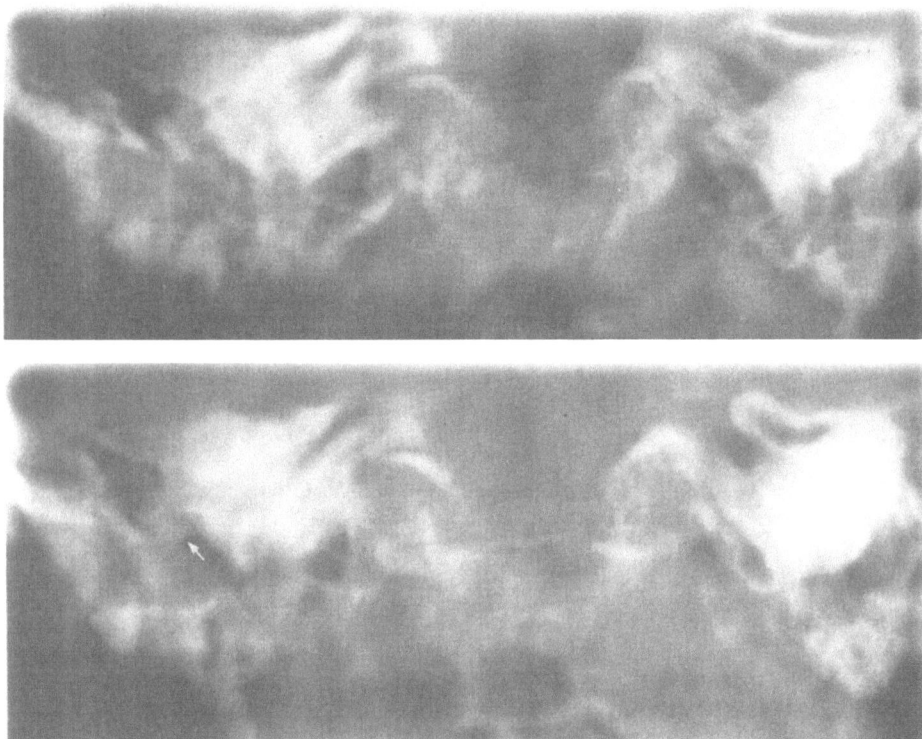

Fig. 4.28. Kniest syndrome. The *arrow* indicates the abnormal thickened stapes.

bone on the ossicles in the attic are also revealed (Fig. 4.27). In cases where tympanometry shows low impedance, imaging may demonstrate the increased bulk of the ossicles. Surprisingly, in some of these cases there is extensive mastoid pneumatisation.

Kniest Syndrome (Spondyloepiphyseal Dysplasia Congenita)

A round flat mid-face, short neck, waddling gait and club feet, characterise this syndrome of dominant inheritance. Radiographs show squat long bones and enlarged metaphyses, although the bone age is normal. The skull may show basilar impression and cleft palate is present in about 50% of patients. Shallow orbits with myopia, retinal detachment and cataracts are frequent and conductive deafness has been reported by a number of authors (Konigsmark and Gorlin 1976).

The authors have seen two patients with the typical features of Kniest disease who had a moderately severe bilateral mixed type of deafness. Tomograms showed tilting and distortion of the petrous pyramids with squat, thickened ossicles, especially the stapes (Fig. 4.28).

Orofacial Digital Syndrome Type II (Mohr Syndrome)

Polydactyly, metaphyseal irregularity and flaring are associated in this condition with hypoplasia of the mandible, median cleft lip and a lobulated tongue. Conductive hearing loss with malformed ossicles has been reported (Gorlin et al. 1976). Note that in the much commoner orofacial digital syndrome type I the hearing is normal.

Otopalato-digital Syndrome

A wide range of skeletal abnormalities accompany hypertelorism, antimongoloid eyes, a small mouth and nose and cleft palate. Abnormalities of the ossicular chain causing conductive deafness have been shown by tympanotomy (Konigsmark and Gorlin 1976) (Fig. 4.29).

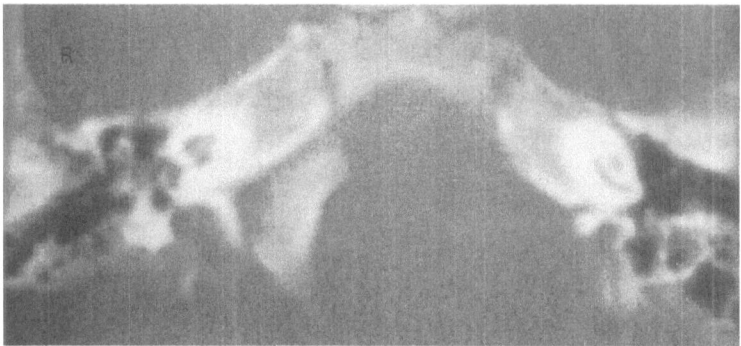

Fig. 4.29. Otopalato digital syndrome. Base CT at the level of the round windows showing bony atresia of the right external meatus.

Other dysplasias where ossicular abnormalities and conductive deafness have occasionally been reported, are dominant symphalangism, multiple synostosis, the EEC (Cockayne) syndrome and achondroplasia.

Chromosome Abnormalities with Ear Malformations

Chromosome Deletion: 4p-Wolf–Hirshorn Syndrome

More than 100 cases have been described and recently Ilino et al. (1987) have reported the histological study of the temporal bones of one case with abnormalities of the ossicles, absence of oval windows and congenital cholesteatoma.

Autosomal Trisomy

Congenital ear deformities have not been considered to be a feature of 21 Trisomy (Down's syndrome) which is the most common type of chromosome abnormality, although there is a well recognised association with chronic suppurative ear disease.

Malformations of the ear are a feature of other autosomal abnormalities, although other extensive and severe deformities mean that survival is often limited.

13–15 or Trisomy "D"

Severe cardiac and neurological abnormalities occur in this condition, as well as cleft palate and lip. The pinnae are low-set and deformed. Temporal bone section of one case showed a normal cochlea but deformities of the semicircular canals (Bergstrom et al. 1972a). Other reports, however, describe cochlea deformities (Kos et al. 1966).

A good review was provided by Tomoda et al. (1983) who describe the temporal bone findings of one case with a flattened cochlea of the Mondini type.

18 or Trisomy "E"

In recent years there have been many reports of individuals with deletions involving chromosome 18. The majority of chromosome deletions are non-familial and parental karyotypes are normal. Cardiac abnormalities with elfish face, low-set ears, ptosis, corneal opacities and glaucoma, often with mental deficiency, are features of these deletion syndromes.

The long arm and ring types (18g and 18r) are associated with structural deformities of the ear in the majority of cases. Atresia of the EAM with ossicular abnormalities but otherwise relatively normal middle ear, is the usual manifestation (Bergstrom et al. 1974) but temporal bone studies have also shown minor labyrinthine anomalies (Miglets et al. 1975).

An adolescent patient of the authors', with 18r abnormality and multiple congenital deformities, had bilateral meatal atresia. Surgical exploration showed that the right middle ear and ossicles were normal except that the handle of the malleus was fused to the atretic plate (Fig. 4.30).

21 Trisomy

Chronic otitis media is a common feature of Down's syndrome. Because of the difficulty of examination

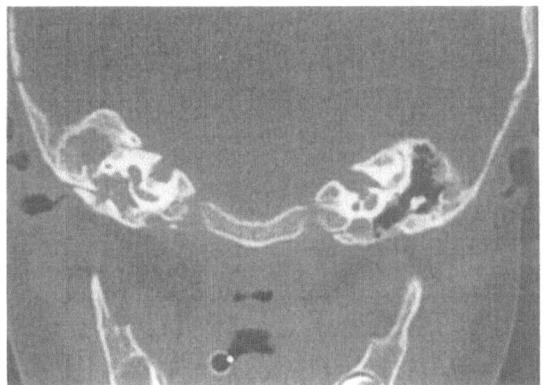

Fig. 4.30. Coronal CT of Trisomy 18. There are bilateral atretic plates, ossicular deformities and fluid in the right middle ear cavity.

however there have been few detailed otological studies on this population. To define the aural manifestations of Down's syndrome, complete otological and audiometric examination was performed on 107 consecutive patients by Balkany et al. (1979). Deficient hearing was found in 64% of these patients and, of these hearing losses, 83% were conductive. Surprisingly, middle ear effusion or tympanic membrane perforation accounted for only 60% of the conductive hearing losses. Five temporal bones of children with Down's syndrome were examined. These histological sections revealed middle ear abnormalities including fixation and superstructure deformity of the stapes and dehiscence of the Fallopian canal. Operative findings in 16 procedures on patients with Down's syndrome and conductive hearing loss, revealed congenital anomalies of the auditory ossicles, especially the stapes, as well as the erosive lesions caused by the cholesteatoma that was often present.

22 Trisomy

Facial abnormalities, with anomalies of the preauricular region and sometimes complete or partial atresia of the EAM are associated with severe deafness (Katano et al. 1979).

Sex Trisomy

Although deafness does occur in XXY trisomy (Klinefelter's syndrome) and the XX anomaly, it is the XO anomaly or Turner's syndrome that has received the most attention.

Turner's syndrome

Webbing of the neck, multiple eye abnormalities, micrognathia and prominent low-set ears, occur in these patients, who are infertile. Otitis media occurs frequently, perhaps due to the abnormal orientation of the middle ear cleft. Abnormalities and fixation of the stapes and sensorineural deafness is common.

Histological section of the temporal bones of a case of Turner's syndrome showed normal middle ears but true Mondini defects of the cochleae (Windle Taylor et al. 1982).

Ear Abnormalities with Endocrine Disorders

Deafness occurs with endocrine disorders and, in particular, hypothyroidism. Structural abnormalities of the ear have, however, not been demonstrated and the hearing loss is usually reversed by appropriate hormone therapy. There is only one condition in which deformities of the bony labyrinth have been shown in association with endocrine disturbances.

Pendred Syndrome

This syndrome is defined as a triad of goitre, positive perchlorate test and congenital sensorineural deafness. There is a recessive mode of inheritance. The enlargement of the thyroid gland begins at puberty and is believed to be a response to a partial block in the synthesis of thyroxine. This enzymatic deficiency results in an abnormal fall of the activity of the gland if perchlorate is given after a tracer dose of iodine-131. The patients are generally euthyroid.

The hearing loss is usually severe. Full tomographic studies of the cochlea with the use of the axial-pyramidal projection have demonstrated Mondini-type defects with deficiency of the modiolus in most patients. The most recent paper by Johnsen et al. (1987) described the Mondini deformity of the temporal bones of five patients with Pendred syndrome studied histologically.

Drug-induced Ear Malformations

Many drugs may produce deafness and tinnitus, usually from temporary or permanent damage to the cochlear end-organ. However, only one has produced structural abnormalities by a tetratogenic effect in utero and it is to be hoped that no similar iatrogenic deformities will occur in the future.

Thalidomide Embryopathy

Ear abnormalities are the second most common result of thalidomide damage to the fetus, and it is estimated that about 10% of the patients affected in utero by thalidomide, administered between 1959 and 1962, have ear lesions. There have been large series reported from Germany (Reisner 1969; Terrahe 1972) and Great Britain (Phelps 1974).

Thalidomide ear deformities have no distinguishing or characteristic feature. They do, however, tend to be bilateral, severe and extensive and often external, middle and inner ears are involved. Terrahe (1972) found inner ear abnormalities in 34 out of 37 cases but in about half of the cases reported by Phelps (1974), where there was a definite history of maternal thalidomide ingestion, middle and external ear lesions were accompanied by normal cochlear function. In some of these cases, a short dilated lateral semicircular canal was present as the only inner ear anomaly. One common and characteristic feature, which is rare in other types of congenital ear deformity, is a complete absence of any vestige of tympanic bone, so that the temporo-mandibular joint abuts directly on the mastoid process. The middle ear cavity is usually present but flattened, distorted and opaque due to glue-like mesenchyme. It may also be markedly narrowed. A deformed and often hyperplastic ossicular mass was the usual operative finding, as well as deformity of the stapes (Fig. 4.31).

Cranial nerve lesions sometimes accompany congenital ear deformities and with thalidomide malformations this association is very common. Of Terrahe's cases 30% had a partial or complete, unilateral or bilateral facial paralysis, 70% of which gave a definite thalidomide history. Phelps (1974) also found that all but one of 19 cases of VIth and VIIth nerve palsies (Moebius syndrome) accompanying congenital ear deformities, were born in the thalidomide era. Such lesions were extensively investigated with electromyographic studies by German authors, whose conclusions were summarised by Phelps and Roland (1977).

Neurofibromatosis (von Recklinghausen's Disease)

This syndrome of i) multiple neuromas ii) cutaneous pigmentation iii) skeletal anomalies and iv) central nervous system involvement, follows an autosomal dominant mode of transmission, with approximately 50% of the cases representing fresh mutations.

The syndrome has protean manifestations. The complexity of the clinical spectrum is compounded by the fact that the disorder may evolve slowly and may present in a variety of different ways. Over 40% of patients demonstrate some manifestations at birth, and over 60% by the second year of life. Incomplete forms are common and may go unrecognised. A sporadic case without neurofibromas and without the requisite number of café-au-lait spots can present great difficulty in diagnosis during childhood (Huson 1987).

Deafness is a common feature of the syndrome and not always due to neuromas of the VIIIth cranial nerve. Nevertheless, bilateral acoustic neuromas are a common feature of neurofibromatosis and are discussed in Chapter 9.

A review of 170 cases of neurofibromatosis was made by Maceri and Saxon (1984). Amongst variable clinical presentations 63 cases had primary involvement of the head and neck. There were 13 cases of optic glioma but only two cases of acoustic neuroma and three of bone dysplasia. Bone dysplasias may result in a very wide IAM without neuromas or deficiencies of other parts of the cranial floor (Fig. 4.32).

The CHARGE Association

In 1981 Pagon et al. applied the acronym CHARGE to an association of congenital defects, which

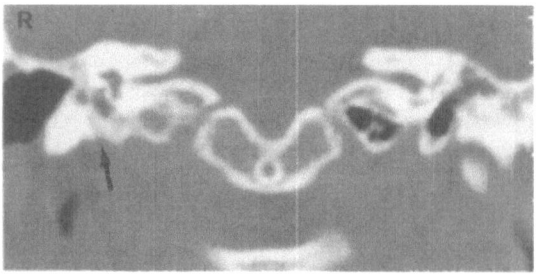

Fig. 4.31. Thalidomide case with right-sided operative cavity. Coronal CT showing a typical combination of inner and middle ear deformities. Note the narrow right IAM, dysplastic lateral semicircular canal, absent ossicles and anterior descending facial nerve canals (*arrow*).

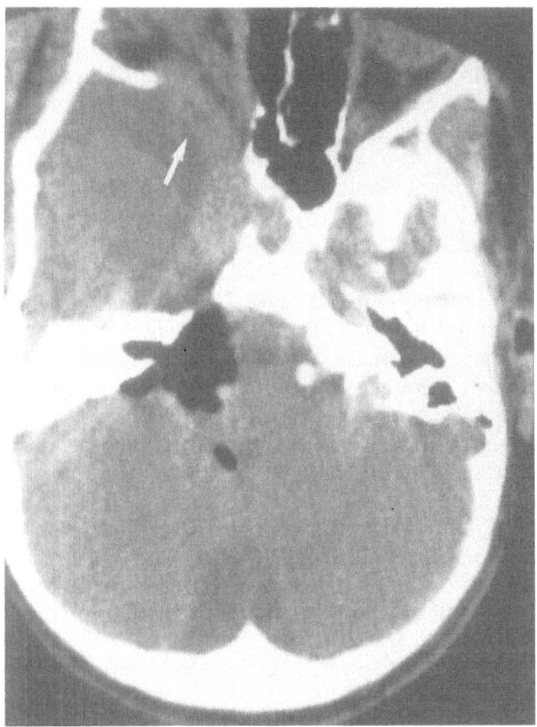

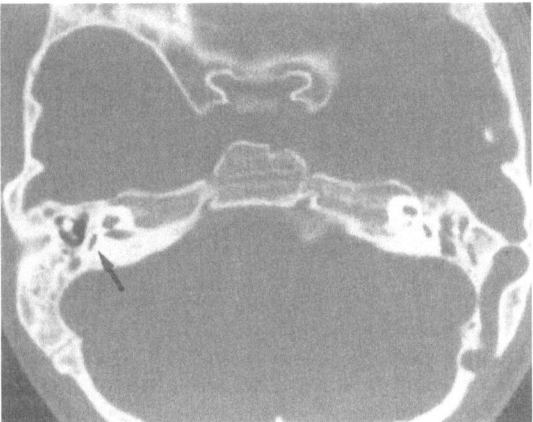

Fig. 4.33. CHARGE association. Base CT showing small vestibules (*arrow*) with no semicircular canals. See also Fig. 3.23.

Fig. 4.32. Neurofibromatosis with skull base defects. The *arrow* points to the defect in the posterior wall of the orbit. There was some right-sided hearing loss but the air-CT meatogram has excluded an acoustic neuroma.

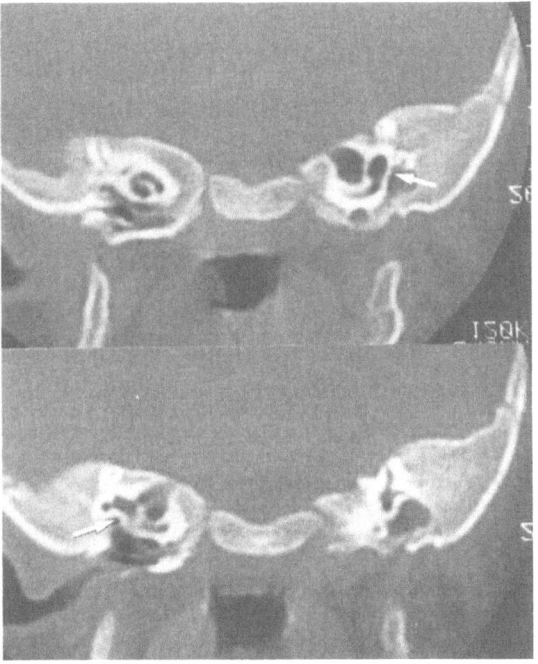

Fig. 4.34. CHARGE association. Bilateral external meatal atresia, absent ossicles and oval windows.

includes coloboma, heart disease, atresia of the nasal choanae, retarded development and/or CNS abnormalities, genital hypoplasia and ear anomalies. There are now several published reports of the external ear malformations and hearing impairment in CHARGE association. Pagon et al. studied 21 patients, 17 of whom had external ear anomalies. Most of these individuals also had hearing loss, which was reported to be predominantly sensorineural and of mild to moderate severity. A number of other congenital anomalies such as micrognathia, cleft palate, facial palsy, swallowing and tracheoesophageal fistula, were also noted but with less frequency. Patients who are included in the CHARGE association must have choanal atresia or ocular coloboma (or both), and a total of at least four of the seven most common anomalies.

We have performed CT scans on 12 deaf children with CHARGE. Six (50%) had structural abnormalities of the hearing organ. The most characteristic feature was absence of the semicircular canals (Fig. 4.33), which occurred in four patients (eight ears). Usually this was associated with a normal cochlea and in only one ear was there a deficiency of the coils compatible with a Mondini deformity. The oval window was absent in two ears (Fig. 4.34) but in several cases could not be adequately assessed, especially when only base views could be obtained.

The patients had atresia of the EAM and minor ossicular abnormalities were present in three. Other problems in CHARGE, and the large sensorineural elements of the deafness, mean that there is little indication for exploratory surgery of the middle ears and none has been carried out on these patients.

Conclusion

The classification above is based on published reports and the authors' own experience. Malformations of bony structures in the hearing mechanism are recorded for syndromes, in which deafness is a feature. Histological section, observations at surgery and imaging appearances provide the basis not only for these descriptions but for future understanding of pathogenesis. Some of the most common minor deformities reported affect the stapes, with congenital fixation in the oval window but, unfortunately, these cannot be reliably demonstrated by current imaging methods. Our classification does not differentiate between conditions in which the hearing loss is static, e.g., craniofacial microsomia and those such as the bone dysplasias, where it is usually progressive. We believe, however, that conventional or computerised tomography should be considered for any patient suspected of having one of these syndromes, preferably at a very early age (see Chap. 3), although priority will obviously have to be given to more important defects of other systems. Important causes of congenital deafness such as rubella embryopathy or degenerative conditions like Usher's syndrome (deafness and retinitis pigmentosa), have not been considered as the lesions seem to be confined to the membranous labyrinth.

Advances in the understanding of congenital deafness and hence, prevention and improved management depend upon work in many fields, including epidemiology and genetics as well as audiology and other clinical investigations. For research purposes, mention has already been made of the great range of ear deformities in anencephalics and studies of animal models for other otocranio-facial syndromes. Poswillo's (1975a) work has helped to differentiate the pathogenesis and subsequent progress of mandibulo-facial dysostosis and craniofacial microsomia. Extensive study of the mouse by mammalian geneticists has resulted in the identification of over 70 different mutations known to affect the inner ear. The mouse is apparently the only species other than man in which mutations lead to morphogenetic abnormalities of the inner ear (Steel and Bock 1983). A wide spectrum of abnormalities has been found, ranging from

absence of any recognisable cochlear or vestibular structures to solitary dysplasia of the lateral semicircular canal in many mutants. The similarity of many of these murine deformities to those occurring in man, suggests a high likelihood of similar developmental mechanisms, although extrapolation from animal models of malformation syndromes to similar patterns of human deformity will not necessarily prove that identical pathogenic mechanisms have been responsible in both cases.

To understand the pathogenesis and type of deformity that may occur in congenital ear abnormalities, it is necessary to correlate scarce postmortem findings and animal model experiments with radiographic appearances and observations at surgery. Surgery and tomography, however, have assessment limitations. Although the surgeon can fully appreciate the state of the ossicles, this assessment is limited to the confines of the hole created by the surgery. Imaging is available for a greater number of ears and gives a better demonstration of the overall anatomy and relations of both inner and middle ear.

References

Balkany TJ, Mischke RE, Downs MP, Jafek BW (1979) Ossicular abnormalities in Down's syndrome. Otolaryngol Head Neck Surg 87: 372–384

Bergstrom LA (1977) Osteogenesis Imperfecta: otologic and maxillo-facial aspects. Laryngoscope 87/9 pt 2, Supp 6

Bergstrom LA, Hemenway WG, Sando I (1972a) Pathological changes in congenital deafness. Laryngoscope 82: 1777–1792

Bergstrom LA, Neblett LM, Hemenway WG (1972b) Otologic manifestations or acrocephalosyndactyly. Arch Otolaryngol 96: 117–123

Bergstrom LA, Stewart JM, Kenyon G (1974) External auditory atresia and the deleted chromosome. Laryngoscope 84: 1905–1917

Booth JR (1982) Medical management of sensorineural hearing loss. J Laryngol Otol 96: 773–795

Calderelli DD (1977) Congenital middle ear anomalies associated with craniofacial and skeletal syndromes. In: Jaffe BF (ed) Hearing loss in children. Baltimore University Park Press pp 310–340

Calderelli DD (1981) Craniofacial anomalies, a perspective for the otolaryngologist. Otolaryngol Clin North Am (14) 47: 763–767

Calderelli DA, Valvassori GE (1979) A radiographic analysis of first and second branchial arch anomalies. In: Symposium on diagnosis and treatment of craniofacial anomalies. Mosby & Co, St Louis, p 45

Chandra Sekar HK, Tokita N, Alexic S, Sachs M, Daly JF (1978) Temporal bone findings in hemifacial microsomia. Annal Otol Rhinol Laryngol 87: 399–403

Converse JM, McCarthy JG, Coccaro PJ, Wood-Smith D (1979) Clinical aspects of craniofacial microsomia. In: Symposium on diagnosis and treatment of craniofacial anomalies. Mosby & Co, St Louis, Ch. 44

Cook JV, Phelps PD, Chandy J (1989) Van Buchem's disease with classical radiological features and appearances on computed tomography. Br J Radiol 62: 74–77

Corey Grey JP, Calderelli DD, Gould HJ (1987) Otopathology in cranial facial dysostosis. Am J Otol 8:14–18

Cremers CWRJ, Fikkers-Van Noord M (1980) The earpits-deafness syndrome. Clinical and genetic aspects. Int J Paed Otol 2: 309–322

Cremers CWRJ, Thijssen HOM, Fischer AJEM, et al (1981) Otological aspects of the earpit-deafness syndrome. J Otorhinolaryngol 43:223–239

Daniilidis J, Magnanaris T, Dimitriadis A, Iliades T, Manalidis L (1978) Stapes Gusher and Klippel-Feil syndrome. Laryngoscope 88: 1178–1183

Goldenhar (1952) Associations malformatives de l'oeil et de l'oreille. J Genet Hum 1:243–282

Gorlin RJ, Pindborg JJ (1964) Syndromes of the Head and Neck. McGraw Hill, New York

Gorlin RJ, Pindborg JJ, Cohen MM (1976) In: Gorlin RJ (ed) Syndromes of the Head and Neck, 2nd Ed. McGraw Hill, New York, p453

Huson SM (1987) The different forms of neurofibromatosis. Br Med J 294: 1113–1114

Ilino Y, Tonyama M, Sarai Y, Hasegawa T, Ishii T (1987) A histological study of the temporal bones and the nose in Wolf-Hirschorn Syndrome. Arch Otolaryngol 113:1325–1329

Johnsen T, Larsen C, Friis J, Jougard-Jensen F (1987) Pendred's Syndrome. J Laryngol 101:1187–1192

Kaban LB, Mullihen JB, Murray JE (1981) Three dimensional approach to analysis and treatment of hemifacial microsomia. Cleft Palate J 18:92–99

Katano K, Yanraoka, Takiguchi T, Kadotani T (1979) Auditory disturbance due to trisomy 22. Lancet i, 276

Kirkham TH (1969) Duane's syndrome and familial perceptive deafness. Br J Opthalmol 55:335–339

Konigsmark B, Gorlin RJ (1976) Genetic and metabolic deafness. Apert syndrome 194. WB Sanders Co., Philadelphia

Kos AO, Schuknecht HF, Singer JO (1966) Temporal bone studies in 13–15 and 18 trisomy syndrome. Arch Otolaryngol 83: 439–445

Kosoy J, Maddox HE (1971) Surgical findings in van der Hoeve's syndrome. Arch Otolaryngol 93: 115–122

Maceri DR, Saxon KG (1984) Neurofibromatomas of the head and neck. Head Neck Surg 6: 842–850

Mafee MF, Valvassori GE (1981) Radiology of the craniofacial anomalies. Otolaryngol Clin N Am 14: 939–988

Miglets AW, Schuller D, Ruppert E, Lim DJ (1975) Trisomy 18: a temporal bone report. Arch Otolaryngol 101: 433–437

Miyamoto RT, House WF, Brachman DE (1980) Neurotologic manifestations of the osteopetroses. Arch Otolaryngol 106: 210–214

Nemansky J, Hageman MJ (1975) Tomographic findings of the inner ears of 24 patients with Waardenberg's syndrome. Roentgenol 124: 250–255

Pagon RA, Graham JM, Zonana J, Young SL (1981) Coloboma, congenital heart disease and choanal atresia with multiple anomalies. CHARGE Association. J Paediatr 99: 223–227

Phelps PD (1974) Congenital lesions of the inner ear, demonstrated by tomography. Arch Otolaryngol 100:11–18

Phelps PD, Lloyd GAS, Poswillo DE (1983) The ear deformities in craniofacial microsomia and oculoauriculovertebral dysplasia. J Laryngol 47: 995–1005

Phelps PD, Poswillo D, Lloyd GAS (1981) The ear deformities in mandibulofacial dysostosis (Treacher Collins Syndrome). Clin Otolaryngol 6: 15–28

Phelps PD, Roland PE (1977) Thalidomide and cranial nerve abnormalities. Br Med J II: 1672

Poswillo DE (1973) The pathogenesis of the first and second branchial arch syndrome. Oral Surg 35: 302–308

Poswillo DE (1975a) Haemorrhage in development of the face. Birth Defects 1: 61–81

Poswillo DE (1975b) The pathogenesis of the Treacher Collins Syndrome (mandibulofacial dysostosis). Br J Oral Surg 13: 1–26

Quisling RW, Moore GR, Jahrsdoerfer RA, Cantrell RW (1979) Osteogenesis imperfecta. Arch Otolaryngol 105: 207–211

Rapin I, Rubin RJ (1976) Patterns of anomalies in children with malformed ears. Laryngoscope 86: 1469–1502

Regenbogan L, Godel V, Goya V, Goodman RM (1982) Further evidence for an autosomal dominant form of oculoauriculovertebral dysplasis. Clin Gen 21: 161–167

Reisner K (1969) Tomography of inner and middle ear malformations. Radiology 92: 11–20

Slack RWT, Phelps PD (1985) Familial mixed deafness with branchial arch defects (earpits-deafness syndrome). Clin Otolaryngol 10: 271–277

Steel KP, Bock GR (1983) Hereditary inner ear abnormalities in animals. Arch Otolaryngol 109: 22–29

Suehiro S, Sando I (1979) Congenital anomalies of the inner ear. Introducing a new classification of labyrinthine anomalies. Ann Otol Supp 59

Terrahe K (1972) Diagnostik der Missbildungen des Ohres und des Ohrachadels. Arch der klinischen experimentellen Ohr, Nasen und Kehlkopp Heilkunde 202: 85–151

Tomoda K, Shea JJ, Shenefelt RE, Wilroy RS (1983) Temporal bone findings in Trisomy 13 with cyclopia. Arch Otolaryngol 109: 553–558

Van Rijn PM, Cremers CWRJ (1988) Surgery for congenital conductive deafness in Klippel Feil syndrome. Ann Otol Rhinol Laryngol 97: 347–352

Wells MD, Phelps PD, Michaels L (1983) Oculo-auriculo vertebral dysplasia. J Laryngol 47: 689–696

Windle-Taylor PC, Buchanan G, Michaels L (1982) The Mondini defect in Turner's syndrome: a temporal bone report. Clin Otolaryngol 7: 75–80

Windle-Taylor PC, Emery PJ, Phelps PD (1981) Ear deformities associated with the Klippel-Feil syndrome. Ann Otol 90: 210–216

Wright JLW, Phelps PD, Friedmann I (1976) Temporal bone studies in anencephaly (1). J Laryngol Otol 90: 919–927

5 Traumatic Lesions of the Temporal Bone

The head is affected in almost 75% of road accidents and if severely injured, the ear is the most frequently damaged sensory organ. Until recently, it was thought that nothing could be done to correct the hearing loss caused by skull traumas. Obviously, hearing loss due to petrous fracture cannot be corrected and radiological examination is concerned with such factors as damage to the facial nerve and the site of a CSF fistula. It is now realised, however, that traumatic hearing loss is often due to disruption of the ossicular chain, and although radiological demonstration may be difficult such an examination can greatly assist reconstruction. Ossicular discontinuity should always be considered

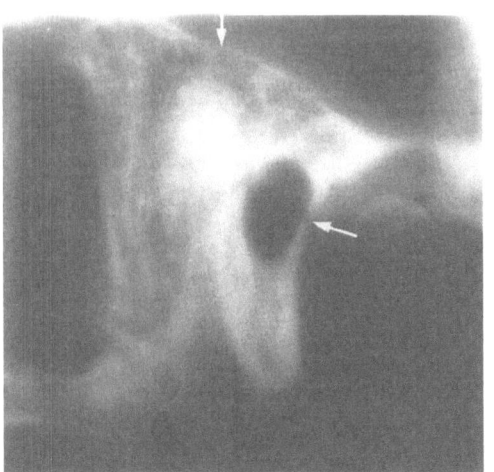

Fig. 5.1. Lateral tomogram showing fracture (*white arrows*) involving the tegmen, external auditory meatus and crossing the facial nerve canal.

where conductive deafness persists following head injury.

Technique

For fractures of the petromastoid, the optimum method of examination combines pluridirectional tomography with CT. CT alone does not provide a totally adequate method of excluding a bony injury in this area. With most CT scanner designs direct sagittal sections are impossible, and reformatted images in this plane lack the spatial resolution to show all longitudinal fractures (Figs. 5.1, 5.2). In practice, transverse fractures may also be missed without the routine use of pluridirectional tomography as a complementary technique.

The following examinations may need to be employed for total evaluation of a petromastoid injury:

1. Plain X-ray examination of the skull to exclude an associated fracture of the calvarium: in particular a linear fracture of the squamous part of the temporal bone is commonly associated with a longitudinal fracture of the petromastoid

2. Conventional pluridirectional tomography in the sagittal and coronal planes

3. Bone studies with the use of high resolution CT in the axial and coronal planes. The former are especially important to show the full extent of both longitudinal and transverse fractures and associated skull base injuries (Fig. 5.3)

4. Patients with a suspected or established CSF leak may need contrast CT cisternography

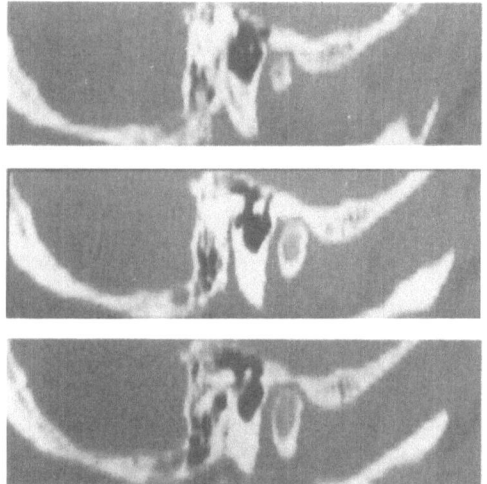

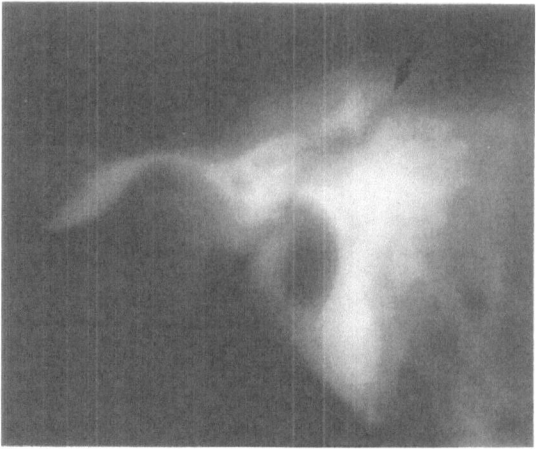

Fig. 5.4. Lateral tomogram showing a longitudinal fracture of the anterior wall of the external auditory meatus and tegmen.

Fig. 5.2. Same patient as Fig. 5.1. The fracture is not demonstrated on reformatted sagittal CT sections.

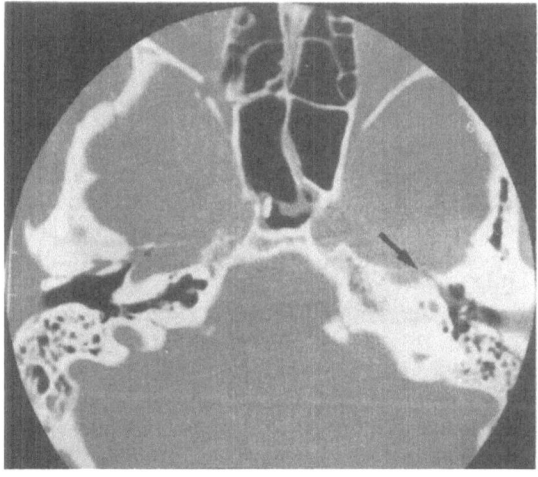

Fig. 5.3. Longitudinal fracture of the petrous bone associated with a fracture of the sphenoid sinus, and greater wing of sphenoid (arrow).

5. The association of temporal bone fractures with severe head injuries means that these patients may need to undergo immediate CT for proof or exclusion of intra or extracerebral haematomas or contusions (Schubiger et al. 1986). In such patients, the finding of an opaque middle ear or mastoid air cells on routine CT should prompt immediate axial high resolution CT of the petromastoid without alteration of the head position. In this way early diagnosis of a petromastoid fracture alerts the clinician to possible complications such as ossicular chain injuries, facial palsy or a CSF leak

6. Magnetic resonance: limited studies of petrous bone trauma examined by this method have shown it to be less useful than CT. Absence of bone signal is the main drawback and although fractures can be visualised either as absence or displacement of the black line of bone, Zimmermann et al. (1987) found that, in comparison with CT, the full extent of fracture was underestimated by magnetic resonance. The technique is, however, superior to CT in the definition of associated epidural, subdural, and intracerebral hemorrhagic lesions.

Classification of Fractures

Although fractures of the petrous temporal bone follow no set pattern, they are usually classified, with reference to the long axis of the petrous pyramid, as longitudinal and transverse.

Longitudinal Fractures

Longitudinal fractures account for 70–80% of petrous bone fractures (Hough 1970). The fracture line is in the long axis of the petrous bone and typically, it extends from the squama across the posterior aspect of the bony external auditory meatus (EAM) and through the tegmen which forms the roof the middle-ear cavity. Harwood-Nash (1970) described two types of longitudinal fracture: one, associated with a fracture of the anterior parieto-temporal region, extends along the anterior aspect of the petrous bone through the tegmen tympani (Fig. 5.4) to the region of the labyrinth capsule; the other involves the superior mastoid complex and the posterior and superior portion of the petrous bone (Fig. 5.5a,b). Both of these tend to converge on the labyrinth and, from this conflu- ence, the fractures proceed either along the roof of the Eustachian tube or to one of the nearby foram- ina, i.e., the foramen lacerum, jugular foramen or IAM. Longitudinal fractures are associated with facial nerve injury in 20% of patients (Hough 1970). Anterior longitudinal fractures tend to involve the horizontal portion of the facial nerve

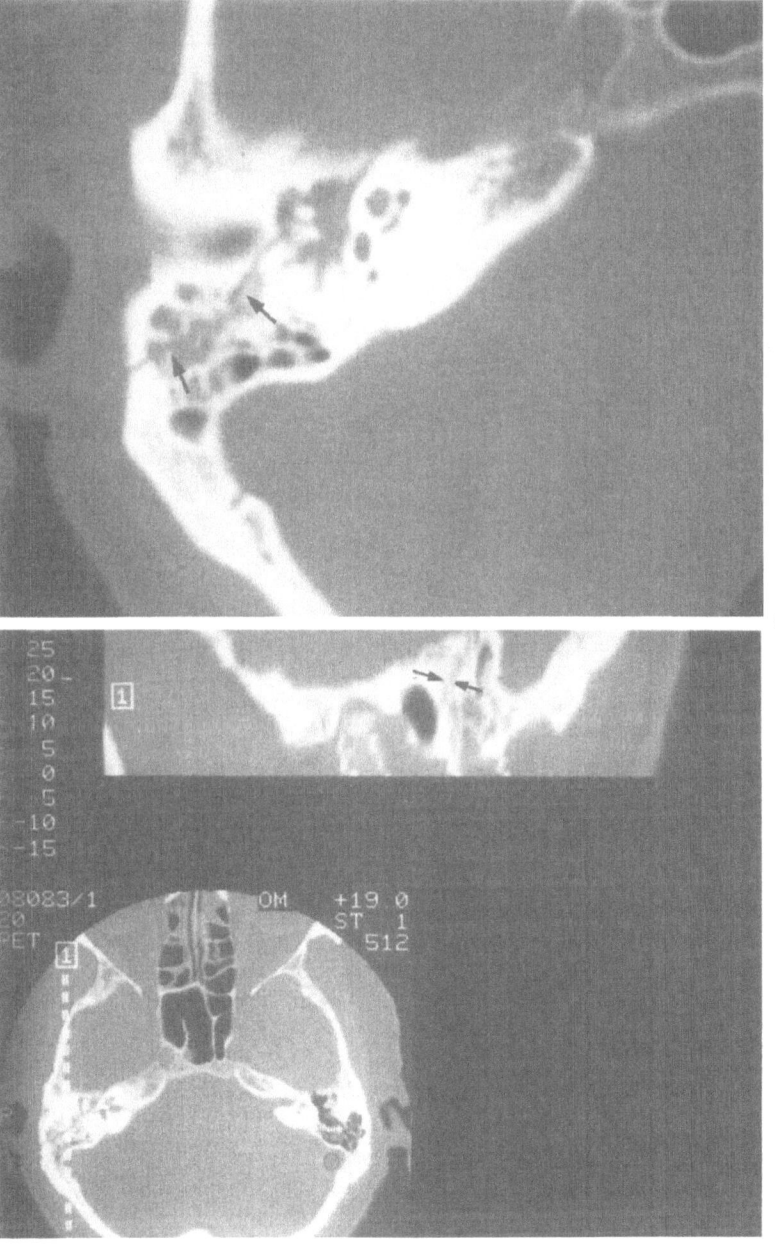

Fig. 5.5 a, b. Axial CT showing a posterior longitudinal fracture of the petrous bone (*arrow*). **b** Same fracture shown on reformatted sagittal sections.

canal in the region of the genicular ganglion. Posterior fractures may involve the vertical portion of the canal or the posterior genu.

To determine the site of injury of the facial nerve in the petromastoid, coronal CT or tomograms are needed to show the involvement of the internal auditory meatus (IAM) and genicular ganglion (Fig. 5.6), and these sections may also be helpful in showing involvement of the descending part of the canal. This is, however, better shown by lateral tomography or reformatted CT. The horizontal portion of the facial nerve lies beneath the lateral semicircular canal, while the vertical portion extends downwards to emerge at the stylomastoid foramen. Posterior longitudinal fractures involving

this part of the canal are readily demonstrated by sagittal tomograms (Fig. 5.7).

Transverse Fractures

The fracture line runs at right angles to the long axis of the petrous bone. As classically described, a transverse type of fracture affects the pyramid, with the fracture line passing across the labyrinth or IAM (Fig. 5.8). This type of fracture, which is much less common, produces facial palsy and sensorineural deafness which may be complete and permanent. It is usually the result of a severe impact on the top of the head or soles of the feet, which fractures the skull base.

Some fractures, however, pass lateral to the pyramid through the middle ear or external meatus and mastoid air cells. Because they are in the same plane, these should strictly be classified as "transverse" although the conductive deafness and other features make them very similar to the longitudinal type.

Complex Fractures These are fractures which combine components of both longitudinal and transverse petromastoid injuries.

Other Fractures Localised fractures of limited extent may occur in the region of the ear. These usually affect the tympanic ring as a result of indirect injury

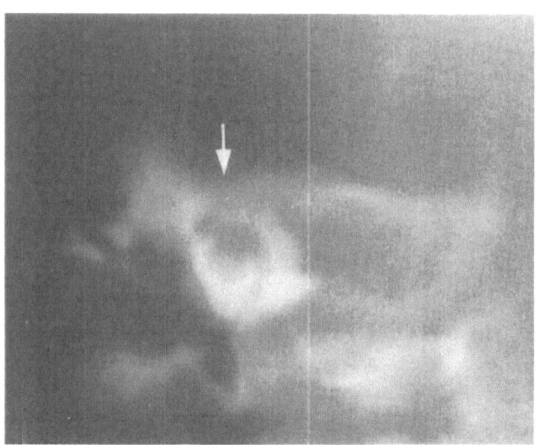

Fig. 5.6. Petrous bone fracture (*arrow*) with facial nerve palsy involving the pit for the genicular ganglion.

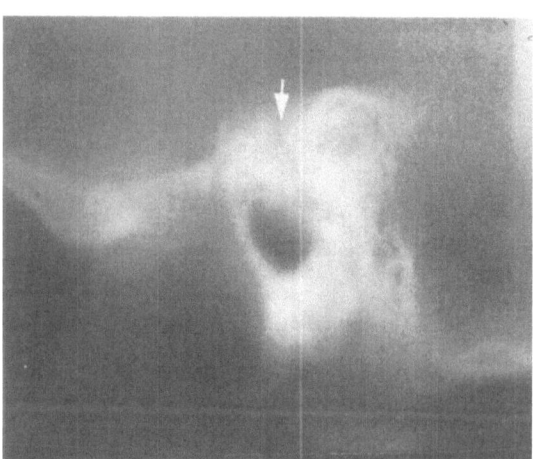

Fig. 5.7. Posterior longitudinal fracture shown on lateral tomography.

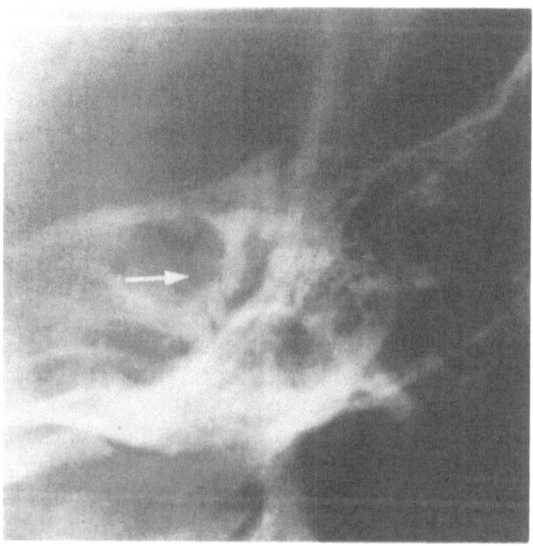

Fig. 5.8. Transverse fracture (*arrow*) shown on Stenver's projection involving the lateral end of the internal auditory meatus.

such as a blow to the chin and may occur as part of injuries to the temporo-mandibular joint.

Complications of Petromastoid Fractures

Uncomplicated fractures of the petromastoid usually do not require surgical treatment. The conductive hearing loss associated with a haemotympanum or ruptured eardrum will resolve with natural healing of the injury; transverse fractures involving the inner ear structures cause permanent sensorineural deafness which is untreatable. On the other hand, the complications of petromastoid fractures, such as discontinuity of the ossicular chain, facial nerve injury and CSF leak, often need surgery.

Trauma to the Ossicles

Ossicular chain injuries were first described in the English literature by Kelemann (1944), who reported the findings in 18 autopsy specimens, but it was not until the publication by Thorburn (1957) that an ossicular discontinuity was reported in the living patient, and a year later Hough (1958) also reported an example. Since that time, numerous reports have appeared.

The majority of ossicular injuries follow skull trauma and are usually associated with a fracture of the vault or skull base, but they can occur in isolation without evidence of a petromastoid fracture. An ossicular chain injury may also be caused by a penetrating injury to the ear via the EAM. Ossicular chain injuries, in common with temporal bone injuries, are generally found in young patients. This bias may be due to the young being more accident-prone, but it has also been attributed to a more malleable petrous bone being more responsive to torsional stress (Hough 1970).

When a head injury is followed by conductive deafness, it is most commonly due to a simple haemotympanum or to a traumatic rupture of the tympanic membrane, and complete recovery of the hearing is to be expected in the majority of cases. However, if hearing loss remains after the drumhead has healed and all signs of a hemorrhagic exudate have disappeared, then disruption of the ossicular chain must be suspected (Ballantyne 1966).

The most common type of injury found is an incudo-stapedial joint separation. Hough (1970) found that this joint was disrupted in 83% of ears operated on for deafness following temporal bone fractures. Isolated fractures of the stapedial arch

also occur. The latter have not yet been demonstrated by any imaging technique but high-resolution CT is now capable of showing isolated incudo-stapedial dislocations. The types of ossicular disruptions encountered are illustrated in Figs. 5.9, 5.10, 5.11, and 5.12.

Massive Incus Displacement

Because of its relative instability, the incus is particularly prone to dislocation and displacement. Separation of the incudomallear joint can be inferred on coronal views, either by conventional tomography or CT, when separated images of the incus and the malleus are seen on the same section (Fig. 5.13). It is often possible to show obvious separation of the incus from the rest of the ossicular chain (Fig. 5.14.a, b). Confirmation of discontinuity can be obtained from axial CT. This is the only projection in which the cartilage space between incus and malleus is clearly seen without obliquity, and is often demonstrable, not only by tomographic techniques but also on a standard submentovertical radiograph of the skull. The relationship of the head of the malleus to the body of the incus is clearly defined and any displacement is readily appreciated (Figs. 5.15, 5.16).

Potter (1969) has described the so-called "molar tooth" sign of incus dislocation on lateral tomograms. In this projection, the normal malleus and incus combine to form a radiographic image resembling a molar tooth. The head of the malleus and the body of the incus form the "crown", the handle of the malleus forms the "anterior root" and the long process of the incus the "posterior root" (Fig. 5.17). The crown should normally appear as a solid shadow and any disruption of this image either in the form of separation of its two components or their non-alignment, indicates a dislocation. The "molar tooth" sign can be demonstrated on reformatted sagittal CT sections (Fig. 5.18), or lateral pluridirectional tomography, and the characteristic shape of the image results from the fact that, with the head in the true lateral plane, the malleus and incus are sectioned slightly obliquely. A truer anatomical representation is given if the head of the patient or the film is angled so that the tomographic cuts are in the true plane of the two larger ossicles. For the same reason, CT sagittal sections should be reformatted with the same slight obliquity.

Dislocation of the Malleus

Fig. 5.19 shows the rare dislocation of the malleus with the remainder of the ossicular chain intact. A

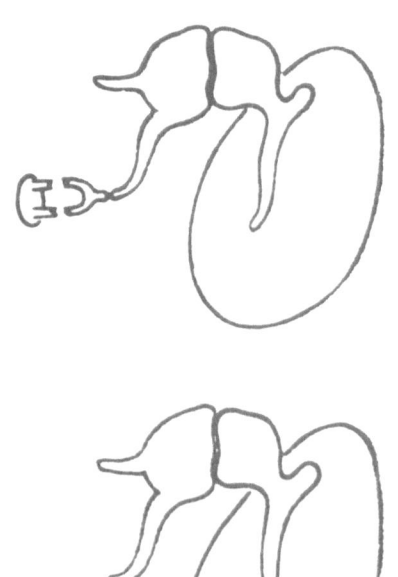

Fig. 5.9

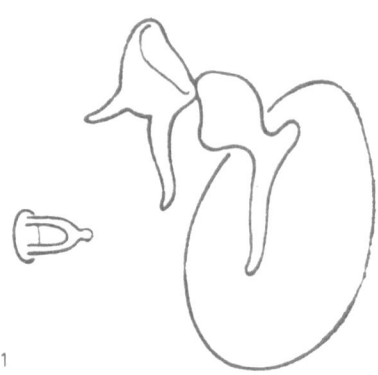

Fig. 5.10

Fig. 5.11

Fig. 5.12

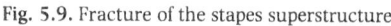

Fig. 5.9. Fracture of the stapes superstructure.

Fig. 5.10. Incudo-stapedial dislocation: the commonest ossicular chain injury.

Fig. 5.11. Massive incus displacement.

Fig. 5.12. Rare dislocation of the malleus with the remainder of the ossicular chain intact.

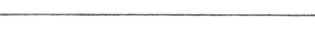

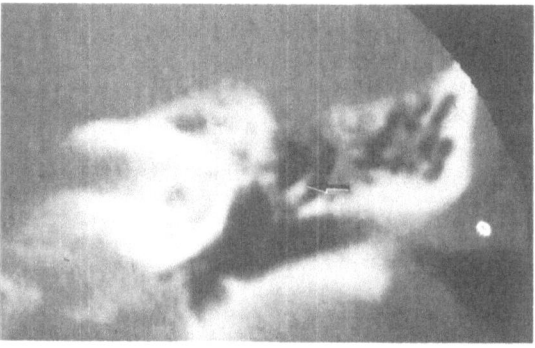

Fig. 5.13. Coronal CT scan showing massive incus displacement following a road traffic accident. The images of the ossicles are completely separate and the incus is lying inverted in the attic (*arrow*).

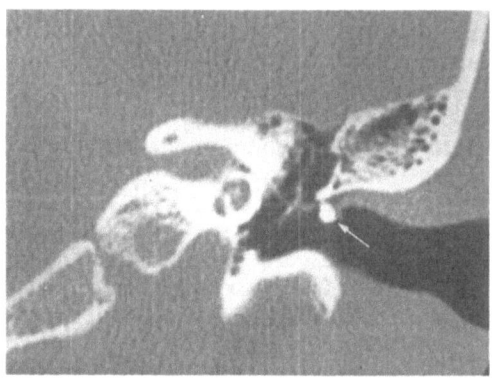

a

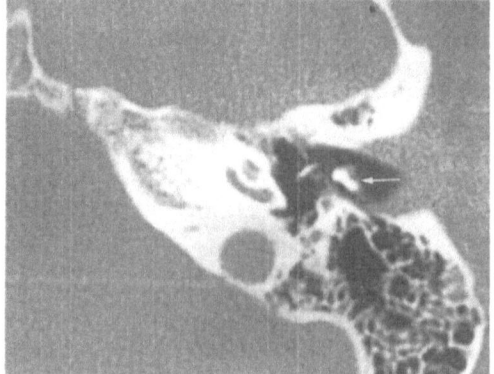

b

Fig. 5.14 a, b. coronal CT; **b** axial CT. Massive incus displacement. The incus (*arrows*) is lying under the epithelium in the roof of external auditory meatus, outside the tympanic membrane.

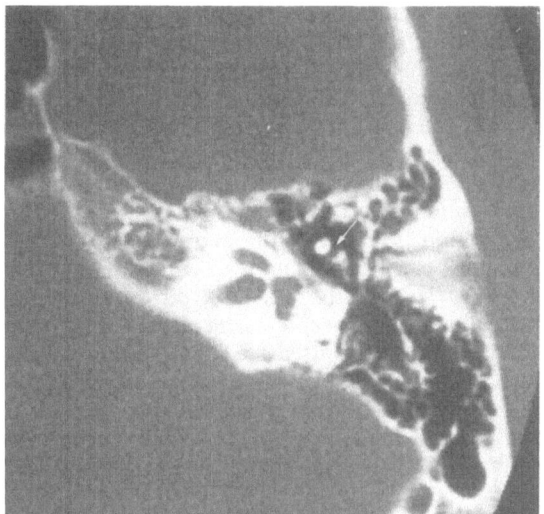

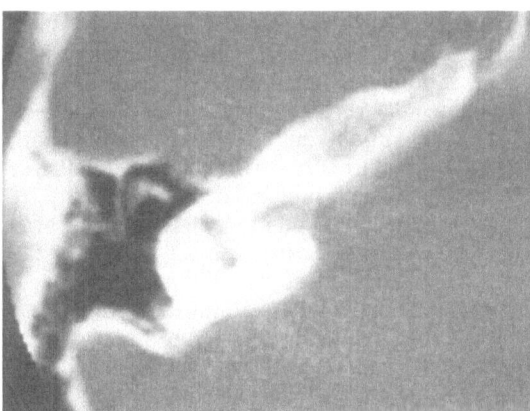

Fig. 5.15. Incudo-mallear dislocation shown on axial CT. There is widening of the joint space between the head of the malleus and the body of the incus (*arrow*).

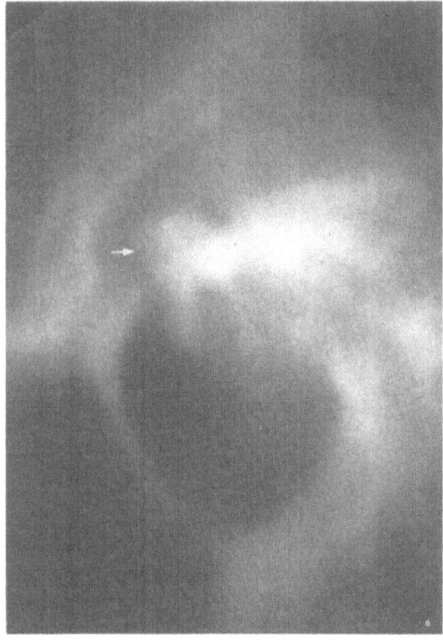

Fig. 5.17. Lateral tomogram showing the incus and malleus in normal position (*arrow*).

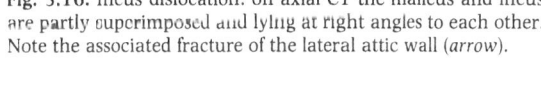

Fig. 5.16. Incus dislocation: on axial CT the malleus and incus are partly superimposed and lying at right angles to each other. Note the associated fracture of the lateral attic wall (*arrow*).

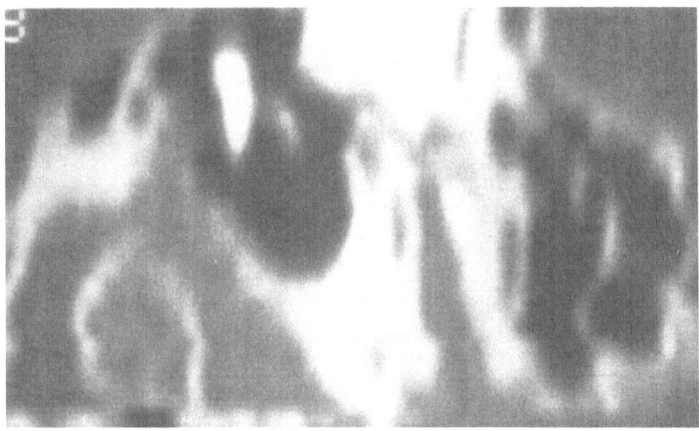

Fig. 5.18. Reformatted sagittal CT, showing incudo-mallear separation.

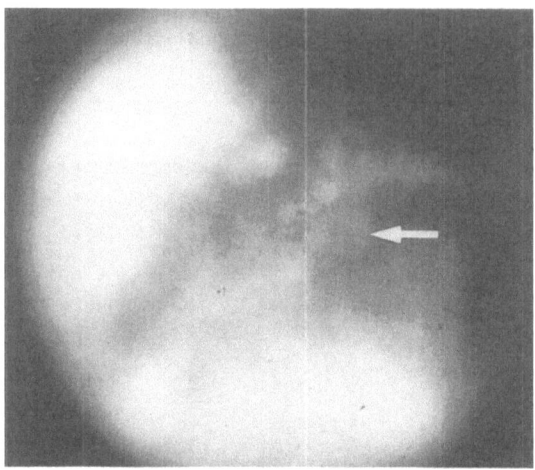

Fig. 5.19. Coronal tomogram showing dislocation of the malleus (*arrow*). The malleus is lying outside the outer attic wall in the external auditory meatus.

single example of this type of injury has been observed by the authors. This was a 40-year-old male patient with a history of previous head trauma and tinnitus, discomfort and severe blockage of the ear. On examination, the head of the malleus was seen to be placed outside the outer attic wall and covered with a false tympanic membrane. This was confirmed on coronal tomographic section and at subsequent surgery.

Facial Nerve Injury

Facial nerve palsy in temporal bone fractures most commonly results from compression of the nerve by an intraneural haematoma. Fisch (1974) reported 50% of cases due to this cause, while total loss of facial nerve continuity was present in 26%. In a minority (17%), a bone fragment impinges directly on the facial nerve. The facial nerve is injured in 10%–20% of longitudinal fractures (Cannon and Jahrsdoerfer 1983). In the vast majority, the perigeniculate section of the nerve is affected (Fisch 1974; Coker et al. 1987); and fewer than 10% are found elsewhere, usually in the area of the posterior genu. The facial nerve may be injured in up to 50% of transverse fractures: usually the labyrinthine part of the nerve is affected but the tympanic segment may also be injured if the medial wall of middle ear is involved in the fracture (McHugh 1963).

Demonstration of the site of facial nerve injury demands radiological display of the whole course of the facial nerve canal. A common site of injury is the region of the genicular ganglion, either in

association with a transverse or an anterior longitudinal fracture. The demonstration of a fracture in this region is difficult and unreliable on axial CT (Schubiger et al. 1986): such fractures are better demonstrated by direct coronal CT or coronal hypocycloidal tomography (Fig. 5.6). The facial nerve may also be injured at the posterior genu or in its descending part in association with a posterior longitudinal fracture of the petrous bone. In this situation, sagittal imaging is essential and in practice this means the use of conventional pluridirectional tomography. The spatial resolution provided by reformatted lateral sections on most currently available CT scanners is sufficient to show all fine fracture lines in this plane (Figs. 5.1, 5.2), and the examination is therefore incomplete without a full set of lateral conventional tomograms.

Cerebrospinal Fluid Leak

This is potentially the most life-threatening of the complications of petromastoid fractures, and usually results from a tear in the dura in the region of the tegmen tympani. It is usually a complication of longitudinal fractures, which frequently traverse the tegmen. The symptoms depend upon the state of the tympanic membrane: if the membrane is ruptured as part of the trauma, CSF escapes through the EAM: if the drum remains intact CSF passes down the Eustachian tube and the symptoms are those of rhinorrhoea.

Radiologically fractures of the tegmen are best demonstrated by lateral conventional tomography and by coronal CT but contrast cisternography may be required to confirm the site of CSF leak: the depressed fracture is often filled by herniated cerebral tissue or dura (Fig. 5.20) with escape of fluid into the middle ear.

Foreign Bodies in the Ear

Prostheses purposely introduced at surgery are the most common cause of foreign bodies in the middle ear. These include stainless steel and tantalum wire for reconstruction of the stapes as well as other forms of wholly or partially radio-opaque replacement parts. The radiologist may be called upon to assess the position of a stapes prosthesis if it is made of radio-opaque material. For example, in a patient with vertigo following stapedectomy it may be possible to show the prosthesis projecting into the ves-

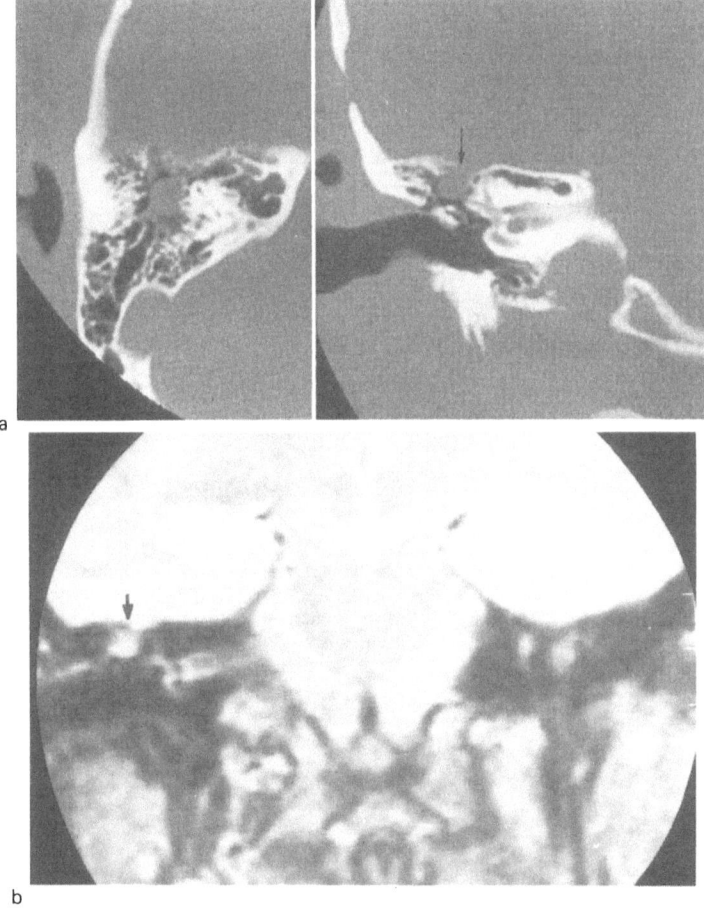

Fig. 5.20 a, b. Traumatic herniation of the dura through a fracture of the tegmen shown on base and coronal CT (*arrow*). **b** Magnetic resonance shows high signal from the herniation on T_2-weighted spin echo sequences indicating the presence of CSF.

tibule (Fig. 5.21). Radiology may also be needed to check the position of the electrode array following cochlear implant surgery. Qaiyumi et al. (1988) investigated 23 patients after implant surgery, who had non-auditory sensations such as pain, or showed malfunction of the electrodes. By the use of plain X-ray and conventional tomography, they were able to correlate these disturbances with dislocation or distortion in the array of electrodes. These authors found that conventional tomography was the method of choice for this investigation and was superior to high-resolution CT, since artefacts

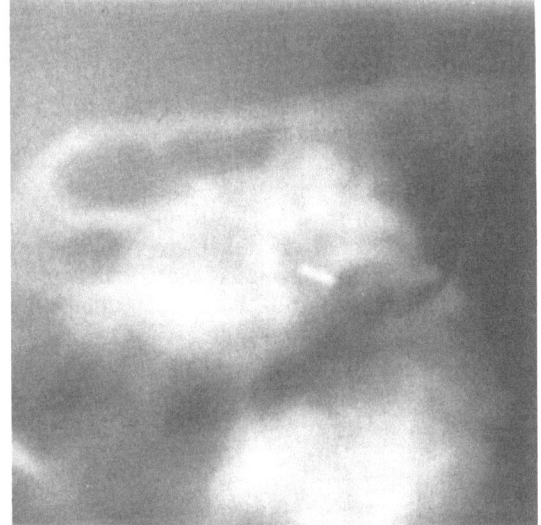

Fig. 5.21. Metal stapes prosthesis projecting through the oval window into the vestibule.

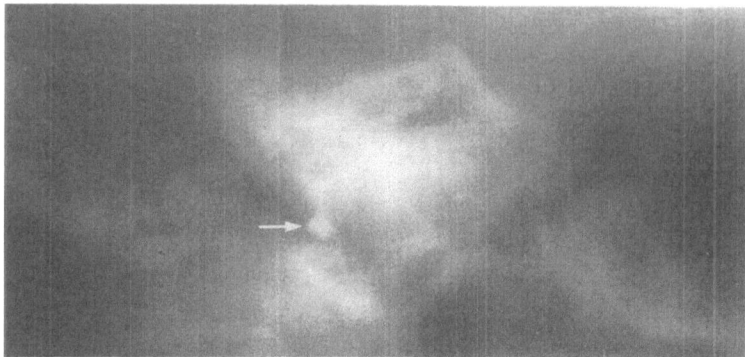

Fig. 5.22. Metallic foreign body lying in the Eustachian tube (*arrow*). The molten metal had entered the middle ear through the tympanic membrane.

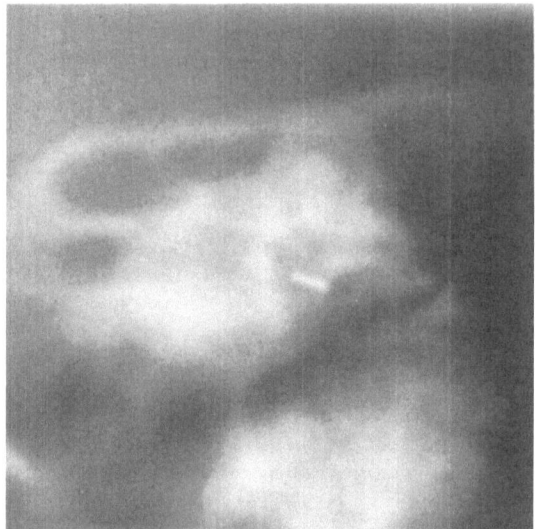

Fig. 5.23. Lateral tomogram showing a bullet lodged in the middle ear.

from the metal electrodes did not disturb the image and the spatial resolution of conventional tomography was superior to CT.

Apart from replacement surgery, industrial accidents account for most foreign bodies in the middle ear. Cutting torches or welding operations may result in fragments of molten metal entering the middle ear (Fig. 5.22). Bullet fragments are the next most common foreign body (Fig. 5.23).

References

Ballantyne JC (1966) Traumatic conductive deafness. Proc R Soc Med 59: 535–542

Cannon CR, Jahrsdoerfer RA (1983) Temporal bone fractures. Arch Otolaryngol 109: 285–288

Coker NJ, Kendall KA, Jenkins HA, Alford AB (1987) Traumatic intratemporal bone injury: management rationale for preservation of function. Otolaryngology – Head and Neck Surgery 97: 262–269

Fisch U (1974) Facial paralysis in fractures of the petrous bone. Laryngoscope 84: 2141–2154

Harwood-Nash DC (1970) Fractures of the petrous and tympanic parts of the temporal bone in children: a tomographic study of 35 cases. Am J Roentgenol 110: 598–607

Hough JVD (1958) Malformations and anatomical variations seen in the middle ear during the operation for mobilisation of the stapes. Laryngoscope 68: 1337–1379

Hough JVD (1970) Surgical aspects of temporal bone fractures. Proc R Soc Med 63: 245–252

Kelemann G (1944) Fractures of the temporal bone. Arch Otolaryngol 40: 333–373

McHugh HE (1963) Facial paralysis in birth injury and skull fractures. Arch Otolaryngol 87: 443–455

Potter G (1969) Trauma to the temporal bone. Seminars Roentgenol 4: 143–150

Qaiyumi SAA, Hendrickz PH, Lasig R, Battmar RD, Bachor E (1988) The value of conventional X-ray tomography in cochlear implant patients. XI International Congress of Head and Neck Radiology, Uppsala p. 62

Schubiger O, Valavanis A, Stuckmann G, Antonucci F (1986) Temporal bone fractures and their complications. Neuroradiol 28: 93–99

Thorburn IB (1957) Post-traumatic conduction deafness. J Laryngol Otol 71: 542–545

Zimmermann RA, Bilaniuk LT, Hackney DB, Goldberg HI, Grossman RI (1987) Neuroradiol magnetic resonance imaging in temporal bone fracture 29: 246–251

6 Inflammatory Diseases of the Temporal Bone

Acute Otitis Media

Acute otitis media is an inflammatory condition of the mucous membrane lining the middle ear cleft, i.e., the Eustachian tube, the middle ear proper and the mastoid air-cell system. It is a condition which predominantly affects children under 8 years of age and arises in association with Eustachian tube obstruction, most commonly following an upper respiratory tract infection. In the past, the condition would seem to have been more severe than in recent years, having been not uncommonly complicated by acute labyrinthitis, acute mastoiditis or intracranial sepsis. The reasons for the decreased severity of the condition are not entirely clear, but factors such as improved social conditions, better general health, lower virulence of responsible organisms and the widespread and early use of antibiotics are almost certainly significant.

The diagnosis of acute otitis media depends essentially on the history and adequate otological examination. Radiology has little part to play in the investigation or management of the condition in its uncomplicated form but loss of translucency of the middle ear cleft, when compared to the normal side, will be seen on mastoid radiographs or CT examination. The infectious and non-infectious complications of otitis media result in significant morbidity. The non-infectious sequelae include perforation of the eardrum, labyrinthine erosion, tympanosclerosis and adhesive otitis.

Acute Mastoiditis

This is the most common complication of acute otitis media and results from the spread of the infective process beyond the mucosal lining of the middle ear cleft into the underlying bone, producing an osteomyelitis. Because of the anatomical arrangement of the region, this phenomenon occurs primarily and predominantly in the mastoid air-cell system and produces clinical signs and symptoms accordingly.

As with acute otitis media, the diagnosis of acute mastoiditis is essentially a clinical one, but radiology may provide supporting evidence. Radiologically, the dominant finding is break-down of the cell wall trabeculations in addition to the loss of translucency found in acute otitis media. However, in conventional plain radiographs, the loss of the normally air-filled spaces, together with possible osteoporosis and swelling of the soft tissues overlying the affected mastoid process (all changes which are also due to the infection), make recognition of the cell walls difficult even if they are intact. This is particularly so in the less highly cellular temporal bone. Again, careful comparison with the normal side, assuming the usual symmetry of mastoid cellularity, is essential (Fig. 6.1).

The improved resolution of the air, soft-tissue and bone boundaries in computerised tomography, makes interpretation of the precise state of the mastoid air-cell system easier but it is not often justifiable to undertake such an examination in the

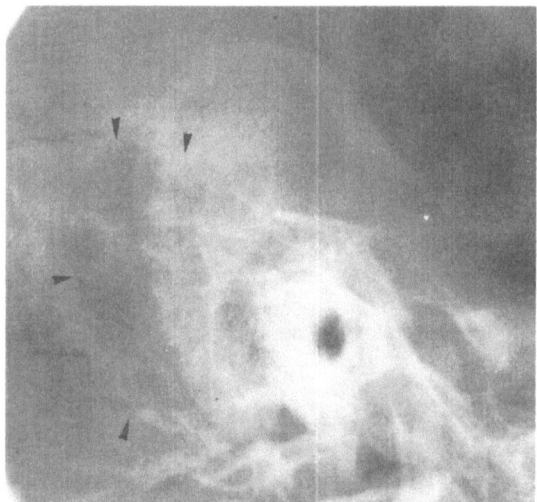

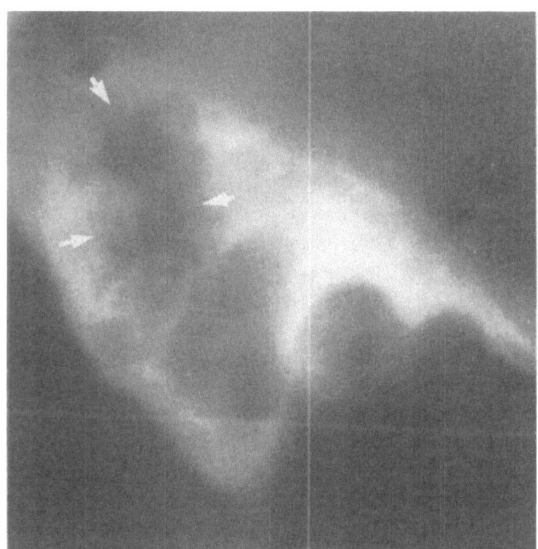

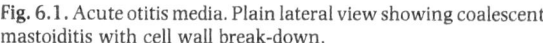

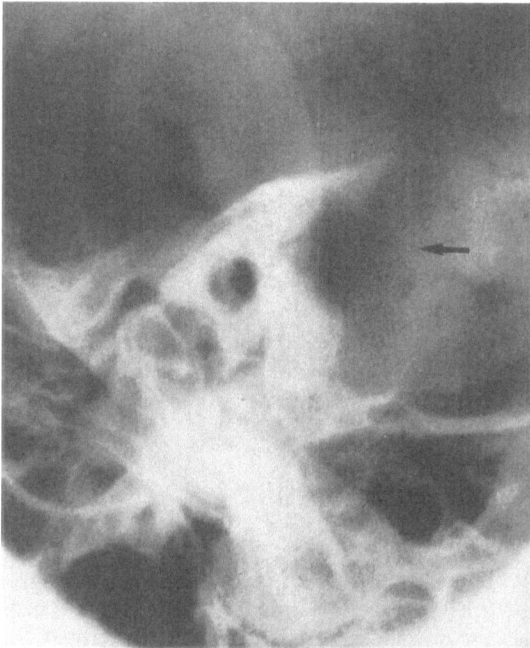

Fig. 6.3. An abscess cavity in a sclerotic mastoid with erosion of the dural plate (*arrow*).

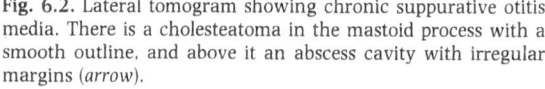

Fig. 6.2. Lateral tomogram showing chronic suppurative otitis media. There is a cholesteatoma in the mastoid process with a smooth outline, and above it an abscess cavity with irregular margins (*arrow*).

average case where, in the end, the management is determined by the clinical findings rather than radiology.

If there is extensive break-down of the cell walls, the resultant abscess cavity may be shown radiologically, with irregular margins (Fig. 6.2). This should not be confused with a large mastoid air cell. It should be noted that radiologically ragged erosions in the mastoid region are produced by histiocytosis and even more so by eosinophil granuloma, both of which are predominantly diseases of childhood, although the clinical picture is usually quite different from that of acute sepsis.

A common clinical feature of acute mastoiditis, the subperiosteal mastoid abscess, may show radi-

ologically as widening of the soft-tissue shadow over the bone of the mastoid process but the presence of a gross defect in the bony cortex, associated with such an abscess, is unusual (Fig. 6.3). A similar abscess may form in relation to air cells at the base of the zygomatic process.

Masked (Latent) Mastoiditis

The widespread use of antibiotics in acute ear infections has resulted in the appearance of a new clinical entity, so-called masked mastoiditis. Typically, the patient is treated for an acute otitis media or mastoiditis, with apparent good effect initially, the result being that treatment may be discontinued prematurely. Subsequently, the symptoms return although most often only to a subacute degree. Lack of awareness of this condition and lack of subsequent treatment place the patient at risk of developing intracranial complications. Histologically, the middle ear cleft will be largely filled with granulation tissue and, radiologically, the findings are those of acute mastoiditis.

Computerised tomography is best able to show cell-wall break-down in the mastoid but is very rarely required, as the decision to proceed to cortical mastoidectomy is almost entirely clinical. Most surgeons are content with single lateral plain views to show the extent of pneumatisation and the position of the sinus and dural plates. Opacity of the air cells is confirmation of the disease process, but neither plain films nor CT are capable of distinguishing the nature of the soft-tissue opacification or type of fluid present. We are at present trying to assess whether magnetic resonance can be more helpful for "tissue characterisation" of pathological contents in the middle ear cleft.

Acute Petrositis

In appropriately pneumatised temporal bones, involvement by infection of air cells in the petrous apex may progress to abscess formation which, if it extends extradurally, gives rise to the classic syndrome of Gradenigo. This comprises pain around the eye due to involvement of the first division of the Vth nerve and lateral rectus palsy due to involvement of the VIth cranial nerve, in addition to the normal signs and symptoms of acute middle ear cleft infection.

Infection from middle ear and mastoid can extend directly into an unpneumatised petrous apex. Proximity to intracranial structures and poor drainage predispose to intracranial extension.

Evidence of apical infection by imaging is often difficult. High resolution CT and isotope bone scans are useful and radiographs showing decalcification of the petrous apex when compared to the normal side will be helpful in confirming the diagnosis (Fig. 6.4). Recalcification may be demonstrated later, following successful treatment of the condition. The role of magnetic resonance for the diagnosis of chocolate cyst of the petrous apex will be described later.

Acute Infections in Infants

The short, wide, Eustachian tube in infants predisposes to the development of otitis media as a common cause of pyrexia and meningeal irritation in this age group, although there may be no obvious symptoms in relation to the involved ears. Although some infants are born with air-cell development already proceeding, it is not until about the age of 12 months that pneumatisation has reached the point where radiology can be of practical use in the diagnosis of infection.

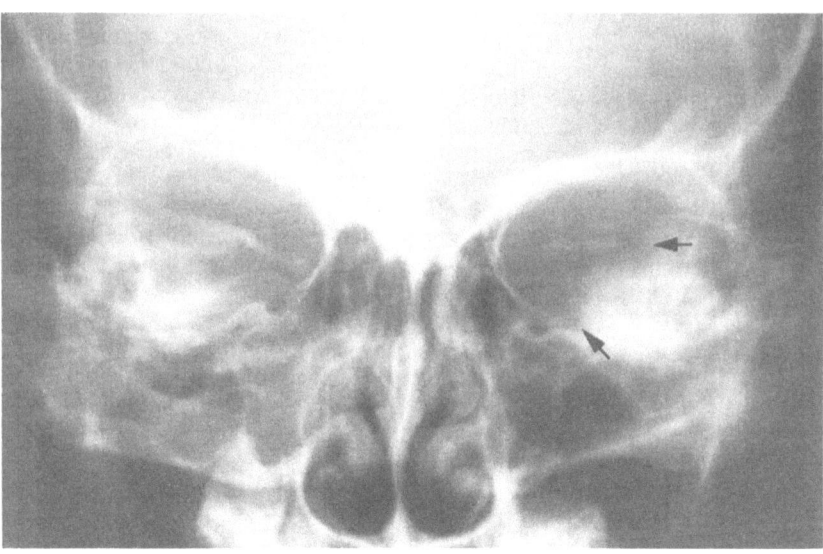

Fig. 6.4. Perorbital view showing decalcification of the petrous apex from apical petrositis (*arrow*). A repeat examination one month later, after antibiotic therapy, showed normal appearances.

Chronic Otitis Media

Chronic Suppurative Otitis Media

Chronic suppurative otitis media is a common oto-logical condition presenting with deafness and/or otorrhoea. The deafness is most commonly the result of destruction of part of the drum or the ossicular chain, but may also have a sensorineural element if the inner ear has been involved by the infective process at some stage in the progress of the disease. The otorrhoea results from infection of the soft tissues and bone in and around the middle ear cleft.

Two main types of CSOM are recognised, i.e., tubotympanic or non-cholesteatomatous and attico-antral or cholesteatomatous.

Tubotympanic Disease

This is associated with a simple central perforation of the tympanic membrane and involves, pre-dominantly, the mucous membrane lining the middle ear cleft; however, secondary osteitis, par-ticularly of the ossicles, may result in defects which significantly affect the function. It is rare for tubotympanic disease to be complicated by lab-yrinthine or intracranial infection or other com-plications normally associated with CSOM.

Radiology is of very limited use in tubotympanic disease, perhaps being helpful in enabling the surgeon to assess the anatomy of the air-cell system and the position of the sinus and dural plates prior to surgical intervention.

The degree of pneumatisation of an ear involved by tubotympanic disease is, commonly, less than that of the normal opposite side in any individual patient and this is apparent on plain radiographs. There has been considerable discussion as to whether the decreased pneumatisation pre-exists or follows the development of CSOM but it is usually the result, at least in part, of the deposition of scler-otic bone around the involved air cells (Friedman 1974).

Cholesterol Granuloma

Yellow nodules are found in the middle ear and mastoid in many cases of chronic otitis media. These are composed of cholesterol crystals surrounded by foreign-body giant cells and other inflammatory cells. Such cholesterol granulomas are almost always found in the midst of haemorrhage in the middle ear mucosa (Michaels 1987). They are indis-tinguishable from the soft tissue opacities by CT but have important characteristics on examination by magnetic resonance, to be dicussed in Chapter 7.

Attico-antral Disease

The typical feature of this type of disease is the acquired form of cholesteatoma, which involves the appearance of keratinising, stratified, squamous epi-thelium in the middle ear cleft. The essential clinical features of this condition, namely discharge and deafness, are indistinguishable from those in the tubotympanic type of CSOM but, because of the erosive nature of cholesteatoma, there is a sig-nificant risk of complications.

Non-suppurative (Secretory) Otitis Media

This is a condition, most common in childhood, in which as a result of Eustachian tube dysfunction, there is the collection of a sterile effusion within the middle ear cleft. The principal clinical feature is a conductive deafness. Radiology is of little use in this condition but will show a non-specific cloudiness of the middle ear cleft indistinguishable from that in otitis media.

Adhesive Otitis Media

This condition of the middle ear cleft involves the development of adhesions and/or tympanosclerosis as a result of previous inflammatory disease, either secretory otitis or suppurative otitis media (Fig. 6.5.). A feature of tympanosclerosis is calcification in areas of hyaline degeneration and plaques of this calcified material may be seen on imaging studies, when it is important not to confuse these dense opacities in the middle ear with normal structures. Post-inflammatory ossicular fixation and erosion may also be shown by CT (Swartz 1986) although the fibrous tissue cannot be differentiated from early cholesteatoma.

Chronic Otitis Media due to Specific Organisms

Tuberculosis otitis media in adults most commonly occurs in association with advanced pulmonary tuberculosis, but in children it may occur in

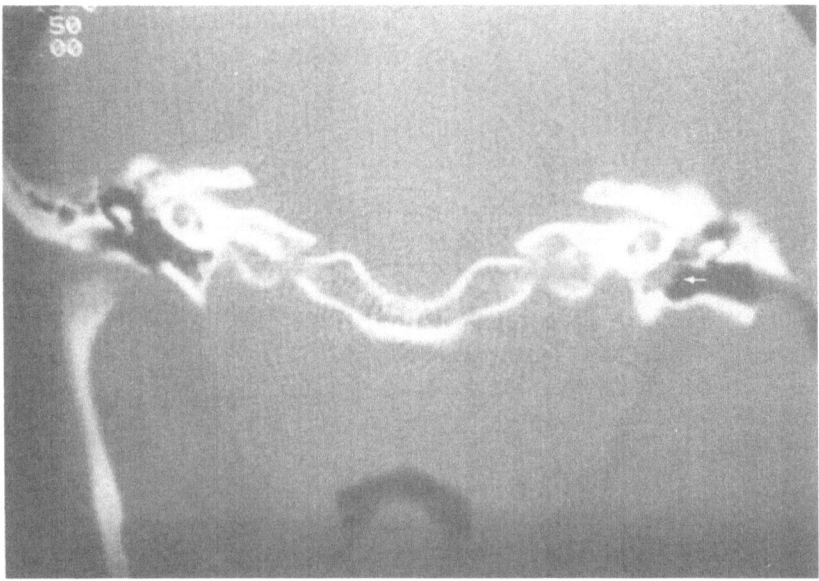

Fig. 6.5. Retracted eardrum with some soft tissue opacification in the meso and hypotympanum (*arrow*). The attic is clear, suggesting residual adhesive otitis but cholesteatoma cannot be ruled out completely on these radiological appearances.

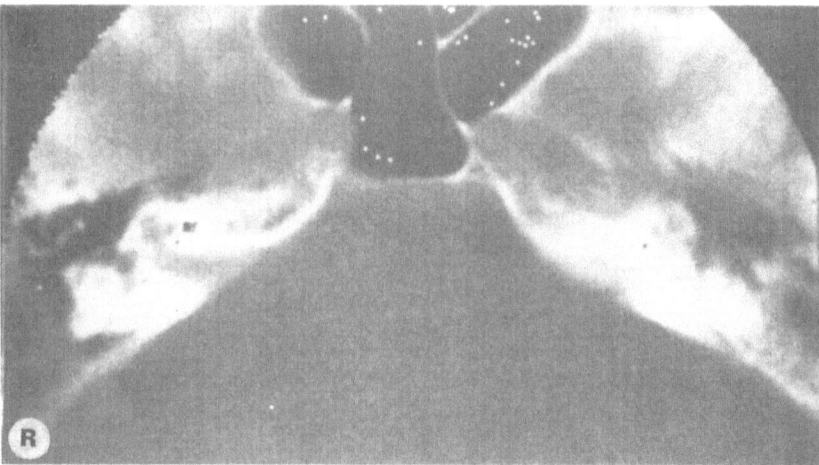

Fig. 6.6. Tuberculous otitis media: base CT shows the opacity of the middle ear cleft and ragged erosion of a large portion of the petrous temporal bone on the left with absence of the ossicles.

isolation. Characteristically, the condition presents with painless otorrhoea and severe hearing impairment but facial paralysis and labyrinthitis or, rarely, tuberculous meningitis, may also be associated. Extensive ragged destruction in the mastoid and middle ear, rather than sclerosis, is the typical radiographic feature (Fig. 6.6).

Actinomycosis may produce a similar picture. The temporal bone may be affected by all types of syphilis but the radiographic findings are indistinguishable from other types of chronic infection unless sequestration of part of the labyrinth occurs.

Syphilis, either congenital or acquired, may affect the capsule in later life causing profound hearing loss. The osteitis may produce sclerosis, but we have seen rarefaction both of the cochlear capsule and its surroundings, presumably due to gumma formation or subsequent fibrosis (Fig. 6.7).

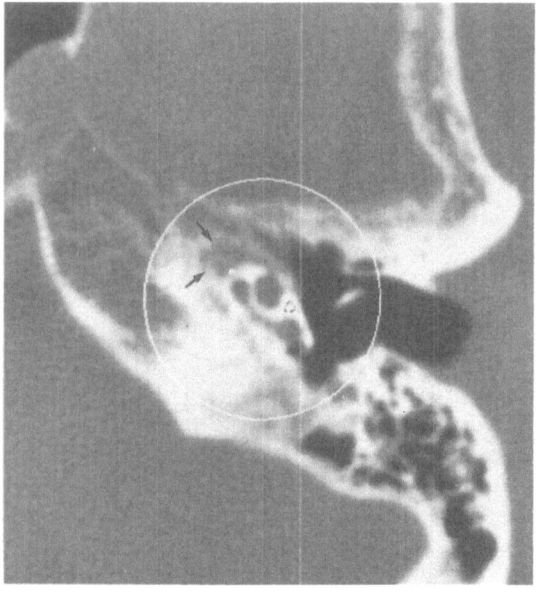

Fig. 6.7. Presumed syphilis of the inner ear. This patient with congenital syphilis and positive serology became profoundly deaf in middle age and a candidate for a cochlear implant. The base CT with densitometry shows rarefaction of the cochlear capsule *and* of the surrounding periosteal bone (*arrow*).

Complications of Middle-ear Infection

These may follow any form of middle ear infection but, most commonly, acute mastoiditis and cholesteatomous CSOM. Samuel and Fernandes (1985) assessed 21 cases with subperiosteal abscess, intracranial abscess, meningitis, sigmoid sinus thrombosis, cerebellitis or facial palsy complicating acute otitis media. All had retroauricular swelling and 90% were below the age of 13 years. In all, the eardrum, although abnormal, was intact and the predominant finding at mastoidectomy was granulation tissue filling the mastoid cavity and antrum.

Labyrinthitis

The symptom of vertigo in the presence of acute or chronic suppurative otitis media indicates the presence of labyrinthitis due to involvement of the labyrinthine fluids in the inflammatory process. Spread of the infection to the labyrinth may be via the intact oval window or the round window

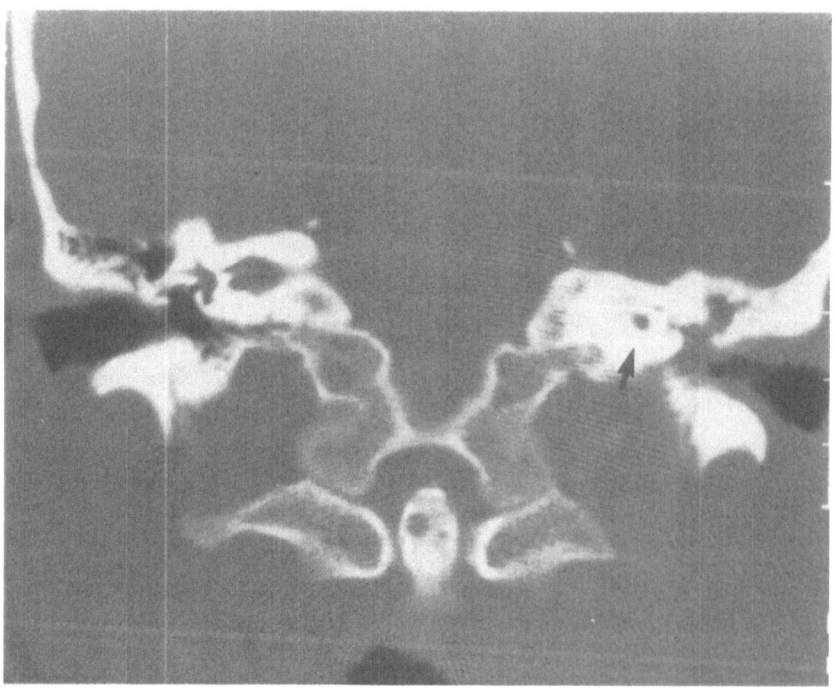

Fig. 6.8. Partial obliteration of the left cochlea by labyrinthitis ossificans complicating middle ear cholesteatoma (*arrow*).

membrane or via an erosion in the labyrinthine capsule, the latter being usually produced by a cholesteatoma. Radiology is likely to be informative only in cholesteatomatous disease, where the most common abnormality is an erosion of the bony capsule of the lateral semicircular canal, demonstrable on base and coronal CT (Chap. 7). Less commonly, CT may show an erosion elsewhere in the labyrinthine capsule, particularly in the vestibule above the horizontal facial canal, the oval window, the posterior semicircular canal or the promontory over the basal turn of the cochlea.

Suppurative labyrinthitis can also result from spread of infection from the bloodstream or meninges.

Following an episode of purulent labyrinthitis, which results in total destruction of the membranous labyrinth, the bony labyrinth may become filled with granulation tissue which often undergoes varying degrees of ossification. This so-called labyrinthitis obliterans is, primarily, a histopathological diagnosis but the ossification is readily detectable by imaging (Fig. 6.8). Other uncommon causes include tumours, advanced otosclerosis, temporal bone fractures and inner ear haemorrhage.

Hoffman et al. (1979) describe four patients with labyrinthitis obliterans following tympanogenic labyrinthitis. In three cases tomograms showed almost complete obliteration of the bony labyrinth, but in the fourth case the ossification affected only part of the labyrinth. The authors have also seen partial obliteration of the bony labyrinth. This is probably a characteristic tomographic feature with a clear-cut margin seen between the parts obliterated by bone and portions seemingly unaffected (Fig. 6.9). This appearance distinguishes post-suppurative labyrinthitis obliterans from advanced otosclerosis, in which the bone encroachment is much more diffuse.

Facial Palsy

Facial palsy is an occasional complication of acute otitis media, probably resulting from involvement of the nerve by infection in an area, usually in the horizontal position of the nerve, where the bony canal is congenitally deficient. In the case of cholesteatomatous disease, facial palsy is usually associated with exposure of the nerve by the erosive process of the cholesteatoma itself.

Basal and coronal CT or tomography, in the semiaxial projection for the horizontal portion, may show a deficiency in the bony wall of the facial canal but, in view of the thinness of the bony walls

of the Fallopian canal, apparent radiological evidence of erosion may not be confirmed by subsequent surgical exploration. The question is, however, largely academic as the treatment of the condition is decompression, whether locally or by full mastoid exploration, being determined by the clinical situation at hand.

Lateral (Sigmoid) Sinus Thrombophlebitis

This condition may be a surprise finding at mastoid exploration for either acute or chronic disease, but may also be suspected clinically pre-operatively, if there is a persistent undulating fever, headache and perhaps tenderness over the line of the internal jugular vein. In the very occasional case where pre-operative demonstration of the lesion may be helpful, this may be achieved either in the late venous phase of a carotid angiogram or by retrograde jugular venography. Irregular filling defects in the sinus may be shown by enhanced CT (de Slegte et al. 1988).

Intracranial Complications

These comprise one or more of the following: extradural abscess, subdural abscess, temporal lobe abscess, cerebellar abscess, meningitis and hydrocephalus. Suspicion of their presence is "par excellence" the indication for computerized tomography in acute or chronic suppurative otitis media. While the incidence of CNS complications of infective ear disease have decreased in absolute numbers, the relative distribution of these complications remains similar to pre-antibiotic days. Gower and McGuire (1983) assessed 100 such cases and found 85% in patients under 20 years old. Meningitis occurred in 76, of whom 9 died. Awareness of these possible complications is therefore essential.

The radiological diagnosis of brain abscess is based on the demonstration of a localised area of low attenuation and, after injection of contrast medium, a surrounding area of high attenuation. The temporal lobe is most frequently involved, followed by the cerebellum. Distortion or displacement of the ventricles may be present if the lesion is large (Fig. 6.10). Serial CT scans allow the development of a lesion to be monitored and give warning of incipient rupture into a ventricle; or CT may be used to assess postoperative progress of the cavity. It is important to remember that up to 15% of brain abscesses of otitic origin are multiple and also interesting to record that, occasionally, an abscess which is clinically silent may be demonstrated (Fig. 6.11).

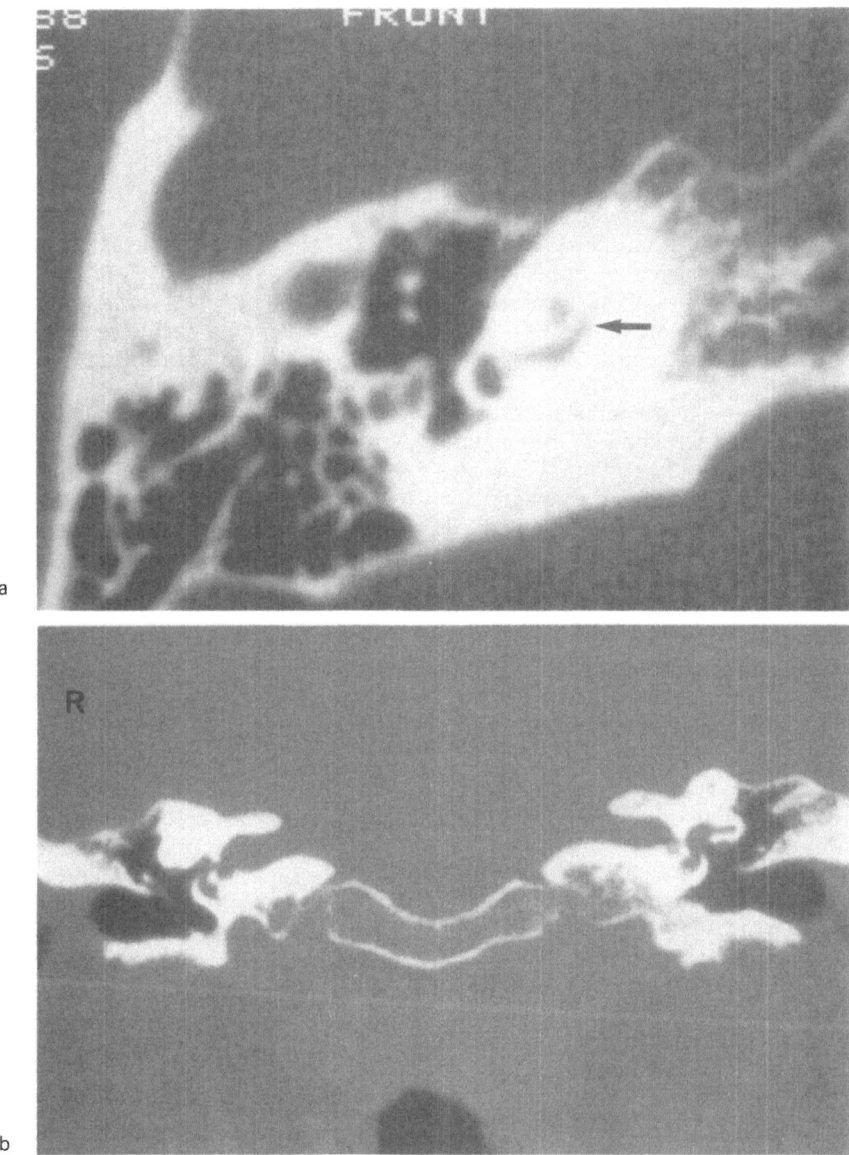

Fig. 6.9 a, b. Labyrinthitis ossificans. **a** base section CT shows the coils of the cochlea partially obliterated (*arrow*); **b** coronal CT shows obliterations of the semicircular canals on the right, although the vestibule is still evident.

Magnetic resonance will also give a good demonstration of a brain abscess, but is seldom necessary because of the accuracy of CT.

Extradural and subdural collections of pus will show a peripheral area of high attenuation rim after contrast enhancement. Not infrequently, however, extradural abscesses are very shallow and not well demonstrated by computerised tomography unless, by chance, a tomographic section passes through the centre of the pathological area. A negative CT scan should not be used by the surgeon as a contra-indication to complete mastoid exploration, if there is clinical suspicion of an extradural abscess.

The CT scan in otogenic intracranial hypertension is normal (O'Connor and Moffat 1978). The pathogenesis of this very rare condition is one of exclusion, but the clinical features of both brain abscess and tumour are similar and a CT scan is, therefore, mandatory. Early eradication of the ear disease is most important.

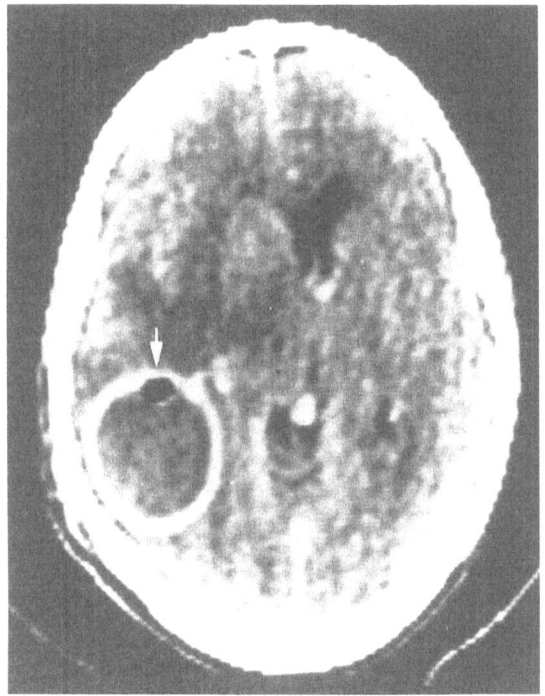
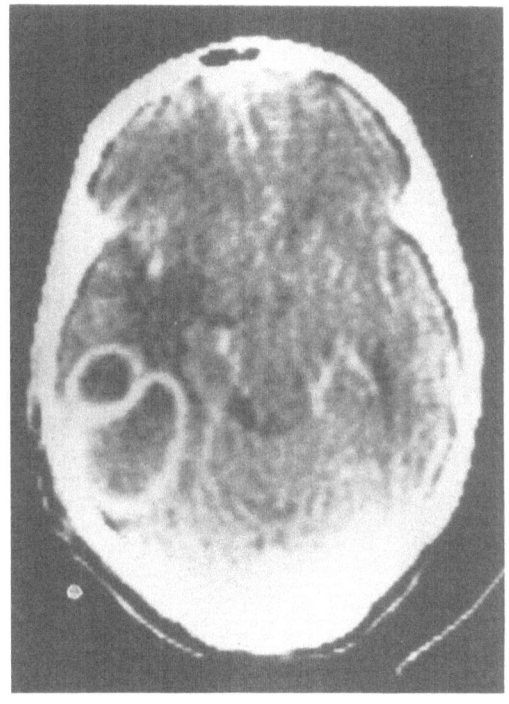

a   b

Fig. 6.10 a, b. Temporal lobe abscess of otogenic origin showing the rim of contrast enhancement and displacement and distortion of the ventricles. **a** Small gas bubble (*arrow*). **b** Bilocular component.

Malignant Otitis Externa

A rare and serious condition, malignant otitis externa is a particularly severe infection of the external auditory meatus occuring almost exclus

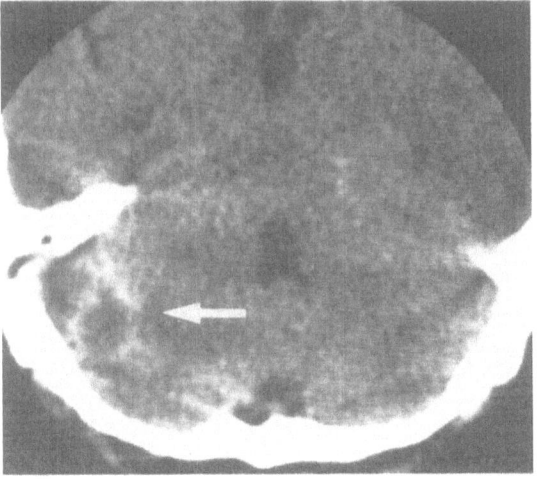

ively in elderly diabetics. The organism is usually *Pseudomonas aeruginosa* and although the disease usually starts insidiously with pain and discharge from the external meatus, there is subsequently centrifugal spread leading to high morbidity and mortality.

Once the infection penetrates the epithelium of the external canal, it involves the underlying cartilage and bone. From this point the infection may extend along one of several pathways. First it may spread anteriorly after destroying the bony external canal, to involve the temporomandibular joint. When this occurs, the mandibular condyle is displaced anteriorly and may be eroded by osteomyelitis (Fig. 6.12). Second, the infection may spread into the mastoid, either by direct posterior extension through the meatal wall or indirectly via the middle ear (Mendelson et al. 1983). Further extension medially affects the petrous apex and the

Fig. 6.11. A small abscess in the cerebellum, with ring enhancement. The patient was admitted with cholesteatomatous ear disease and, at exploration, was found to have an extradural abscess. The small cerebellar abscess was clinically silent and had disappeared on a repeat scan two weeks later.

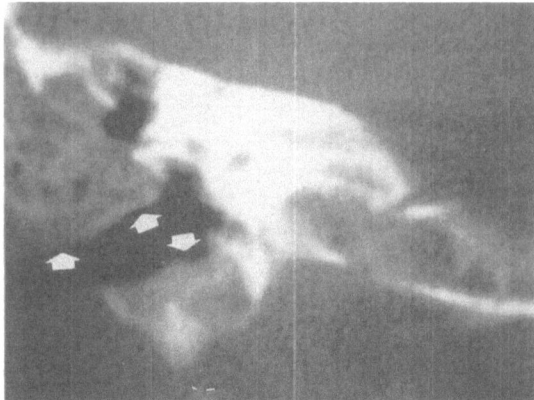

a

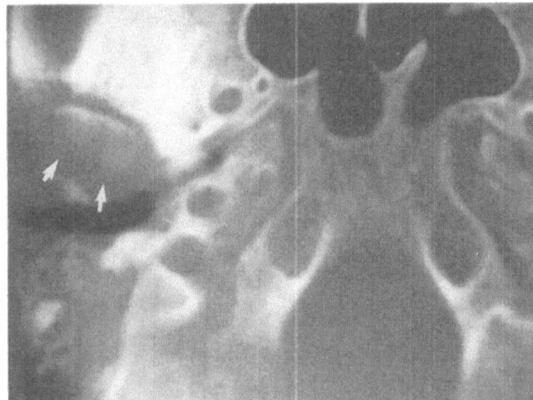

b

Fig. 6.12 a, b. Malignant otitis externa. a Coronal showing necrosis of bone in the roof and floor of the external meatus. b Base showing erosion of back of mandibular condyle (*arrows*).

skull base and the soft tissues in the infratemporal fossa to give parotid swelling and trismus. Intracranial complications are the ultimate phase and include meningitis and brain abscess. The VIIth cranial nerve is usually affected first, and indicates spread beyond the external auditory meatus. Spread inferiorly causes paralysis of the lower cranial nerves, and Mendez et al. (1979) found that when there was a unilateral facial palsy or a jugular foramen syndrome, bone destruction was always demonstrable (Fig. 6.13). Five of their nine cases had evidence of jugular fossa destruction, but only one had a jugular foramen syndrome. Retrograde jugular venography confirmed the presence of a high degree of venous obstruction at the jugular bulb.

Imaging Investigation

The extent of the bone destruction and associated soft tissue abnormalities are best shown by high-resolution CT (Fig. 6.13). Occasionally, lateral poly-

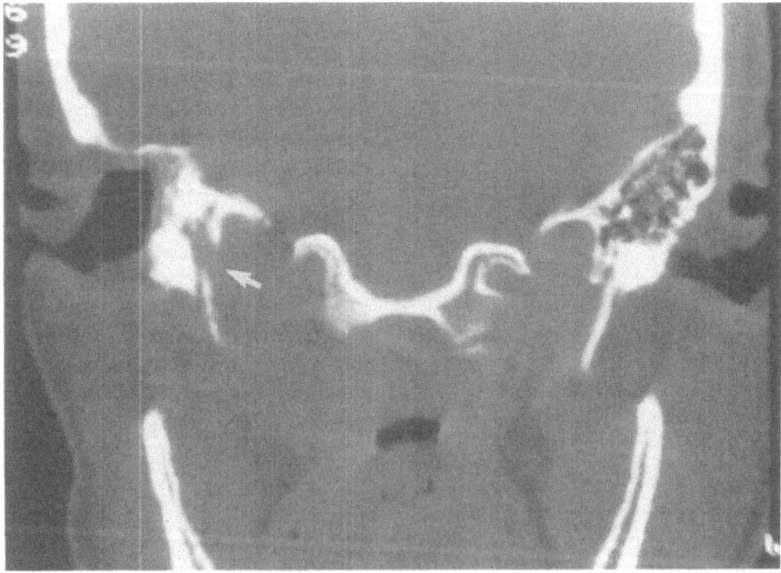

Fig. 6.13. Malignant otitis externa with facial palsy. The *arrow* shows the erosion crossing the descending facial canal and extending to the jugular fossa on this coronal section.

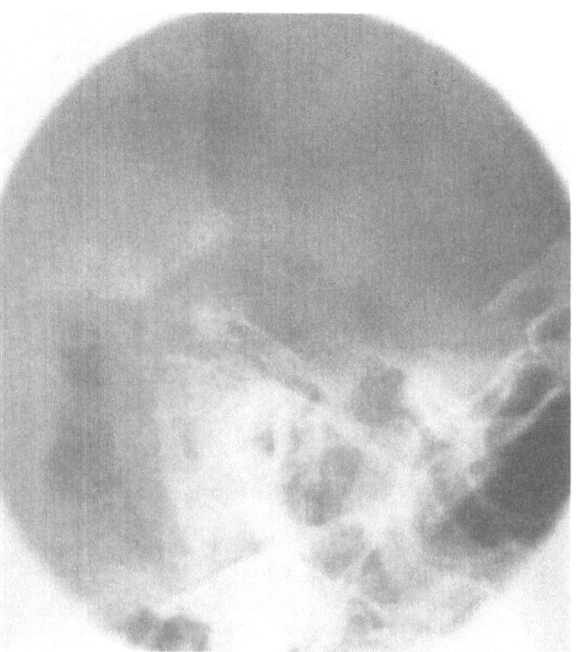

Fig. 6.14. Malignant otitis externa in a diabetic patient. Plain lateral views showing spreading erosion from the external auditory meatus into the squamous temporal bone.

tomography may help in showing destruction of the external meatus, and if the destruction is widespread it can be seen on plain films (Fig. 6.14).

Intracranial complications and extension into the infratemporal fossa are also well shown by CT, although the latter may only appear as obliteration of the soft tissue planes. However, although CT gives the best anatomical demonstration, it needs to be supported by isotope studies in the initial assessment and for monitoring the course of the disease (Mendelson et al. 1983). Tc-99m bone scanning has proved useful in the early detection of the disease. It is clear that this study may be positive well before radiographically detectable demineralisation occurs (Fig. 6.15).

Gallium-67 citrate scanning is the preferred technique for assessing resolution of infection. This radionuclide is bound by granulocytes and thus accumulation of this agent occurs only when the inflammatory process is active. The improvement or return to normal of this scan correlates well with the clinical inactivity of the infection.

References

Friedman I (1974) Pathology of the ear. Blackwell Scientific Publications, Oxford, p 56

Gower D, McGuire WF (1983) Intracranial complications of acute and chronic infectious ear disease: a problem still with us. Laryngoscope 93: 1028–1033

Hoffman RA, Brookler KH, Bergeron RT (1979) Radiologic diagnosis of labyrinthitis ossificans. Ann Atol 88: 253–257

Mendelson DS, Som PM, Mendelson MH et al. (1983) The role of computed tomography and radionucleides in evaluation of malignant otitis externa. Radiology 149: 745–749

Mendez G, Quencer RM, Donovan Post MJ, Stokes NA (1979) Malignant external otitis: a radiographic clinical correlation. Am J Roentgenol 132: 957–961

Michaels L (1987) Ear nose and throat histopathology. Springer-Verlag, Heidelberg, p 45

O'Connor AFF, Moffat DA (1978) Otogenic intracranial hypertension. J Laryngol Otol 92: 767–775

Samuel J, Fernandes CMC (1985) Otogenic complications with an intact tympanic membrane. 95: 1387–1390

de Slegte RGM, Kaiser MC, van der Baan S, Smit L (1988) Computed tomography diagnosis of septic sinus thrombosis and their complications. Neuroradiology 30: 160–165

Swartz JD (1986) Imaging of the temporal bone. Thieme Medical Publishers, New York, p 50

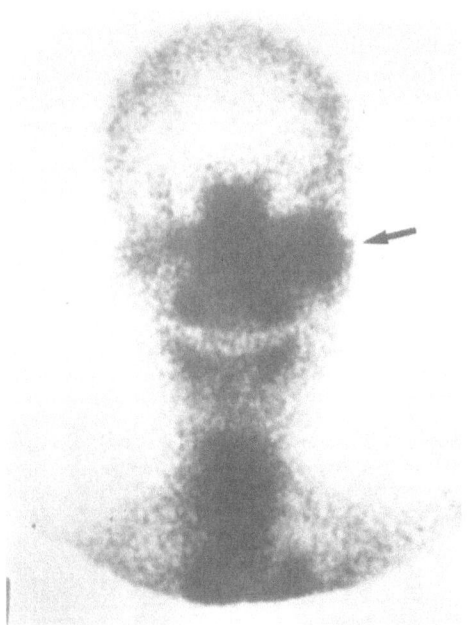

Fig. 6.15. TC-99m bone scan showing a "hot" area in the region of the right ear.

7 Cholesteatoma

The characteristic feature of cholesteatoma is the presence in the middle ear cleft of keratinising, stratified, squamous epithelium. This epithelial layer forms a matrix which constantly desquamates sheets of keratin. The accumulation of keratin in a confined space is called a cholesteatoma, although the term is a misnomer as the mass is not a neoplasm and bears no relation to cholesterol granuloma. The aetiology of this "skin-bag in the wrong place", also called an epidermoid or pearly tumour, is controversial and largely irrelevant to the present discussion. It is pertinent however to divided cholesteatomas into two groups:

1. Congenital cholesteatoma originating from ectodermal cell rests. This may arise in any of the cranial bones, the petrous temporal being the most commonly affected, or within the cranial cavity
2. Acquired cholesteatoma, associated with disorders of the middle ear cleft and involving the attic, with or without preceding infection

This categorisation is not always clearly defined or dependant on whether or not the eardrum is intact. A congenital cholesteatoma in the middle ear cavity can burst through the eardrum, or alternatively the eardrum may heal over an acquired cholesteatoma. Histologically the two types are indistinguishable.

Congenital Cholesteatoma

Peron and Schuknecht (1975) reviewed all previously reported cases of congenital cholesteatoma affecting the petrous temporal bone. There were 36 cases affecting the petrous apex, 11 affecting the middle ear and mastoid and 20 cases occurring in association with congenital atresia of the external auditory meatus, of which eight were medial to a bony atretic plate and three were medial to an atretic cartilagenous canal.

There have since been other series published of congenital cholesteatoma, both intracranial (Valavanis 1987) and intratemporal (Latack et al. 1985).

Cholesteatoma with Congenital Ear Deformity

The external auditory meatus develops by recannulation of a solid plug of ectodermal cells of the first branchial arch. This process begins at the medial end, with the membrane separating the primitive meatus from the tubotympanic recess developing into the eardrum. Failure of recannulation will result in congenital atresia of the external auditory meatus, potentially with the epidermis trapped medial to the atretic plate. This situation would seem to have all the potential for development of a cholesteatoma, especially if, as is often found at operation, a vestigial eardrum is present.

Congenital atresia of the external auditory meatus is not rare but, surprisingly, cholesteatoma beyond the atresia is most unusual. The authors found only four cases of cholesteatoma of retained squamous desquamation in 270 congenital deformities of the middle and external ear (Phelps et al. 1977). Of these four cases, two were due to stenosis of the external auditory meatus and two were true soft-tissue atresia. Unfortunately, because the cholesteatoma is radiologically indistinguishable from soft tissue, these could not have been diagnosed even in retrospect. Others have had similar experience with cholesteatoma in association with congenital ear malformations (Hoenk et al. 1969; Ombredanne and Porte 1962).

Primary Congenital Cholesteatoma

Congenital cholesteatoma can arise anywhere within the petrous temporal bone but may be conveniently classified into (a) cholesteatoma of the cerebello-pontine angle, (b) cholesteatoma arising deep within the petrous pyramid, (c) cholesteatoma arising in the jugular fossa region and (d) congenital cholesteatoma of the middle ear cleft. Classically, these lesions present in middle age with severe sensorineural deafness and facial spasm or weakness. This involvement of the facial nerve is a characteristic feature. Facial palsy is a most unusual presenting sign of acoustic neuroma, although it may be an early feature of glomus tumours.

In the Cerebello-pontine Angle

Cholesteatoma is the third most common tumour of the cerebello-pontine angle after acoustic neuroma

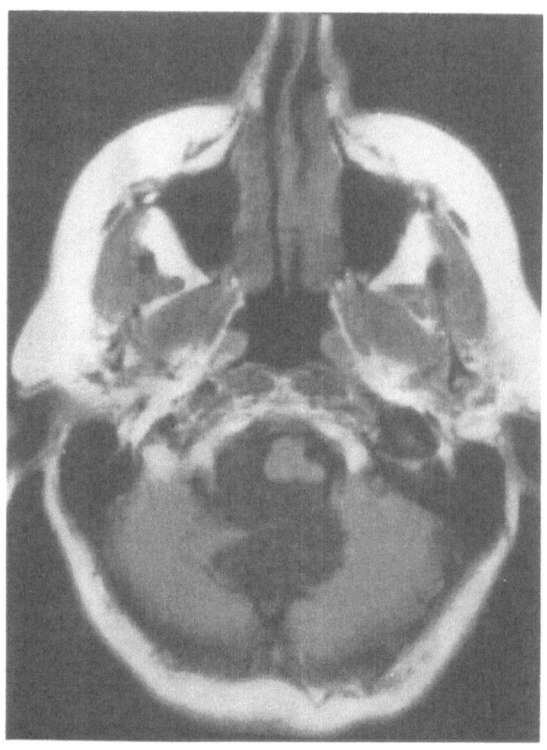

a

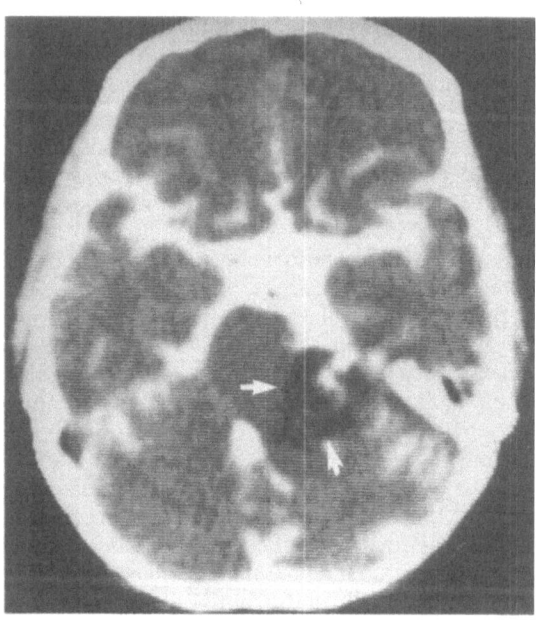

Fig. 7.1. Congenital cholesteatoma (epidermoid) of the cerebellopontine angle appears as a mass of low attenuation in this Niopam study of the posterior cranial fossa.

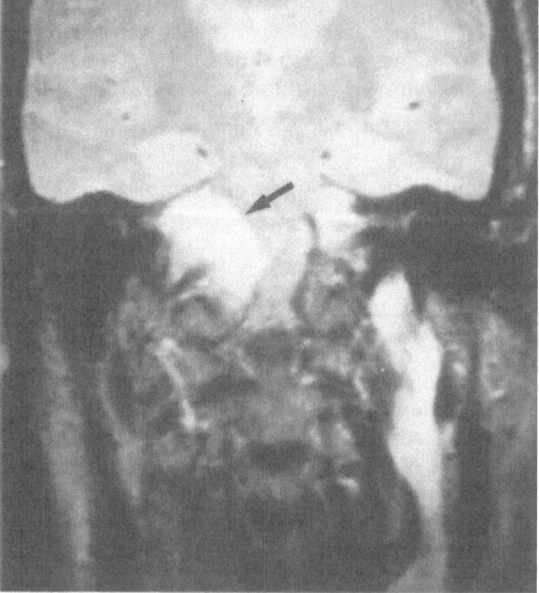

b

Fig. 7.2 a, b. A very extensive cholesteatoma (epidermoid) in the posterior cranial fossa wrapped around the brainstem. It has similar signal characteristics to CSF appearing rather dark on these T_1-weighted base sections (a: SE 560/26) at the level of the IAM (*arrow*) and below but brighter on the T_2-weighted coronal CT (b: SE 1500/80). The IR sagittal sections showed a low signal but a pronounced displacement and compression of the cerebellum and are shown in the next chapter as the patient presented with dizziness and balance problems.

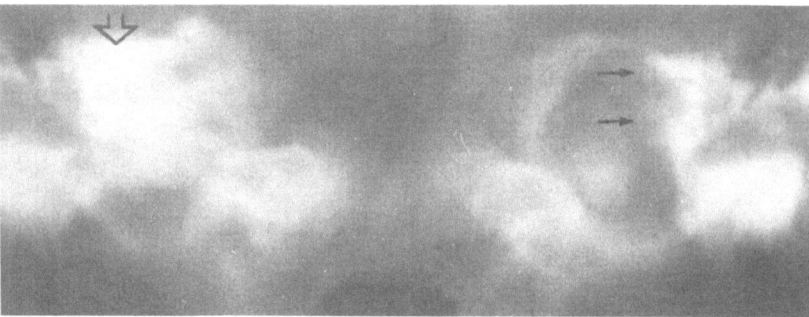

Fig. 7.3. Coronal section showing clearly defined erosion which has partially destroyed the cochlea (*arrows*). The *open arrow* indicates the cochlea on the normal side.

and meningioma. In a review of 208 patients presenting with cerebello-pontine angle syndrome, there were 122 acoustic neuromas and 10 cholesteatomas (Kendall and Symon 1977). Only one of the cholesteatomas was associated with erosion of the IAM, although another had eroded the petrous apex.

Computerised tomography will demonstrate a non-enhancing mass of low attenuation (Fig. 7.1). Although not a constant finding, negative Hounsfield unit values in the tumour on CT are virtually pathognomonic of a cholesteatoma (Kendall and Symon 1977). The epidermoids may occasionally show ring enhancement of the capsule surrounding the mass (Valavanis 1987). Their mass effect will be clearly shown by magnetic resonance but the signal intensity varies with the chemical composition. The higher the fat content, the higher the signal intensity on T_1-weighted images (Fig. 7.2).

In the Petrous Pyramid

A large erosion is usually evident on plain films in a patient with cholesteatoma of the pyramid or petrous apex. Tomograms show a clearly defined "punched-out" area of bone destruction (Fig. 7.3). The clear-cut margins may be scalloped and the labyrinth is destroyed by a "steam roller" effect, although individual coils of the cochlea and the modiolus may be identified after invasion of the cochlea has taken place. There may be thinning and elevation of the superior petrous ridge. Computerised tomography will demonstrate a non-enhancing mass of low attenuation and a typical, smoothly outlined expansile appearance on the bone studies (Fig. 7.4).

Previously, it was thought that this characteristic appearance always indicated a cholesteatoma. However, recently, Lo et al. (1984) have reported 12 cases of cholesterol granuloma in the petrous apex in the short space of 3 years. These were confirmed surgically. The cystic lesions were filled with brownish fluid containing cholesterol crystals. In most cases there was pneumatisation into the petrous apex and these authors believe that obstruction to drainage of the air cells is most important in the development of these cholesterol granulomata, otherwise called Giant Cholesterol Cyst or Chocolate Cyst. Confusion in terminology probably accounts for the paucity of previous descriptions.

The lesions are characteristic on CT examination but indistinguishable from cholesteatoma. Magnetic resonance, on the other hand, can clearly distinguish the two types of pathology (Fig. 7.5). Cholesterol granulomas have a high signal intensity on both T_1- and T_2-weighted protocols (Amedee et al. 1987), probably due to the presence of fluid rich in cholesterol crystals in the cyst, or to the presence of free methaemoglobin within the cyst, formed from the break-down of red blood cells and acting as a paramagnetic contrast agent. For the space-occupying lesions of the petrous apex, a sound knowledge of the relevant anatomy and comparison with the CT scans is essential to avoid confusion with the strong signal from marrowfat on the T_1-weighted images. In this respect, fat suppression STIR sequences can be helpful (Fig. 7.5 d).

Cholesteatoma and cholesterol granuloma may be progressive or remain relatively dormant and the decision regarding the necessity for surgery depends on the clinical features and evidence of progressive expansion by CT. However, the importance of pre-operative differentiation concerns the type of surgery. Cholesteatoma ideally needs total excision; cholesterol granuloma will respond to an adequate

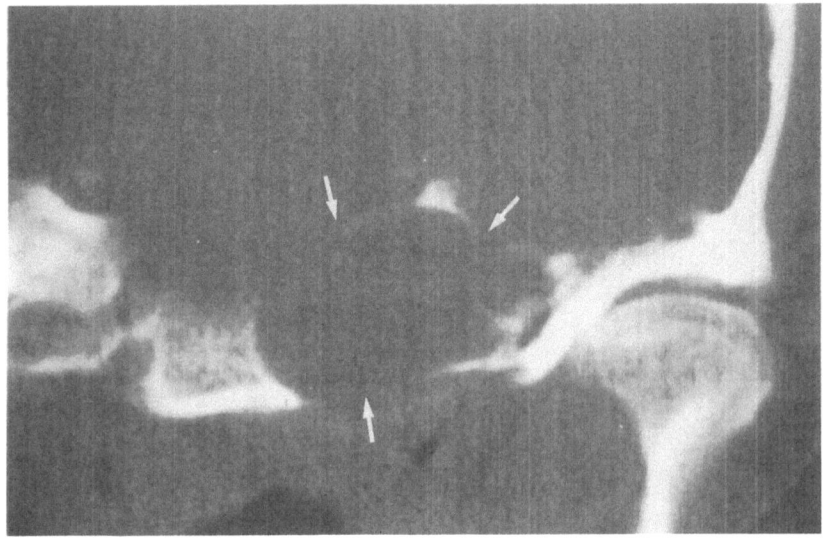

Fig. 7.4. Coronal section of a CT scan, showing the smooth expansile appearance of a cholesteatoma in the petrous apex (*arrow*).

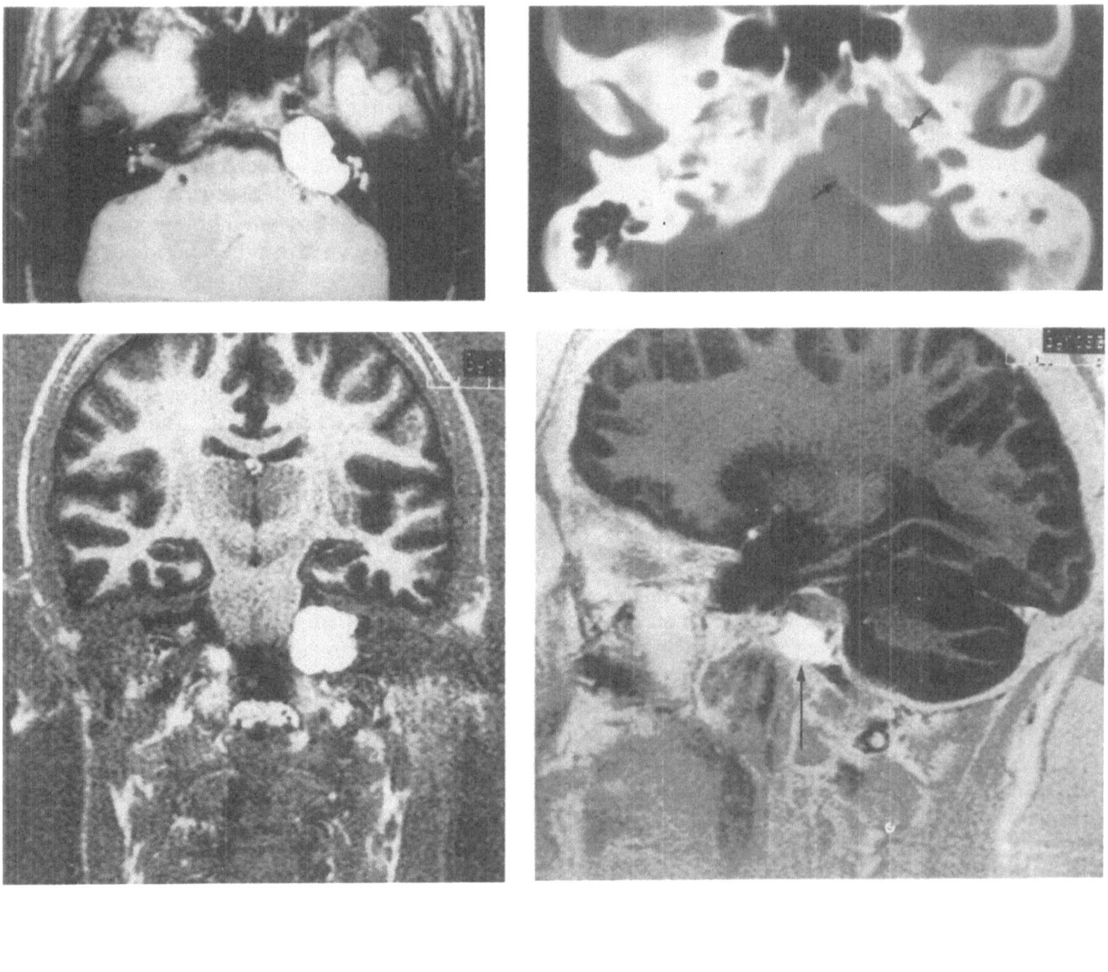

a

c

b

d

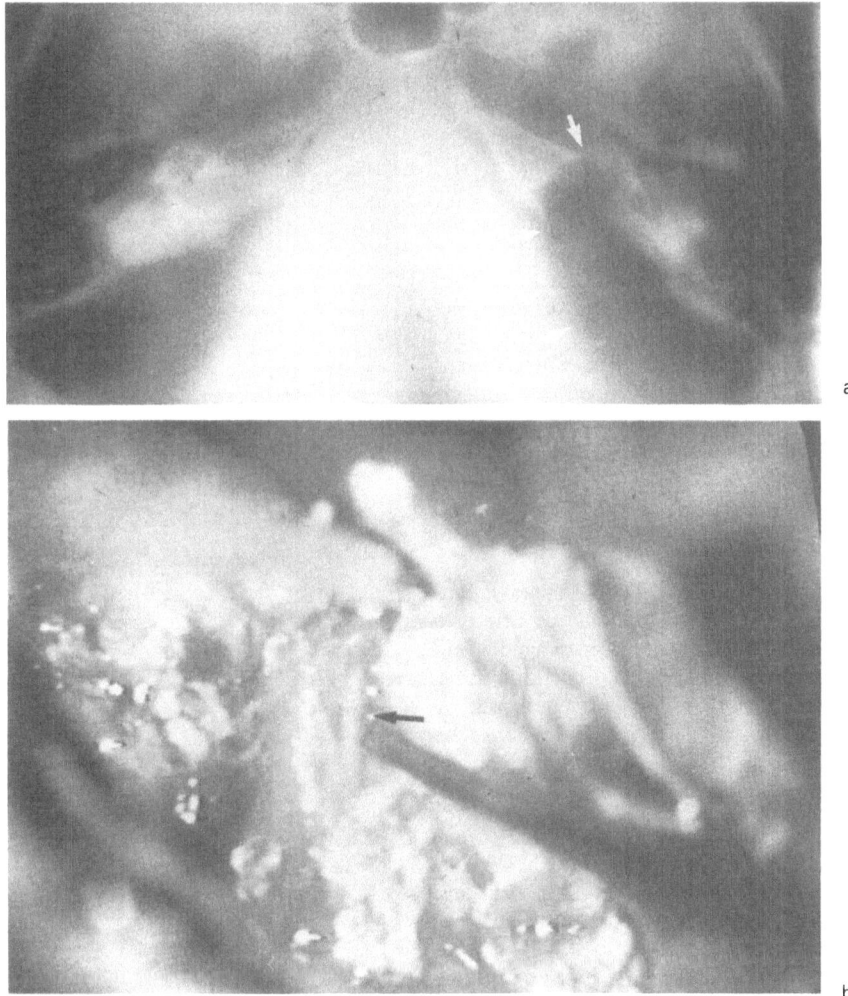

Fig. 7.6 a. Extensive cholesteatoma involving the jugular fossa, IAM and extending into the medial side of the cochlea (*arrow*). Note the smooth outline. b The picture taken at operation via a suboccipital approach shows the VIIth and VIIIth nerve bundle (*arrow*) surrounded by cholesteatoma.

drainage procedure. Given the problems of surgical access to the petrous apex, the value of examination by magnetic resonance to discriminate is paramount.

Fig. 7.5 a–d. Expansile lesion in the petrous pyramid giving a very strong signal on both, **a** T$_2$-weighted protocol (SE 2000/50); and, **b** on coronal inversion recovery sequence (IR 1400/400/80). Cholesterol granuloma. **c** shows the characteristic but non-specific expansile lesion shown on the base section; **d** the fat suppression sagittal STIR sequence shows high signal from the cholesterol granuloma only (*arrow*).

In the Jugular Fossa

A cholesteatoma arising in the region of the jugular fossa or skull base may mimic a glomus tumour, both radiologically and clinically. Although the destruction may be extensive (Fig. 7.6), it is usually less ragged than that caused by a glomus tumour. A CT scan should differentiate between the two lesions if intravenous contrast enhancement is used, but magnetic resonance or angiography will be decisive.

In the Middle Ear and Mastoid

It is uncertain what proportion of the much more common cholesteatomas arising in the attico-antral region have a congenital origin, but the percentage is probably small and they are, subsequently, indistinguishable from acquired cholesteatomas.

Valvassori (1974) considers that there are two criteria which distinguish a cholesteatoma of the middle ear cleft which has a congenital rather than an acquired origin. These are (i) an intact eardrum with no evidence of a perforation and (ii) an intact scutum or spur, with erosion of the attic walls higher up and not involving the site of attachment of the eardrum. This gives a scooped-out appearance to the outer attic wall. Caution should be used when ascribing a congenital origin to any cholesteatoma of the petrous temporal bone, as in many of these cases there is previous history of otitis media, and a perforation of the eardrum may heal with minimal scarring.

Sanna and Zini (1982) described 11 cases of congenital cholesteatoma of the middle ear out of a total of 429. Nine of these were children aged 3 and 10 years. No case had a history of infectious otitis, the eardrum was normal and all were confirmed by exploratory tympanotomy. These authors noted the following characteristics of congenital cholesteatoma in the middle ear:

1. They look like cysts
2. The surrounding mucosa is normal
3. They show no relation to the pars flaccida and occur mainly in the mesotympanum (Fig. 7.7). Localisation around the incudo-stapedial joint may occur, with a resultant conductive deafness through bone erosion. One case of ours was "hearing through pathology" and the post-surgical air–bone gap had to be improved by an ossiculoplasty

Acquired Cholesteatoma

The vast majority of cholesteatomas arise in the attic. From here they extend into other parts of the middle ear cleft, into the rest of the tympanic cavity and backwards into the mastoid antrum and air cells. There is associated erosion of the walls of the cleft. Typically, there is an attic perforation or a marginal perforation in the postero-superior aspect of the eardrum.

The most important single radiographic projection in the management of typical cholesteatoma

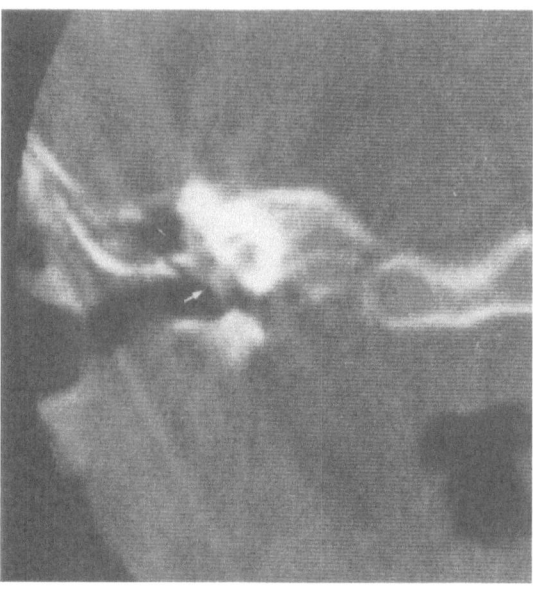

Fig. 7.7. Congenital cholesteatoma in the mesotympanum (*arrows*). Note the clear attic and normal outer attic wall.

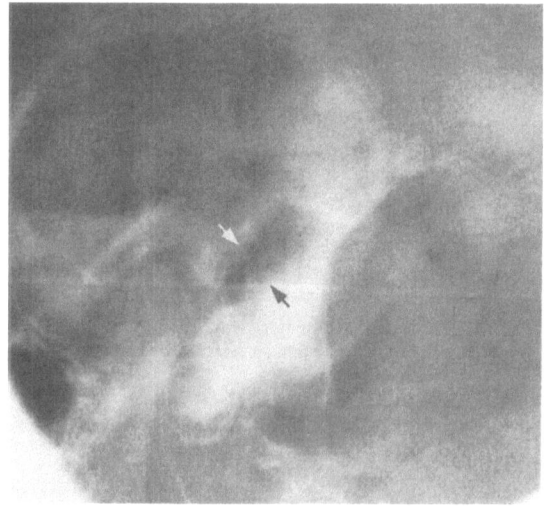

Fig. 7.8. Tilted lateral view, showing typical appearances of an attico-antral cholesteatoma which has eroded the "bridge" (*arrow*). There is a sclerotic unpneumatised mastoid.

is the lateral, with the incident beam tilted 20% caudally. This will show the extent of pneumatisation and the position of the sinus and dural plates. On this view, erosion of the attic and antrum may be seen. Loss of the normal "bridge" appearance of the superior aspect of the external auditory meatus indicates erosion of the outer attic wall (Fig. 7.8). The other mastoid projections will only

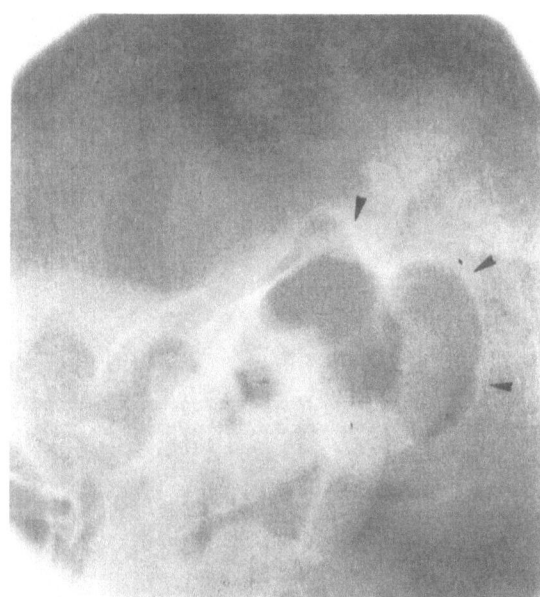

Fig. 7.9. Lateral view of large cholesteatoma.

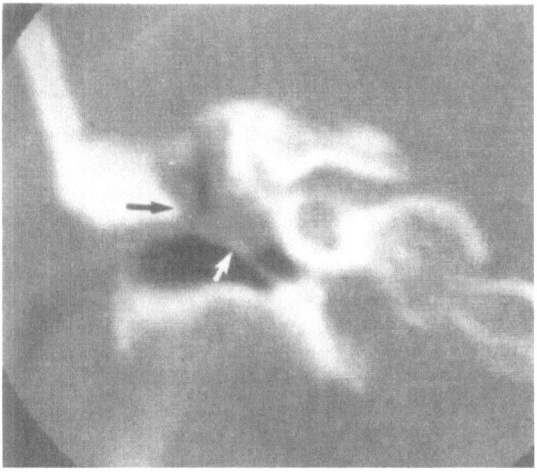

Fig. 7.10. Coronal CT section at the level of the cochlea. There is a small cholesteatoma at the upper middle ear cavity with blunting of the spur (*black arrow*). Only the handle of malleus remains of the ossicles (*white arrow*).

cholesteatoma may, if clearly defined, appear exactly like an operative cavity and details of any previous mastoid surgery must be obtained (Fig. 7.9).

Computerised tomography in the coronal plane is the optimum method for demonstrating small cholesteatomas in the attic and antrum and is based on the detection of bone erosion and soft-tissue changes in the middle ear and mastoid. Of the two findings, only the first is reliable, since radiographic density of a cholesteatoma is the same as that of granulation tissue and other soft-tissue masses.

In the attic the following signs indicate the presence of a cholesteatoma:

1. Destruction of the lateral spur of bone formed by the junction of the lateral boundary of the attic and the roof of the external auditory canal (Fig. 7.10)
2. Bone destruction of the lateral attic wall
3. Destruction of the ossicles
4. Erosion of the medial attic wall. This is a less common sign but may lead to involvement in the facial canal or a labyrinthine fistula

Blurring or blunting of the normally sharp tip of the spur is often the earliest sign of the attico-antral cholesteatoma but also occurs in chronic otitis. Complete or partial destruction of the malleus and incus (Fig. 7.11) and sometimes displacement, medially or laterally, by the cholesteatoma, may be demonstrated, but the most usual finding is a slight downward displacement of the malleus (Fig. 7.12). Demonstration of this displacement and of the cholesteatoma as a clearly defined soft-tissue mass above the isthmus with an air-containing hypotympanicum are typical features of acquired cholesteatoma. The isthmus is the narrowest part of the middle ear cavity.

Cholesteatoma in the antrum is characterised by cavity formation. These cavities are smooth walled (Fig. 7.9). A cavity with irregular boundaries is usually due to chronic otitis with osteitis. It is important to differentiate a cavity due to a cholesteatoma from a normal mastoid antrum.

demonstrate large erosions. Pneumatisation is usually poor or absent and the mastoid is sclerotic, but cholesteatoma may be encountered, with minimal bone destruction, in an extensive air-cell system. The radiographs of such a case will show opaque air cells suggesting exudate and the extent of the cholesteatoma is usually a surprise finding at the operation. On the other hand, erosion due to

Cholesteatoma in Children

Clinically a more extensive and rapid growth in the middle ear and mastoid is characteristic of cholesteatoma in children and early diagnosis is rare. In a series of 117 operated cases, Jahnke (1982) found 90% were in the age group 6–14 years. Most had

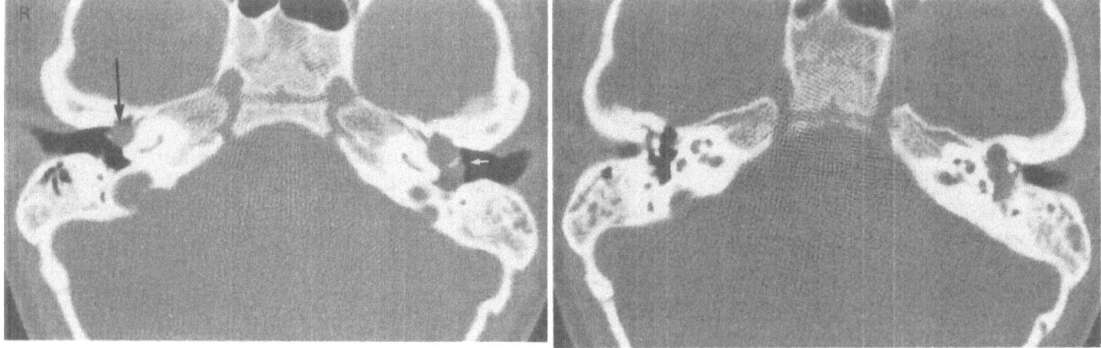

Fig. 7.11. Two base CT sections showing a small congenital cholesteatoma in the anterior hypotympanum on the right (*arrow*). The ossicles are unaffected. On the left is a larger cholesteatoma which has eroded the ossicles leaving only the malleus (*white arrow*).

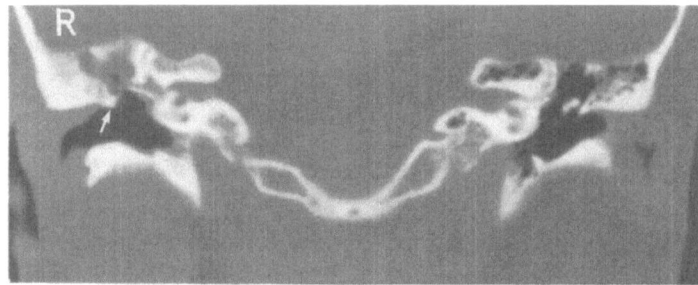

Fig. 7.12. Coronal CT section showing a cholesteatoma in the right attic. There is partial erosion of the malleus head (*arrow*).

purulent discharge for more than 1 year and more than 50% had an extensive air-cell system. The eardrum perforations were usually small and attic or postero-superior. This study showed a high incidence of ossicular erosion, but this was usually not extensive and most commonly involved the incudo-stapedial region. Hearing loss was usually not great. House and Sheehy (1980) reported 41 cases of cholesteatoma behind an intact eardrum, of whom 50% were under the age of 20 years. Complications were rare, and duration of disease related. Only one case had a labyrinthine fistula. Another series of 20 congenital cholesteatomas of the middle ear in children (Levenson et al. 1986) found two thirds to be manifested as antero-superior masses that seemed to arise from the region of the processus cochleariformis and could be removed by an extended anterior tympanotomy approach.

Our experience is broadly in agreement with the above. Most of our cases occupied the whole of the middle ear and well pneumatised mastoid but two cases discovered at an early stage by otoscopy and myringotomy were confined to the mesotympanum with a clear attic (Fig. 7.10). The possibility of congenital middle-ear cholesteatoma should therefore be considered whenever there is persistent, unexplained, unilateral hearing impairment.

Invasion of the Labyrinth by Cholesteatoma

The labyrinthine capsule is the hardest bone in the body and relatively avascular yet it is easily eroded by an adjacent cholesteatoma. The mechanism of erosion is uncertain and much discussed (Michaels 1988) but there appears to be always a thin layer of granulation tissue between the capsule of the cholesteatoma and the bone. Extensive erosion of the labyrinth will inevitably lead to a "dead ear" and this may be confirmed radiologically by the presence of air in the labyrinth.

This propensity for clear-cut erosion of the labyrinthine capsule is entirely different from the type of erosion caused by neoplasms such as chemodectomas or carcinomas. Such tumours infiltrate, affecting the periosteal bone first and eroding the labyrinth only at a late stage. Moreover, erosion of the capsule by a cholesteatoma exposing the membranous labyrinth is not necessarily followed by immediate loss of function. The lateral semicircular canal is the part of the labyrinth closest to the usual attic cholesteatoma and hence this is the part most often eroded. This gives rise to the well-known "fistula sign" whereby stimulation of a functioning but exposed membranous external canal by use of a Siegel's speculum causes intense vertigo. A positive fistula sign in the presence of cholesteatoma is therefore an indication for immediate surgical exploration to save the hearing. Nevertheless, imaging confirmation by CT may be helpful. Ideally, the erosion should be demonstrated in both base and coronal planes (Fig. 7.13).

Preservation of cochlear function in the labyrinth invaded by cholesteatoma, first described by Phelps in 1969, is now a well-recognised, though unusual, phenomenon. Bumsted et al. (1977) reviewed 14 cases described in the literature and added four more with extensive destruction of the bony and membranous labyrinth and loss of caloric function

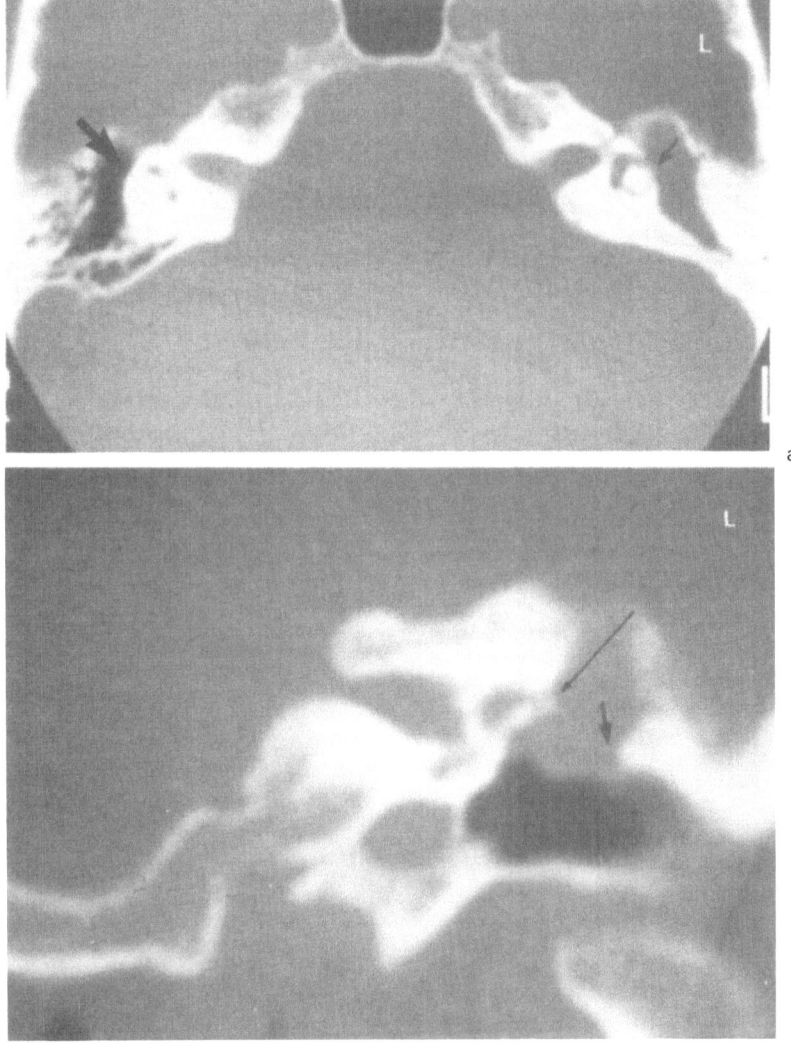

a

b

Fig. 7.13 a, b. Attic cholesteatoma eroding the lateral semicircular canal. **a** Base; **b** coronal views – the *small arrows* indicate erosion to the external semicircular canal and outer attic wall on the left. The *large arrow* points to the normal lateral semicircular canal on the other side.

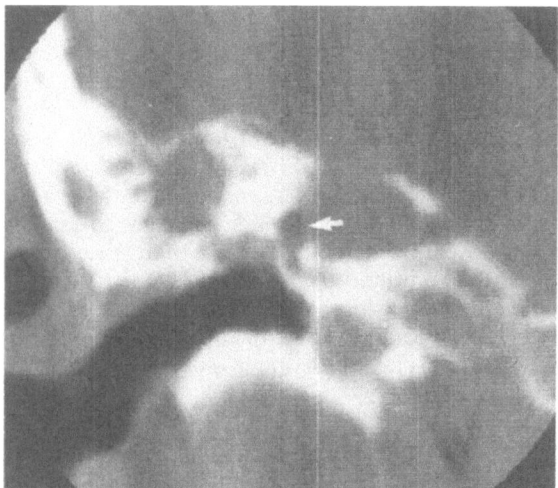

Fig. 7.14. Coronal CT at the level of the vestibule showing cholesteatoma in the attic extending into the petrous pyramid to erode the medial wall of the vestibule (*arrow*).

but with retention of hearing. Their cases are unique in that hearing was preserved after surgical removal of the disease in the inner ear itself in one instance.

We have since reported three cases of intra-cochlear cholesteatoma (Bagger-Sjoback and Phelps 1985). All three ears had some degree of auditory function before surgical treatment. All three patients presented with partial or total facial nerve palsy on the affected side. After surgery none of the patients has any hearing in the operated ear and the basal and possibly the middle coils were eroded. One case was of a man aged 37 years who developed a right facial weakness. He had had persistent otorrhoea until the age of 14 years, but none since. The eardrum was scarred but intact. An audiogram with full masking showed 80dB air conduction and 30dB bone conduction levels in the affected ear. Pluridirectional tomography and high resolution CT scan showed the typical appearances of an attico-antral cholesteatoma, which had extended anteriorly around the labyrinth and had invaded the medial aspect of the vestibule (Fig. 7.14) and the top of the cochlea (Fig. 7.15). This was confirmed at operation when cholesteatoma was found in the top of the cochlea.

Cerebrospinal otorrhoea is an uncommon complication of chronic suppurative otitis media, but when it does occur it is usually secondary to surgical treatment of a cholesteatoma. More rarely it may arise spontaneously from tissue destruction due to the disease itself and Walby (1988) describes a case with extensive cholesteatomatous erosion of the labyrinth and internal auditory meatus resulting in profuse CSF drainage over a long period. Previously reported cases of CSF leak caused by petromastoid cholesteatoma are described. The intracranial complications of cholesteatoma are mostly those of infection and have been described in the previous chapter.

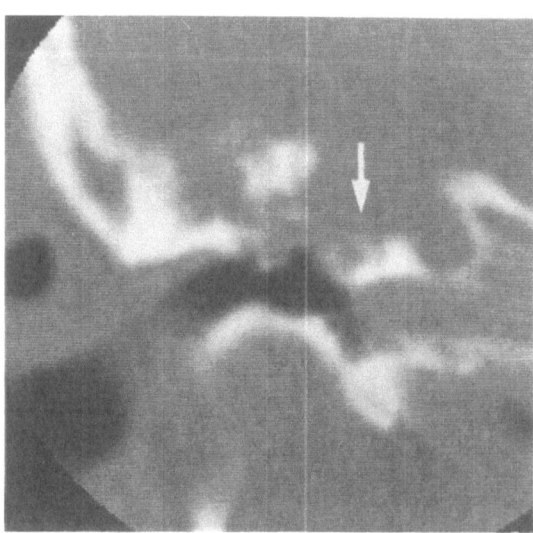

a

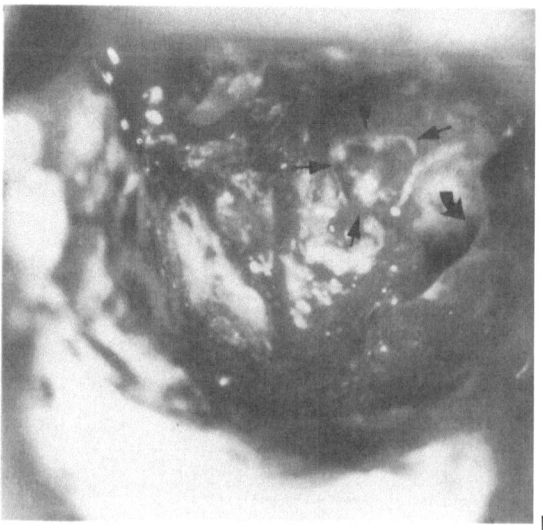

b

Fig. 7.15 a. Coronal CT of the same case at the level of the cochlea which has been eroded from above. The *arrow* points to the remains of the central bony spiral. Note also the lateral displacement of the malleus by the cholesteatoma in the attic. **b** Operative picture showing the rim of the bony cochlea (*small arrows*) after removal of the cholesteatoma. This view down the operating microscope, from above and behind, looks into the eroded cochlea. The *curved arrow* points down the Eustachian tube.

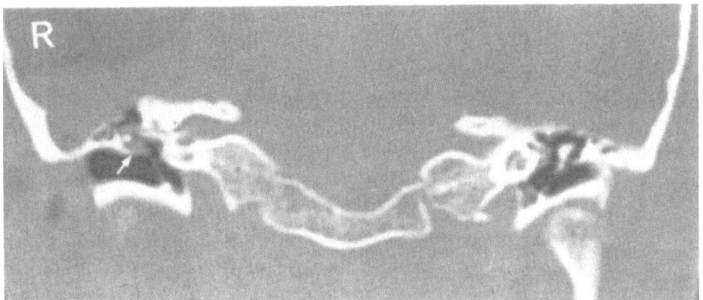

Fig. 7.16. Coronal CT showing a small attic cholesteatoma (*arrow*).

Investigation

How then should cholesteatoma be investigated by imaging? This will depend on whether the presence of cholesteatoma is known from the appearance of the eardrum or whether it is suspected from clinical features such as a persistent or progressive facial palsy. We do not believe there should be any "routine" regime of investigation and in a straightforward uncomplicated cholesteatoma of the middle ear cavity with attic perforation any extensive imaging constitutes a waste of money and unnecessary irradiation. However *plain views* may have limited value for pre-operative "mapping". These will show the general anatomy, the extent of pneumatisation, the state of the air cells and, maybe, bone erosion indicating unusual extension of the disease process. From the position of the sinus and dural plates, the surgeon will know how much "room" there is between the external auditory meatus and the middle ear fossa dura above and the lateral sinus, behind, when making his approach to the mastoid antrum. The potential hazard of a high jugular bulb will also be demonstrated. Only relatively gross bone erosion will be demonstrated (Fig. 7.8). Some surgeons require only a lateral view.

A cholesteatoma may not, however, always be apparent on inspection. It may also be associated with a central type of perforation, usually a feature of the safe tubotympanic type of disease. Often polyps or granulation tissue obscure both types of disease.

Although conservative treatment may be tried for a small attic pocket, surgery is nearly always necessary when squamous epithelium is demonstrated in the middle ear cavity. Wright and Benjamin (1968) have listed the following reasons for not relying on radiology:

1. Nearly all attic perforations are associated with cholesteatoma and most cholesteatomas are associated with attic perforations. The otologist, thereore, rarely requires the radiologist to make the diagnosis unless the eardrum is obscured

2. Operation must be exploratory as the extent of disease can only be assessed by surgery

3. Radiology will not exclude cholesteatoma and the dangers of leaving a cholesteatoma unexplored are such that it is usually right to operate on suspicion

Demonstration of the site of imminent complications, such as damage to the facial nerve or invasion of the labyrinth by the disease process, are sometimes given as reasons for an elaborate tomographic investigation. However, these signs only stress the necessity for immediate surgery. The extent of involvement of the facial nerve will be apparent following removal of the cholesteatoma matrix.

Computerised tomography is now the imaging investigation of choice and its ability to demonstrate fine bone detail and erosion along with the morphology of a soft tissue mass (Fig. 7.16) makes it superior to polytomography, which is now redundant for the investigation of cholesteatoma.

It must be stressed that demonstration of a small cholesteatoma in the middle ear cavity by CT depends on two things:

1. Bone erosion, particularly of the outer attic wall or scutum, and erosion and displacement of the ossicles.

2. The morphology of a soft tissue mass, typically in the attic and only extending down to the isthmus of the middle ear cavity (Fig. 7.17). However, if the middle ear and mastoid are filled with cholesteatoma without obvious bone erosion, this cannot be discriminated from serous fluid or anything else of soft tissue density such as granulation tissue or cholesterol granuloma. This is a particular problem in children.

For congenital cholesteatoma not involving the middle ear cavity, CT is of great value. The clear-cut margins of the lesions may indicate the likely diagnosis. The extent of a congenital cholesteatoma of the petrous pyramid can be accurately defined by computerised tomography. This information is essential to the surgeon, who must decide upon

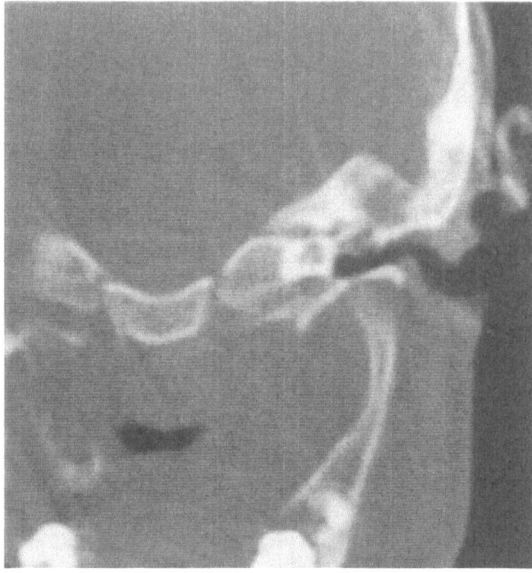

Fig. 7.17. A more extensive cholesteatoma reaching down to the isthmus.

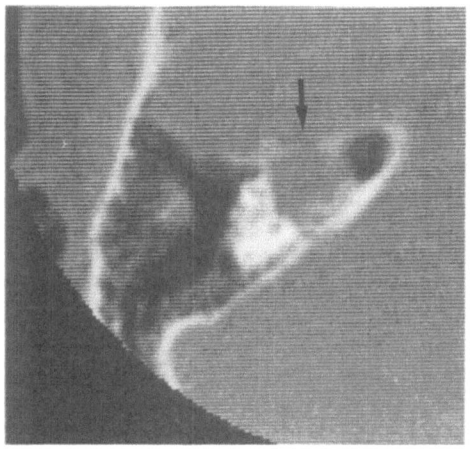

Fig. 7.18. Base CT of a well-pneumatised petrous pyramid. A congenital cholesteatoma lies medial to the superior and posterior semicircular canals. It had eroded into the IAM causing complete loss of function of the VIIth and VIIIth cranial nerves on this side.

which of several otological and neurosurgical routes to use to remove the lesion (Fig. 7.18).

Magnetic resonance will not demonstrate the bone erosion produced by a cholesteatoma or the situation in the petromastoid nearly as well as CT. Does MR have a role in tissue characterisation? The evidence so far is conflicting. Latack et al. (1985) found variable signal characteristics in three cholesteatomas studied by MR. Signal patterns similar to those of fatty tissue were found in six patients by Koenig et al. (1986). Such has not been our experience with patients with cholesteatoma. These were studied by MR as part of a research project to try to assess tissue characterisation and therefore the means of discriminating cholesteatoma from other soft tissue opacities in the petromastoid. A preliminary assessment has shown the following features:

1. Cholesteatoma is best shown by its bright signal on long spin echo T_2-weighted sequences (Fig. 7.19a). This is not as bright as fluid but differentiation can be difficult, especially as the mass usually appears non-homogeneous
2. The appearance of short spin echo T_1-weighted protocols is variable. Usually a grey appearance similar to CSF is found (Fig. 7.19b), but the signal may be stronger, presumably depending on a higher fat content. However we have not seen the characteristics of fat in our small series and the signal was different from the marrow fat in the petrous apex except for one case. Cholesteatoma usually appeared black on the few inversion recovery sequences used (Fig. 7.20).

Thus the MR appearances of cholesteatoma are usually characteristic but non-specific and difficult to differentiate from fluid such as serous otitis. Moreover, the signal from granulation tissue (Fig. 7.21) also seems variable and in one surgically proven case the characteristics described above seemed to be applicable to the granulation tissue in the middle ear rather than the cholesteatoma. Moreover, the other ear, where a fascial obliteration of the operative cavity had been undertaken previously, seemed identical to the cholesteatoma/granulation tissue mixture in the ear under investigation. This particular cholesteatoma most closely corresponded to marrow on the T_1- and T_2 protocols but the most noticeable feature was two small areas of intense signal corresponding to fluid in necrotic areas within the cholesteatoma mass (Fig. 7.22).

It would appear, therefore, that the role of MR for acquired cholesteatoma of the middle ear is going to be very limited, not only because of the restricted need for any imaging but because of the mixture of

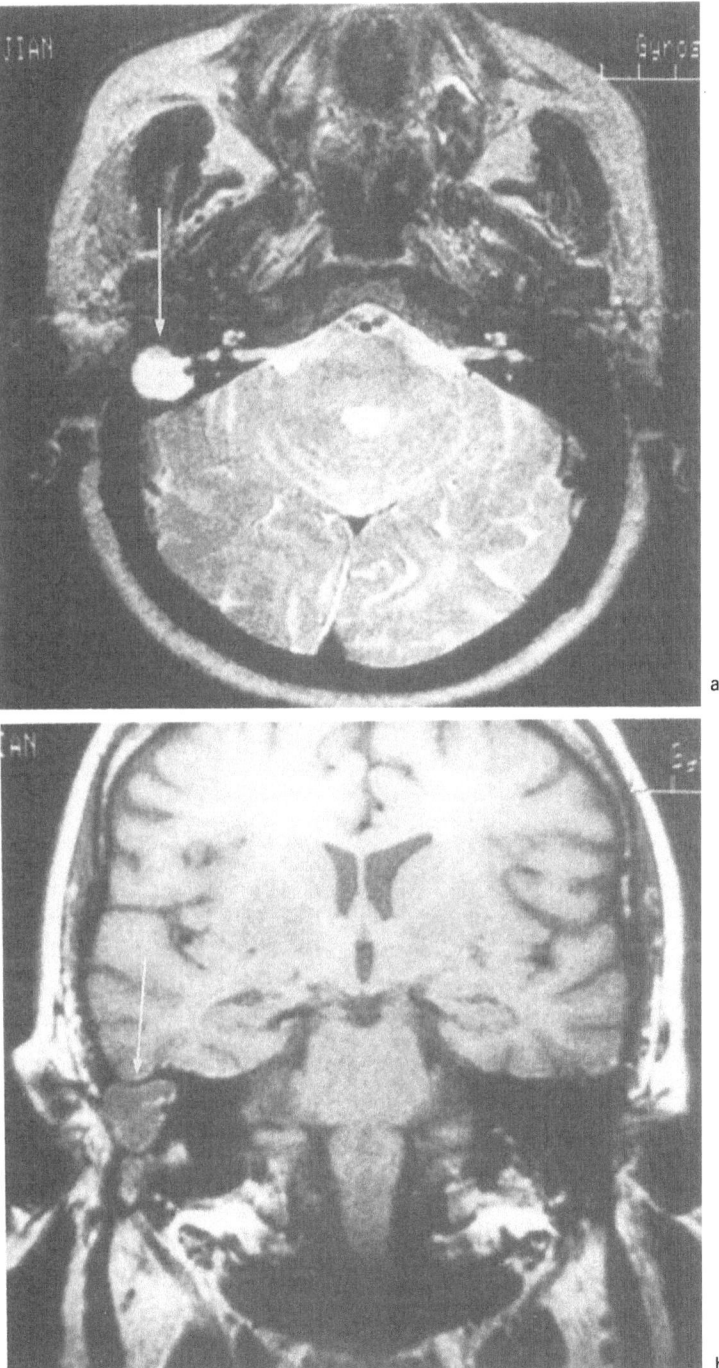

Fig. 7.19 a, b. Acquired cholesteatoma in a large cavity. **a** The T_2-weighted base section (SE 2000/100) shows a strong signal from the lesion (*arrow*), but of a similar intensity to CSF and the fluids of the labyrinth. **b** The T_1-weighted coronal section (SE 450/30) shows a non-homogeneous lesion, again with a similar intensity to CSF. This is very different from the signal characteristics of cholesterol granuloma (see Fig. 7.5).

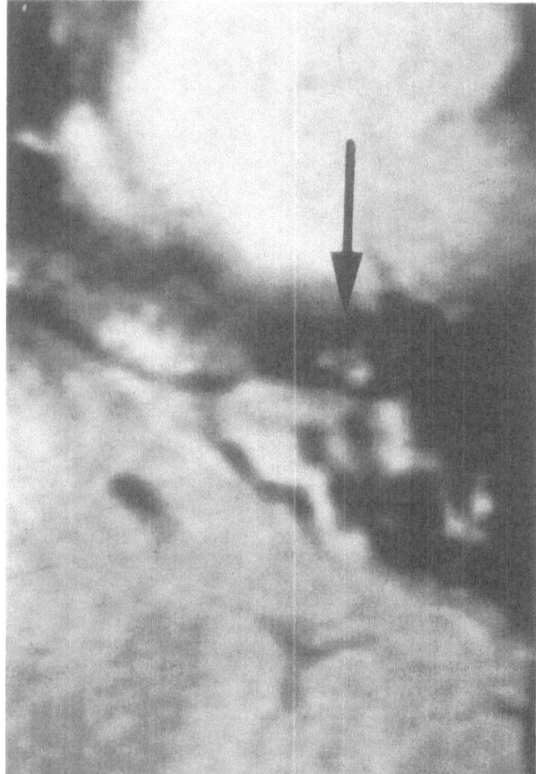

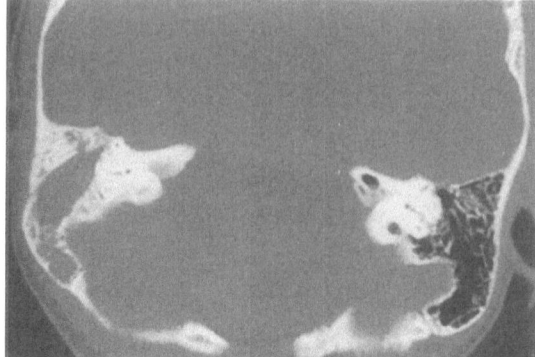

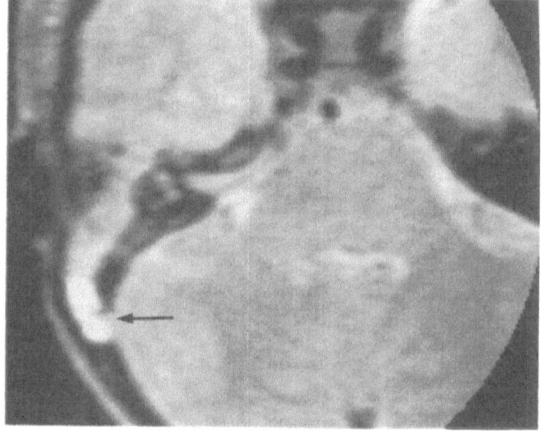

Fig. 7.21 a, b. Base CT (a) and T₁-weighted MRS (b) (SE 1500/80) of a large cholesteatoma in the mastoid. The cholesteatoma has similar signal intensity to brain but the granulation tissue behind it is much brighter (arrow). This information is not of any practical value to the surgeon.

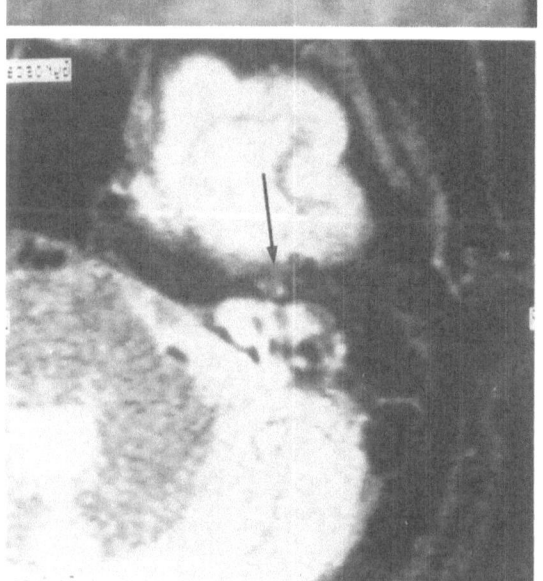

Fig. 7.20 a, b. Base section (a) proton density weighted (SE 2000/50) and (b) STIR (1400/30/190) of a congenital cholesteatoma behind the cochlea (arrow). This appears bright on both sequences. The STIR sequence eliminates the signal from the marrowfat in the petrous apex.

pathological entities usually defying analysis even at surgery. An expansile lesion of congenital origin in the petrous pyramid is a different matter. As described above, there are clear MR features to enable cholesteatoma to be distinguished from cholesterol granuloma and probably other fluids and mucocoeles and aneurysms. Magnetic resonance is therefore a most valuable adjunct to CT for lesions of the petrous apex (Amedee et al. 1987).

Imaging the Post-operative Ear

Computerised tomography may occasionally have a limited role in the assessment of a mastoid cavity. Previous surgery should always be recorded on the request card as an operative cavity can look just like

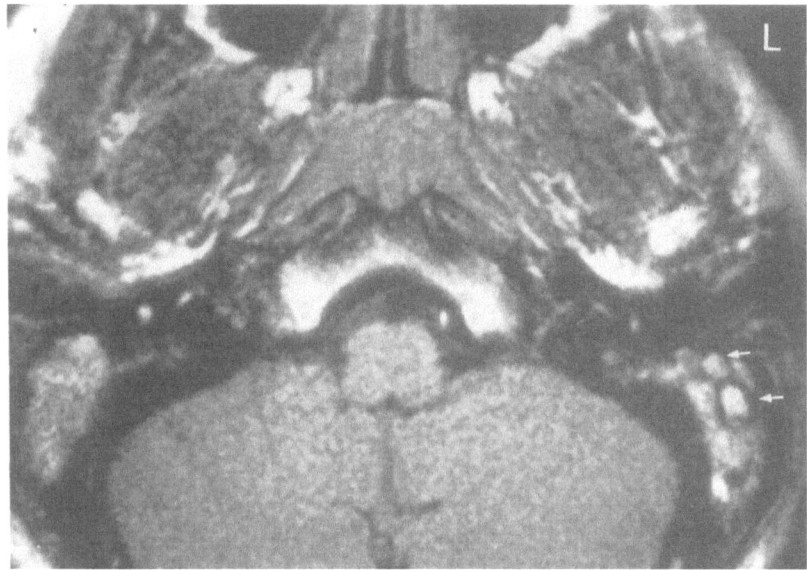

Fig. 7.22. The non-specific features of an acquired cholesteatoma on a T_1-weighted base MR section (SE 450/30). The cholesteatoma on the left has a similar appearance to the fascial pack inserted previously when a similar cholesteatoma was removed from the other ear. The two areas of brighter signal represent zones of necrosis in the cholesteatoma and gave a much stronger signal on the T_2-weighted sequences.

one produced by the cholesteatoma. Assessment to exclude residual disease depends on showing a cavity that is entirely air-containing with no evidence of further deep erosion (Fig. 7.23). An air-containing sinus tympani and facial recess are reassuring but, unfortunately, the usual fibrous tissue and thickened lining post-operatively cannot be differentiated from residual cholesteatoma, although a large soft tissue mass would seem to

confirm recurrent disease. Recurrences in the region of the genicular ganglion may produce a facial palsy and mimic a facial neuroma (Fig. 7.24; and see Chap. 8). Herniation of brain into the cavity to give a meningoencephalocoele is not a rare post operative feature and is difficult to exclude by CT (Fig. 7.25). Presumably magnetic resonance would be able to distinguish from residual cholesteatoma and this has been recorded (Mafee et al 1988).

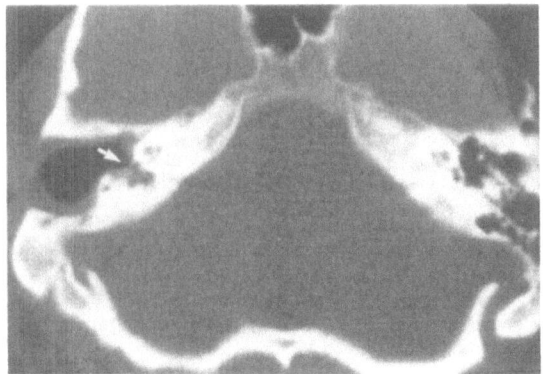

Fig. 7.23. Base CT at round window level. An operative cavity on the right but with residual or recurrent cholesteatoma extending medially through the labyrinth (*arrow*).

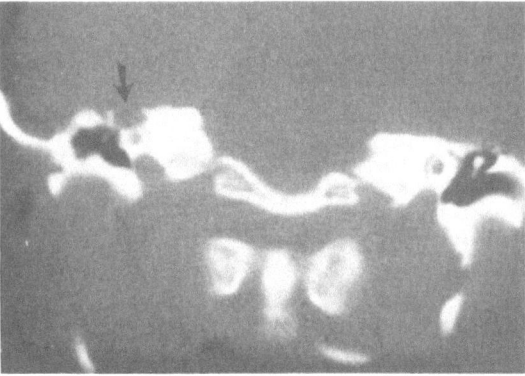

Fig. 7.24. Coronal section at the level of the cochlea showing a residual cholesteatoma causing a facial palsy by affecting the genicular ganglion (*arrow*). Compare with the normal sulcus for the genicular on the other side.

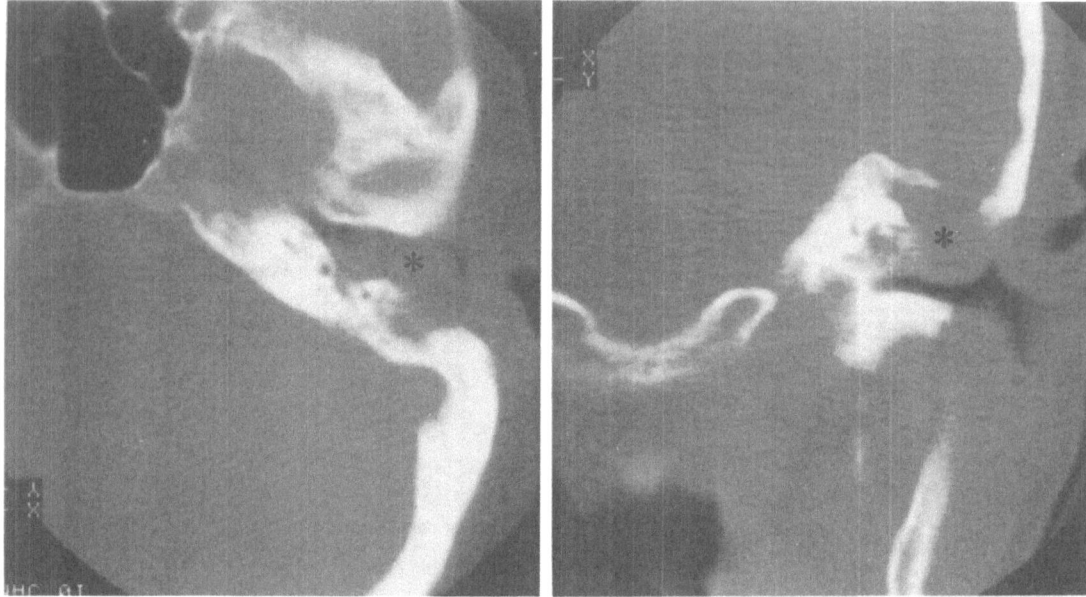

Fig. 7.25. A soft tissue mass in the upper aspect of a mastoid cavity (*asterisk*). This was a herniation of cerebral contents through the defect in the tegmen but only magnetic resonance would be able to differentiate from a recurrent cholesteatoma.

Closed technique tympanoplasty with intact canal wall means that direct observation of the mastoid cavity is not possible. CT has therefore been advocated as a useful procedure in the follow-up of such cases (Voorhees et al. 1983). However, closed technique is at present in disrepute because of the large number of recurrences and the necessity for second or even third look procedures when residual disease is found in a high percentage of patients, often as small solitary pearls (Smyth 1985). Careful consideration is, therefore, given to the suitability of open or closed procedures. Some authorities favour a closed technique in children (Wayoff et al. 1987) but with a routine planned "second look" procedure subsequently.

References

Amedee RG, Marks HW, Lyons GD (1987) Cholesterol granuloma of the petrous apex. Am J Otol 8: 48–55

Bagger-Sjoback D, Phelps PD (1985) Cholesteatoma with extension to the cochlea. Am J Otol 6: 338–343

Bumsted RM, Sade J, Dolan KD, McCabe BF (1977) Preservation of cochlear function after extensive labyrinthine destruction. Ann Otol Rhinol Laryngol 86: 131–138

Hoenk BE, McCabe BF, Anson BJ (1969) Cholesteatoma auris behind a bony atresia plate. Arch Otolaryngol 89: 470–478

House JW, Sheehy JL (1980) Cholesteatoma with intact tympanic membrane: a report of 41 cases. Laryngoscope 90: 70–76

Jahnke V (1982) Clinical pathological and therapeutic aspects of cholesteatoma in children. Kugler Publications, Amsterdam, p 25

Kendall P, Symon L (1977) Investigation of patients with cerebellopontine angle syndromes. Neuroradiology 13: 65–84

Koenig H, Lenz M, Sauter R (1986) Temporal bone region: High-resolution MR imaging using surface coils. Radiology 159: 191–194

Latack JT, Kartush JM, Kemicnk JL, Graham MD, Knake JE (1985) Epidermoidomas of the cerebellopontine angle and temporal bone: CT and MR aspects. Radiology 157: 361–366

Levenson MJ, Parisier SC, Chute P, Wenig S, Juarbe C (1986) A review of twenty congenital cholesteatoma of the middle ear in children. Otolaryngol Head Neck Surg 94: 560–567

Lo WWM, Solti-Bohman OG, Brackmann GE, Gruskin P (1984) Cholesterol granuloma of the petrous apex: CT diagnosis. Head Neck Radiol 153: 705–711

Mafee MF, Bevin BC, Applebaum EC, Campos M, James CF (1988) Cholesteatoma of the middle ear and mastoid in diagnostic imaging. Otolaryngol Clin North Am 2112: 265–293

Michaels L (1988) Origin of congenital cholesteatoma from a normally occurring epidermoid rest in the developing ear. Int J Paed Otorhinolaryngol 15: 51–65

Ombredanne M, Dorte L (1962) Cholesteatoma primitif de la caisse et aplasie mineuvre. Ann Otolaryngol 79: 427–430

Peron DL, Schuknecht H (1975) Congenital cholesteatoma and other anomalies. Arch Otolaryngol 101: 499–505

Phelps PD, Lloyd GAS, Sheldon PWE (1977) Congenital deformities of the middle ear and external ear. Br J Radiol 50: 714–727

Phelps PD, LLoyd GAS (1980) The radiology of cholesteatoma. Clin Radiol 31: 501–512

Sanna M, Zini (1982) Congenital cholesteatoma of the middle ear. In Cholesteatoma and Mastoid Surgery. Kugler Publications, Amsterdam, p 29

Smyth GDL (1985) Cholesteatoma surgery: The influence of the canal wall. Laryngoscope 95: 92–96

Valavanis A (1987) Clinical Imaging of the Cerebello-pontine angle. Springer Verlag, Berlin, p 77

Valvassori GE (1974) Benign tumours of the temporal bone. Radiol Clin North Am 12: 533–542

Voorhees RL, Johnson DW, Lufkin RB, Hanafee W, Canalis R (1983) High resolution CT scanning for detection of cholesteatoma and complications in the postoperative ear. Laryngoscope 93: 589–595

Walby AP (1988) Cerebrospinal otorrhoea – a temporal bone report. J Laryngol Otol 102: 399–402

Wayoff M, Charachon R, Roulleau P, Lacher G, Deguine Ch (1987) Surgical treatment of middle ear cholesteastoma. Advances in Oto-Rhino-Laryngology 36: 215–221

Wright JT, Benjamin B (1968) Cycloidal tomography of the temporal bone. J Coll Radiol Aust 12: 320–332

8 Tumours of the Middle Ear and Petrous Temporal Bone

Neoplasms may involve the middle ear, the mastoid and the temporal bone, metastatically or by extension from adjacent sites such as the postnasal space, external auditory meatus (EAM), parotid gland or even from structures within the cranial cavity. Nager (1967) has reported five forms of glioma which produced temporal bone erosion. Acoustic neuroma is the most common tumour to erode the temporal bone but it is most unusual for this neoplasm to cause any radiological abnormality of the temporal bone, other than expansion of the IAM. Tumours in the VIIIth nerve and arising in the IAM and region of the cerebello-pontine angle will be considered in Chapter 9.

Primary tumours of the middle ear region are extremely rare, the most common benign lesion being a glomus jugulare neoplasm and the most common malignant tumour, a squamous-cell carcinoma.

Benign Neoplasms

Osteoma

A compact osteoma appears as a well-defined, usually single, although occasionally lobulated, bony mass of high density. Cancellous osteomas are more rare and present as less dense and defined masses (Fig. 8.1). Denia et al. (1979) reviewed 53 reported cases of osteomas of the temporal bone, the majority of which arose from the mastoid or squama. We recently described three osteomas arising from different sites in the petrous pyramid (Beale and Phelps 1987). Osteomas occur in the following places:

1. External auditory canal, where they are asymptomatic unless they become large enough to cause obstruction, with consequent hearing loss or retention of cerumen and skin debris

2. Squama of the temporal bone, where they cause a hard bulge above and behind the pinna

3. Mastoid, where they are asymptomatic unless encroaching upon the facial nerve canal, when they cause paralysis

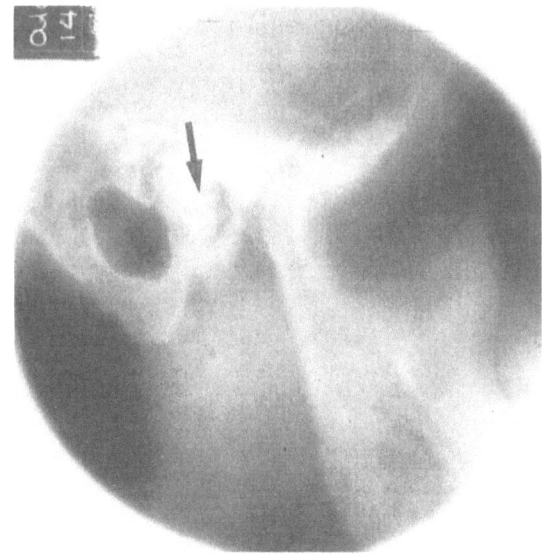

Fig. 8.1. Large osteoma (*arrow*) in the external auditory meatus.

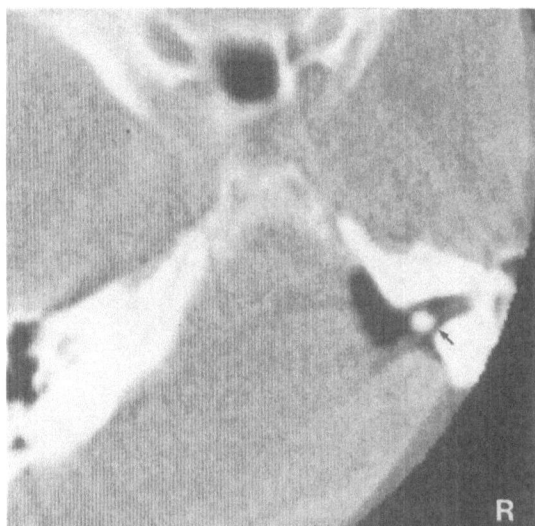

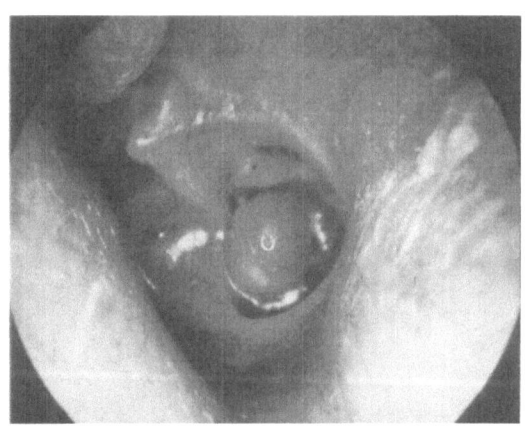

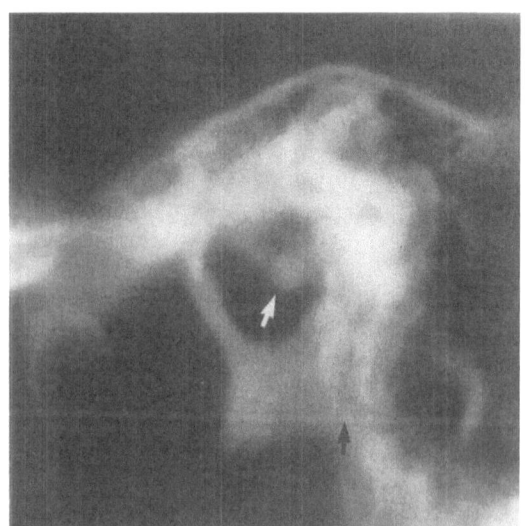

a

b

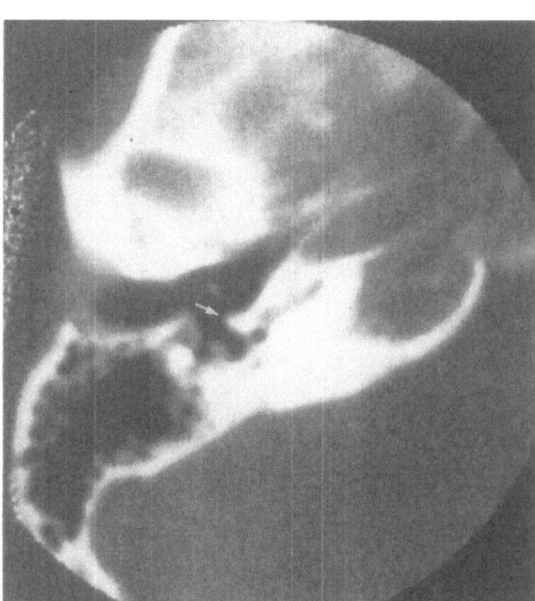

Fig. 8.2. Osteoma in the IAM surrounded by air on a base CT. Air meatogram study (from Beale and Phelps 1987).

Fig. 8.4. The same case as shown in Fig. 8.3. The situation of the osteoma on the promontory is shown clearly on the base CT scan.

4. Petrous pyramid, where they are not unusual in the region of the porus of the IAM (Fig. 8.2)
5. Middle ear, where they may impinge upon the ossicular chain, causing conductive hearing loss (Figs. 8.3, 8.4). We have also seen an apparently unique case of osteoma of the incus. The ossicle was ten times the normal size and the normal bone had been replaced completely by the tumour which was less dense radiographically (Fig. 8.5)

Exostoses in the EAM, usually multiple and bilateral, represent areas of hyperostosis from prolonged and repeated stimulation by cold water ("swim-

Fig. 8.3a, b. Osteoma on the promontory of the middle ear cavity. (a) Otoscopic appearances; (b) equivalent lateral tomographic section from Scott Brown's *Otolaryngology*, Vol. 3, 1986).

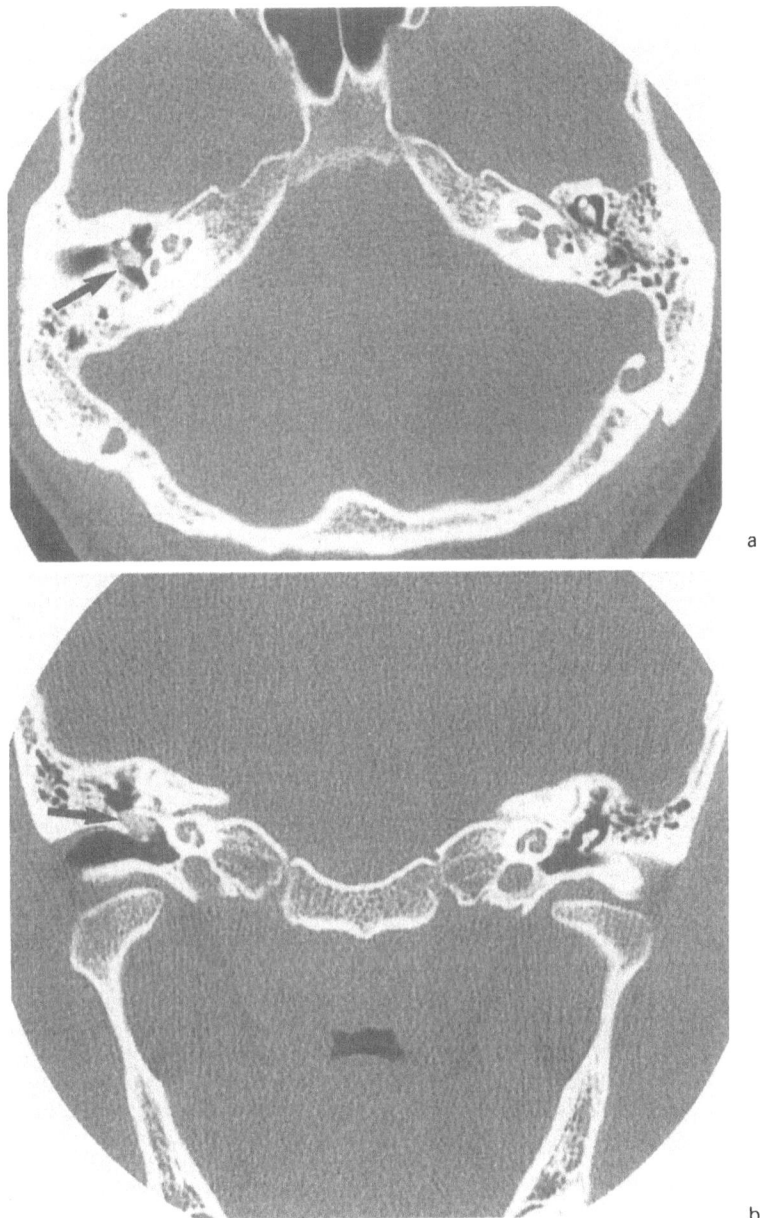

Fig. 8.5 a, b. Osteoma of the incus (*arrow*). Base (**a**) and coronal (**b**) CT.

mer's ear") (Fig. 8.6). If large enough, they cause obstruction of the canal.

Giant-cell Tumours

Giant-cell tumours or osteoclastomas of the skull, are rare. They are, on the whole, benign and rarely metastasise but they have a high rate of recurrence. A few cases of giant-cell tumour of the temporal bone have been reported (Livingstone 1974; Wolfowitz and Schmaman 1973). Radiographically, they are expansile tumours with poorly defined margins and they can arise anywhere within the temporal bone. We have seen an example of this tumour which presented radiologically with

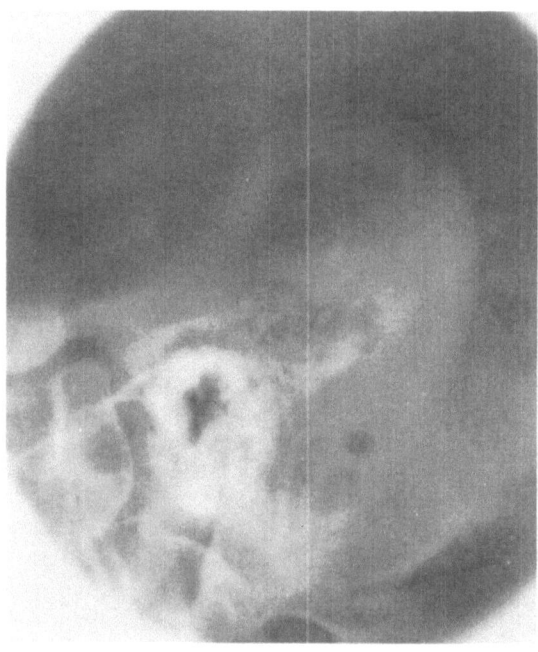

Fig. 8.6. Multicentric compact osteomas narrowing the external auditory meatus – "swimmers' ear".

enlargement of the jugular fossa (*see also* Moyes et al. 1970).

Chondroma

Cartilagenous tumours may arise from the skull base. Chondromas are slow-growing, avascular tumours which often show some patches of calcification (Phelps et al 1970) (Fig. 8.7). They may erode the petrous apex, the posterior surface of the temporal bone or the basisphenoid.

Chordoma

This rare, slowly growing destructive tumour is believed to be derived from notochordal remnants. These cranial tumours usually destroy the clivus, but may occur or extend more laterally to produce bone destruction in the petrous apex (Fig. 8.8), in the cerebello-pontine angle or jugular foramen (Valavanis et al. 1987). They appear as hyperdense masses with variable enhancement on CT but are best shown by MR which reveals clearly the extent of the tumour. There is usually a characteristic mixed signal without enhancement by Gadolinium.

Haemangioma

Areas of radiolucency with typical spoke-like trabeculations may be apparent but, usually, haemangioma, which is very rare in the temporal bone, appears as a poorly defined mass in the middle ear or EAM. Angiographically and even histologically it may be difficult to differentiate from glomus tympanicum. However, haemangiomas do seem to occur rarely along the course of the intratympanic facial nerve when they mimic neuromas (Curtin 1986). At least two haemangiomas arising from the chorda tympani have been reported (Dayal et al 1983) and recently Mazzoni et al. (1988) described two cases, one in the roof of the IAM and the other at the genicular ganglion.

Glomus tumours

Glomus tumours, sometimes called chemodectomas or paragangliomas, arise from small structures called glomus bodies. These have been found in the so-called normal location, adjacent to the dome of the jugular bulb, along the tympanic branch of the glossopharyngeal nerve (Jacobsen's nerve) where it extends through the bony floor of the middle ear, on the medial wall of the middle ear cavity and along the auricular branch of the vagus nerve (Arnold's nerve). They are similar, histologically, to carotid body and other chemoreceptor organs. Although the function of the carotid body in the neck is chemoreceptive, there are no indications that the glomus jugulare has this, or indeed any other, function (Rosenwasser 1974) and, therefore, the term "chemodectoma" for tumours arising from these structures would seem inappropriate.

The tumours are usually classified as glomus jugulare, vagale or tympanicum, depending on the site of origin. Glomus tympanicum may be entirely confined to the middle ear cavity but, usually, these tumors have reached such a size on presentation that it is difficult to determine exactly where in the base of the skull or upper part of the neck the tumour has arisen. In rare instances, glomus jugulare tumours may be associated with signs and symptoms of a phaeochromocytoma and any case with hypertension should be carefully investigated. Glomus tumours rarely metastasise but recurrence in a more malignant form may occur.

Their clinical presentation results from expansion into areas around the site of origin, and, in an area so complicated anatomically as the skull base, this results in a wide range of symptoms. Tumours arising in the middle ear have tinnitus and conductive deafness as their presenting problems,

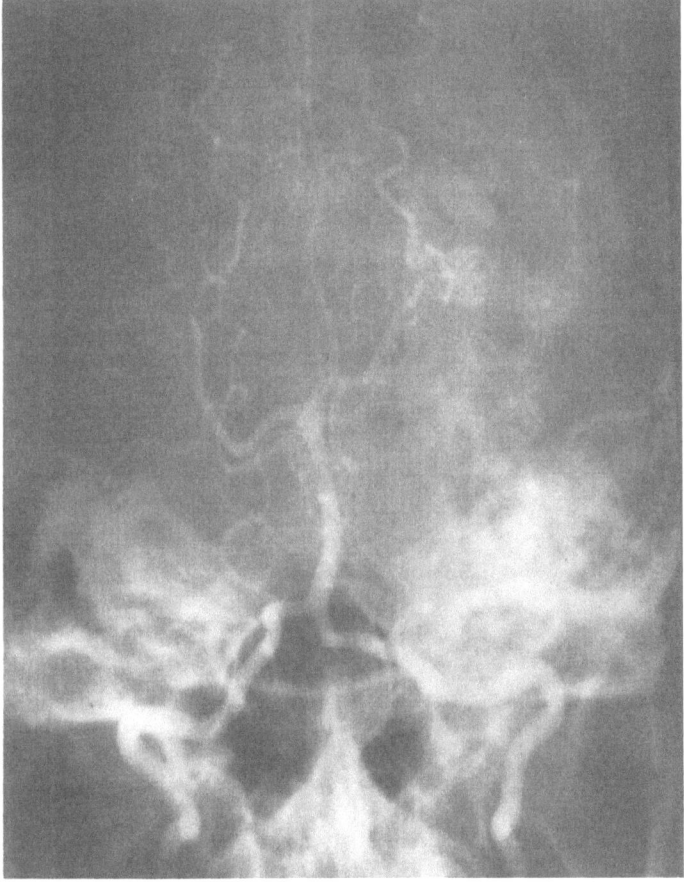

Fig. 8.7. A large chondroma arising from the superior surface of the petrous pyramid.

whilst those arising from the jugular bulb may present in the same way, with lower cranial nerve lesions, as a mass in the upper neck, or with symptoms and signs of intracranial extension. However, for jugulotympanic glomus tumours, the VIIth cranial nerve is the one most often affected initially. There may be bleeding from the ear or a protruding polyp in the EAM.

The treatment of glomus tumours is by radiotherapy or radical surgery, the latter, where technically feasible, now being recognised by most authorities as the preferred treatment, at least in the younger patient. Microsurgical techniques and cooperation between otologists, head and neck surgeons, and neurosurgeons, now permit the removal of even very large glomus tumours with limited morbidity. However, the surgical approach to any individual tumour is determined by its precise extent. Thus, a small glomus tympanicum may be removable via a limited transmeatal tympanotomy, whilst a large glomus jugulare may be manageable only by an extensive infra-temporal fossa approach, such as that described by Fisch (1982). Intermediate-sized tumours may be removed by a transmastoid approach.

If such surgery, or even the alternative of radiotherapy, is to be planned optimally, an accurate pretreatment assessment of the extent of the tumour is necessary, and, in particular, the roof of the jugular fossa, the segments of the carotid canal, the foramen lacerum, the IAM and the intracranial space. This has led to the classifications of jugulotympanic glomus tumours proposed by Glasscock et al (1978) and Fisch (1982). The assessment of these tumours is largely radiological and the most critical area from the surgeon's point of view is the dome of the jugular fossa, where anything more than the most minor involvement by tumour means

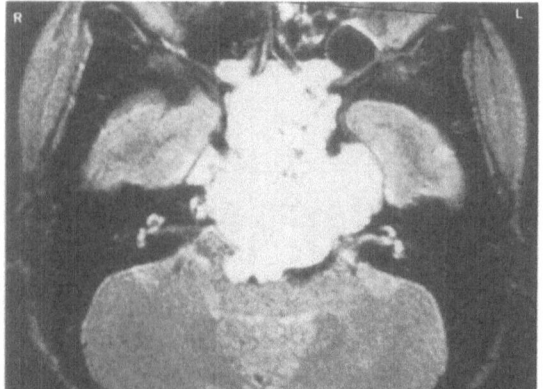

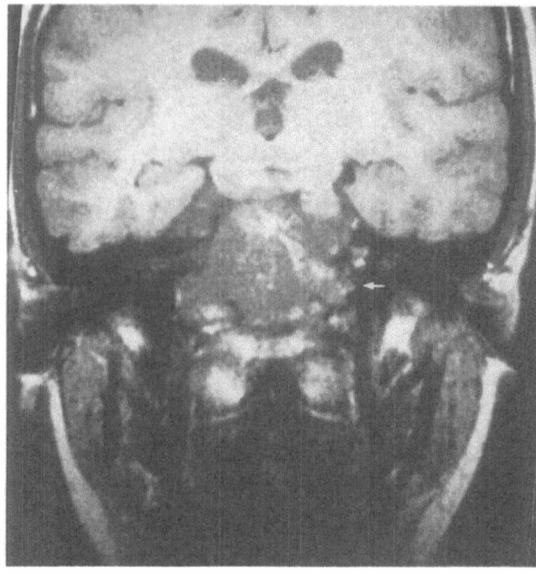

Fig. 8.8 a, b. A large chordoma of the clivus encroaching upon the left petrous apex. **(a)** Base proton-density-weighted MR scan (SE 2000/50); **(b)** Coronal T_1-weighted (SE 450/30). Note the non-homogeneous appearance of the tumour.

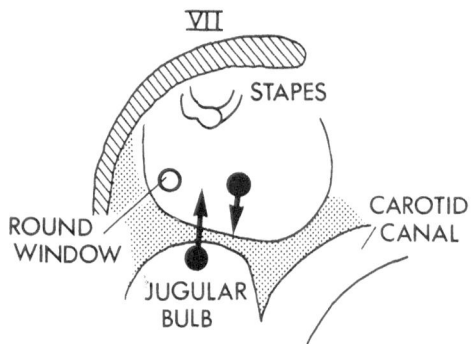

Fig. 8.9. Progression of small glomus tumours through the floor of the middle ear. (Phelps and Stansbie 1988).

that the more major infratemporal surgical approach is necessary, instead of the relatively minor tympano-mastoid approach. This, in essence, means that there is a need to distinguish between the larger glomus tympanicum, which has spread downwards to involve the jugular bulb, and the small glomus jugulare, which has spread upwards into the middle ear (Fig. 8.9). In the situation where the bony plate forming the dome of the jugular bulb is clearly visible, no problem arises but, unfortunately, the variable thickness, position and shape of this partition often makes it difficult to demonstrate reliably, even by sectional imaging. Partial volume averaging, soft tissue silhouetting, and the limits of the resolving power of the techniques inhibit the reliability of CT; in particular, in assessing whether or not a thin bony lamina is intact (Phelps and Stansbie 1988).

Radiological Investigation

Imaging of glomus tumours in and around the middle ear depends on showing the following pathological features:

1. Bone destruction
2. A soft tissue mass
3. Abnormal vascularity

The relevant investigations and their value in assessing the various aspects of the lesions are shown in Table 8.1.

Conventional Imaging. We believe that conventional imaging still has a role in the initial investigation. Ragged erosion and loss of the outline of cortical bone in the jugular fossa is the most important plain film sign of a glomus tumour, and this is well shown on a special jugular foramen view, either a modified submento-vertical with the baseline at 45°, or a modified occipito-mental, with the mouth open. It is important on these films not to confuse erosion with the usual asymmetry of the jugular foramina in any individual.

Glomus jugulare tumours located in the jugular bulb have ready access to various parts of the temporal bone and the foramina at the base of the skull, since these tumours spread along the lines of least resistance. Intracranial extension, therefore, can be along the carotid artery, through cranial nerve foramina, into the nasopharynx, intravascularly into the sigmoid sinus and inferior petrosal sinus, through the temporal bone air-cell system to the petrous apex, or retrofacially into the mastoid process.

Table 8.1 Signal strength from structures in the petrous temporal bone.

	T_1 Protocols	T_2 Protocols Short TE	Long TE	$T_1 + Gd$
1 Carotid artery		No signal = black		
2 Jugular vein		No signal = black		
3 Labyrinth fluids	+	+ +	+ +	−
4 CSF	−	+	+ +	−
5 Marrowfat	+ +	+	+	+ +
A Glomus tumour	+	+ +	+	+ +
B Serous otitis	+	+ +	+ +	+

TE, time to echo

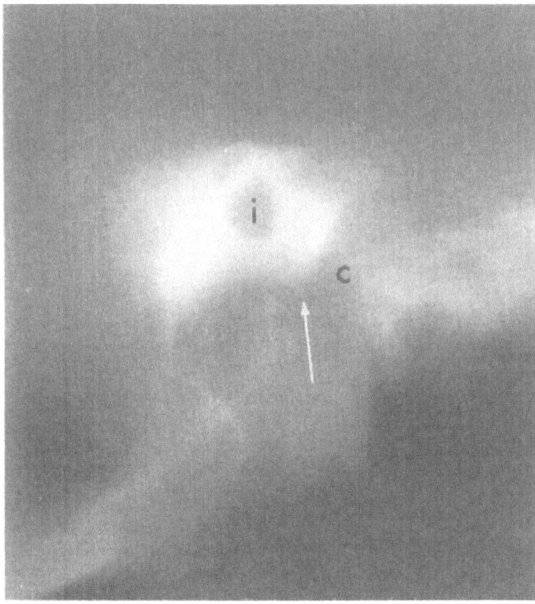

Fig. 8.10. Erosion of the jugular fossa and crest of bone anteriorly (arrow). Lateral tomogram. Compare with Fig. 8.1. I, IAM; C, carotid canal.

One of the first parts of the jugular fossa to be eroded may be the small crest of bone between the fossa posteriorly and the carotid canal anteriorly (Phelps and Lloyd 1986). This crest is best shown by lateral hypocycloidal tomography (Fig. 8.10). Lateral tomography may also show erosion of the thin bony plate of the dome of the jugular fossa, but in view of the variable thickness and contour of the plate, interpretation of minor changes is difficult.

Computerised Tomography. Computerised tomography is currently the investigation of choice for glomus tumours. Erosion of the jugular fossa is well shown (Fig. 8.11) as is the extension of the mass into the middle ear (Fig. 8.12). Contrast enhancement is mandatory to show intracranial spread, but only gross extension into the infra-temporal fossa

is clearly depicted (Fig. 8.13). We have not found contrast enhancement helpful for small lesions of the middle ear, but others have; even dynamic scanning has been recommended (Mafee 1983).

The greatest contribution of high resolution CT is the morphological demonstration of the soft-tissue mass in the middle ear and its position relative to patterns of bone destruction. Also, the demonstration of a clear air boundary between the tumour mass and the jugular bulb immediately identifies the lesion as a glomus tympanicum (Fig. 8.14). However, tissue characterisation of the glomus tumour is not possible, and a completely opaque middle ear cleft may be due to an extensive tumour, to fluid, or to granulation tissue associated with it. Coronal sections are usually considered to be the most sensitive for demonstrating glomus tympanicum masses as small as 3 mm (Larson et al, 1987), but most authorities use thin section base CT as well (Fig. 8.15).

Lateral high-resolution CT sections should demonstrate well the thin bony plate of the dome of the jugular fossa, as well as the jugulo-carotid crest. However, in our experience, hypocycloidal tomography is more satisfactory in this regard as the CT must be obtained either in a position which is difficult for the patient to maintain, or by reformatting from multiple base sections, which results in inferior bone detail, even discounting the considerably higher radiation dose involved.

One of our cases of a true glomus tympanicum which almost filled the middle ear was shown by base and coronal CT to have calcific densities within the tumour mass (Fig. 8.16). Histological examination showed extensive deposits of bone, lamellar and woven, which could represent overgrowths from the walls of the middle ear.

Calcification in a glomus tumour is extremely rare. Valavanis et al. (1987) noted microscopic calcification in several specimens, but only one case appears to have been reported previously of calcification apparent on imaging investigations and confirmed histologically (Moody et al. 1976). This large tumour had eroded the petrous pyramid, and

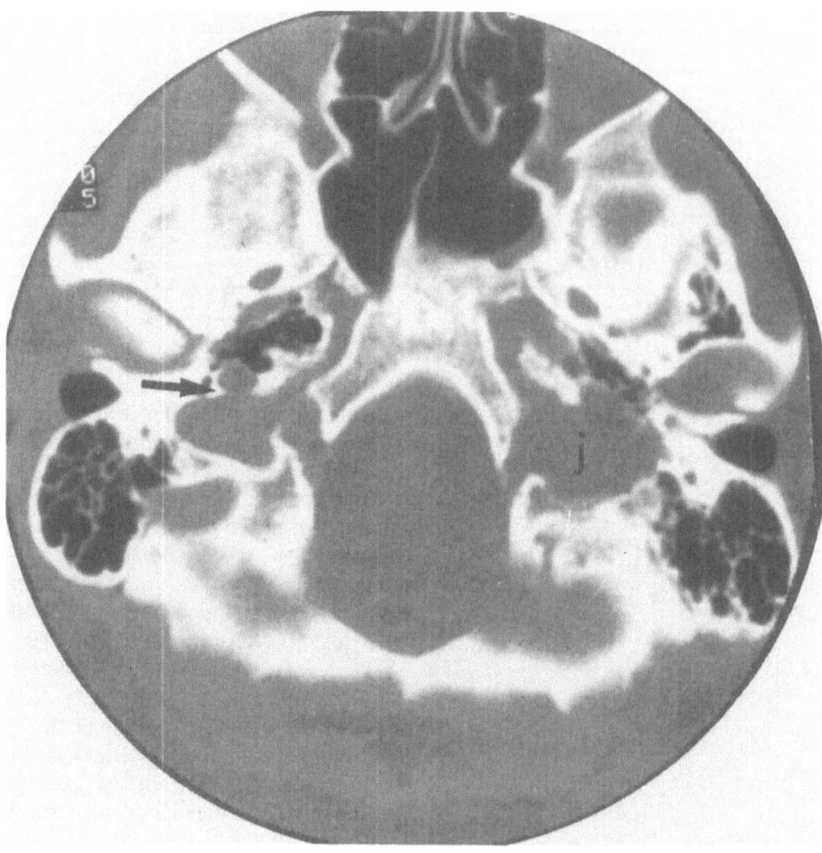

Fig. 8.11. Base CT showing erosion of the margins of the jugular fossa (*j*) by a glomus tumour. Compare with the normal fossa and intact crest of bone (*black arrow*).

extensive calcification had spread intracranially, although, at autopsy, the tumour was found to be extradural. Calcification is much commoner in primary adenocarcinomas of the temporal bone, which may mimic a glomus tumour, and Goebel et al. (1987) found intralesional calcification in the CT scans of three patients with adenocarcinoma, and considered this to be a point of distinction from glomus tumours.

Angiography. Transfemoral super-selective arteriographic catheterisation provides the definitive demonstration of the pathological circulation, blood supply and tumour blush. Common carotid injection is usually satisfactory for showing glomus tympanicum tumours (Larson et al. 1987). The stain of a small glomus tympanicum located on the promontory of the middle ear may be demonstrated with external carotid angiography (Latchaw 1986), but this is only necessary if embolisation is contemplated and is therefore not required for small

tumours confined to the middle ear. Moreover, there is a risk of not opacifying the ascending pharyngeal artery. Various views and projections have been described and Hesselink et al. (1981) recommended a trans-canalicular view, with the head rotated 20° contralaterally and titled 20° away from the side of the lesion. This view projects the middle ear cavity slightly anteriorly and superior to the jugular fossa. These authors, however, make the point that the inferior tympanic artery, a branch of the ascending pharyngeal branch of the external carotid, supplies both the middle ear and the jugular fossa. Therefore, extension of a tumour from the jugular fossa to the middle ear or vice versa cannot be determined from the arterial pedicle alone.

The angiographic appearance is nearly always characteristic (Fig. 8.17) with large vascular spaces, arterio-venous connections and dense homogeneous tumour stain. The blood supply is principally from the ascending pharyngeal artery, which is the first branch of the external carotid.

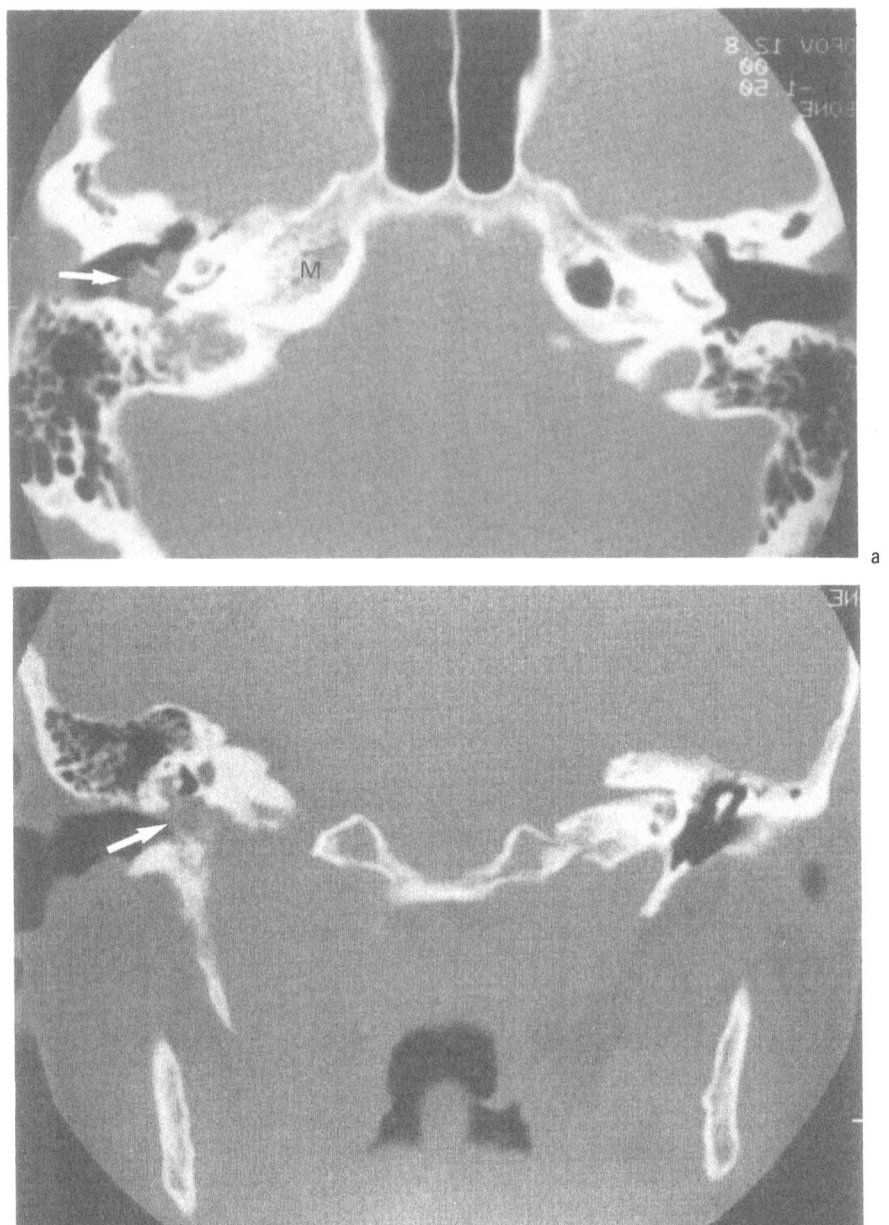

Fig. 8.12 a, b. Glomus jugulare extending into the middle ear (*arrow*). (a) Base; (b) coronal CT sections. Note that the tumour reaches to the round window and fills the facial recess but not the sinus tympani. *m*, marrowfat in the petrous apex.

Other collaterals, from both external and internal carotid systems (Fig. 8.18) develop as the tumour enlarges and eventually there may be an additional supply from the vertebral system (Fig. 8.19). The initial injection, therefore, should be into the common carotid artery, with subsequent selective catheterisation and vertebral injection as required. Subtraction films are necessary.

Recently, percutaneous catheter embolisation has been used for large tumours. Embolisation aims at blocking the vascular bed of the tumour, causing thrombosis and preventing the establishment of col-

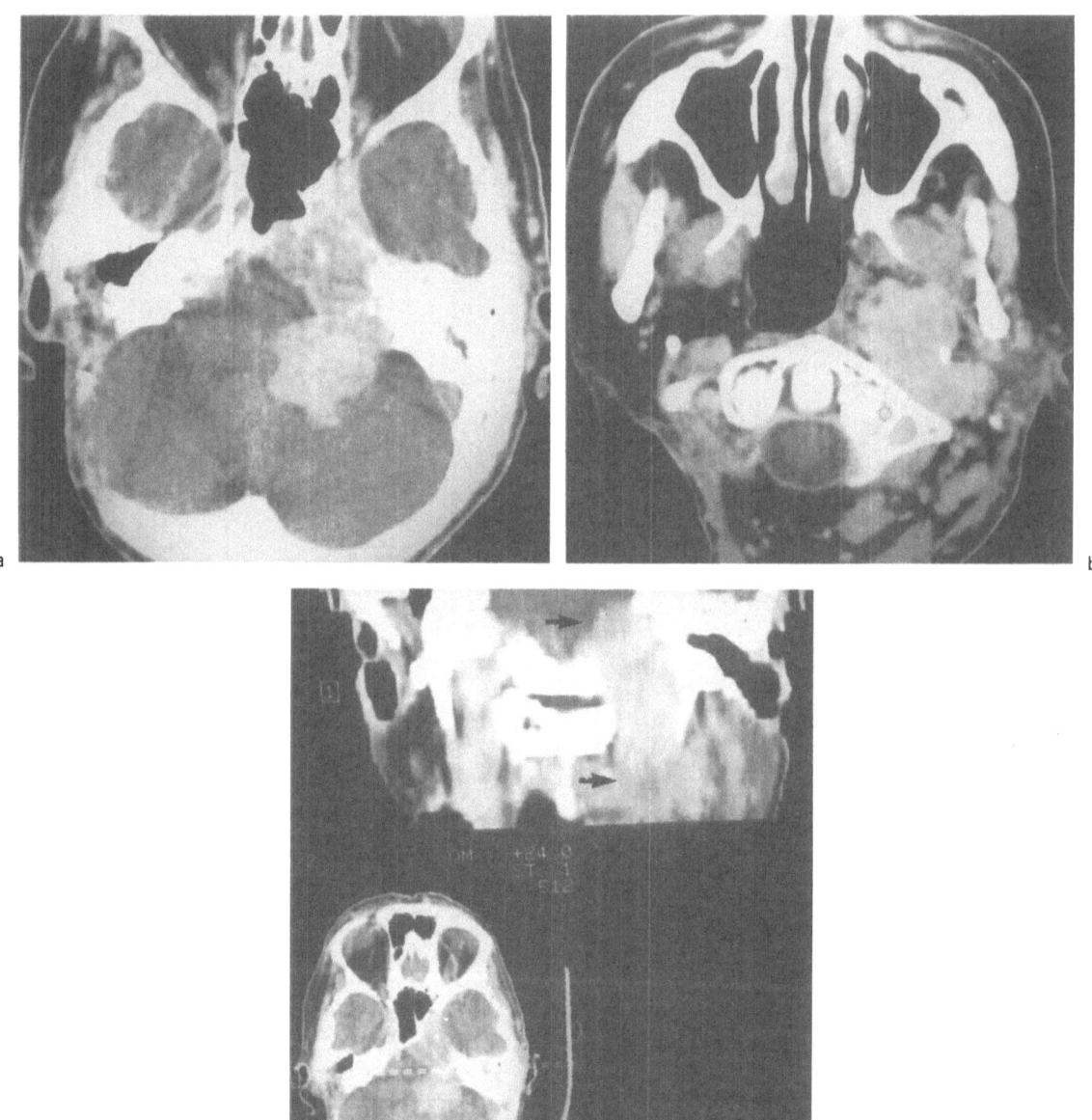

Fig. 8.13 a, b, c. Infusion CT with reformatting in the coronal plane. A large glomus jugulare extends intracranially and into the infratemporal fossa (*arrows*).

lateral channels as long as obliteration of the vascular bed is maintained. Selective angiography of the external carotid artery is an indispensable prerequisite to embolisation. The vessels feeding the tumour are identified. The catheter should be advanced as close as possible to the lesion before emboli are introduced. This will reduce the chances of reflux of emboli back into the carotid bifurcation

where stray emboli may enter the internal carotid artery. Embolisation can produce significant preoperative reduction in the blood supply to glomus jugulare tumours (Fig. 8.20).

Digital Vascular Imaging. Intravenous digital subtraction angiography can show the characteristic tumour blush and its relationship to the major

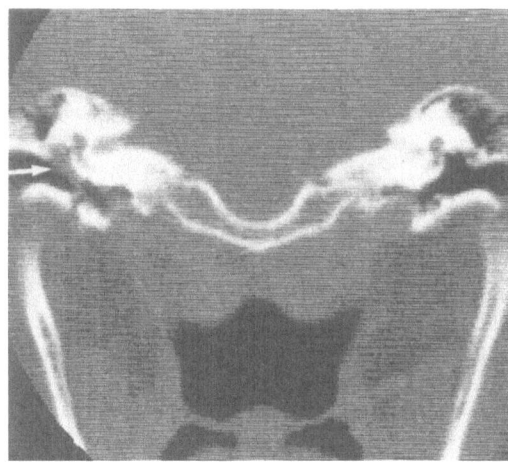
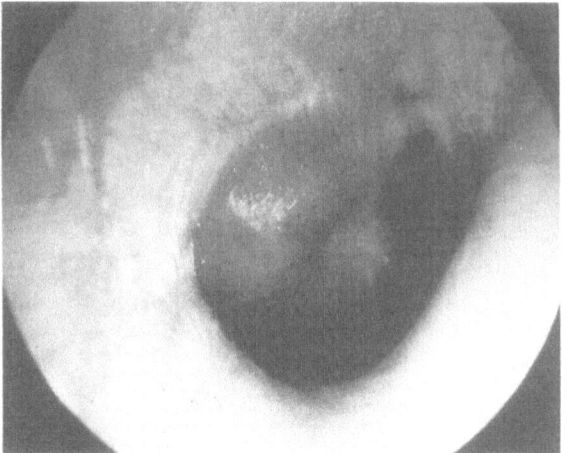

Fig. 8.14 a. Coronal CT of a small glomus tympanicum in the mesotympanum of the right middle ear. (b) This could be diagnosed by otoscopy but the air above and below could only be appreciated by CT.

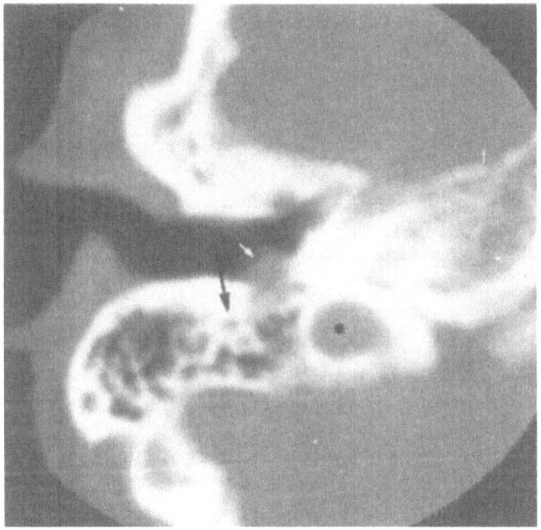
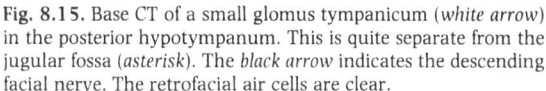
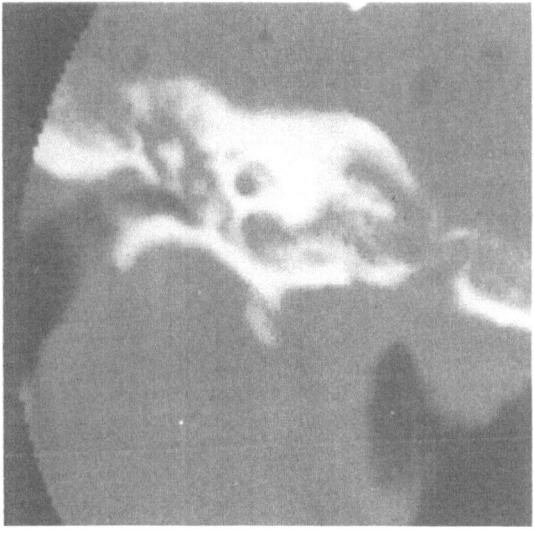

Fig. 8.15. Base CT of a small glomus tympanicum (*white arrow*) in the posterior hypotympanum. This is quite separate from the jugular fossa (*asterisk*). The *black arrow* indicates the descending facial nerve. The retrofacial air cells are clear.

Fig. 8.16. Coronal CT of a glomus tympanicum with bony excrescences in the hypotympanum.

vessels. The examination can be done on an outpatients basis, with the injection being usually made after catheterisation of the superior vena cava, and demonstration of a normal jugular bulb in the venous phase will help to exclude the presence of a jugulare tumour (Fig. 1.34). If the contrast is injected intra-arterially, a smaller amount of contrast medium than is used for angiography can produce a high quality image, a minor advantage over the conventional technique.

Retrograde Jugulography. Catheterisation of the internal jugular vein with retrograde injection will demonstrate the jugular bulb well (Fig. 8.21), but is now rarely required, as subtraction angiography, either via transfemoral catheterisation or digital vascular imaging, usually demonstrates the jugular bulb equally well in the venous phase.

Magnetic Resonance Imaging. The role of magnetic resonance imaging for glomus tumours is in its

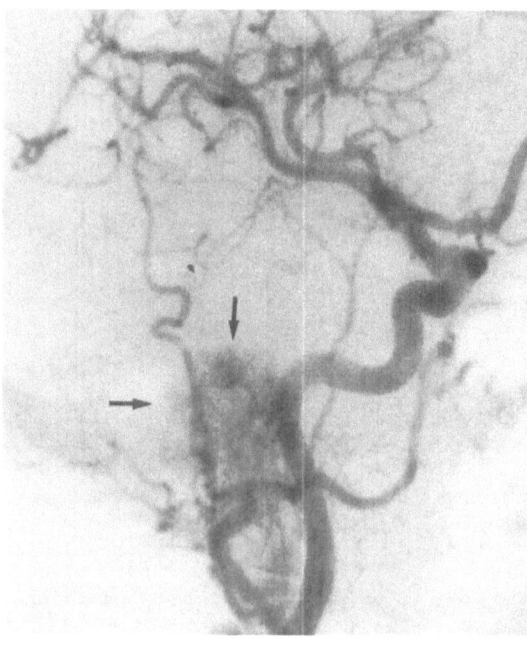

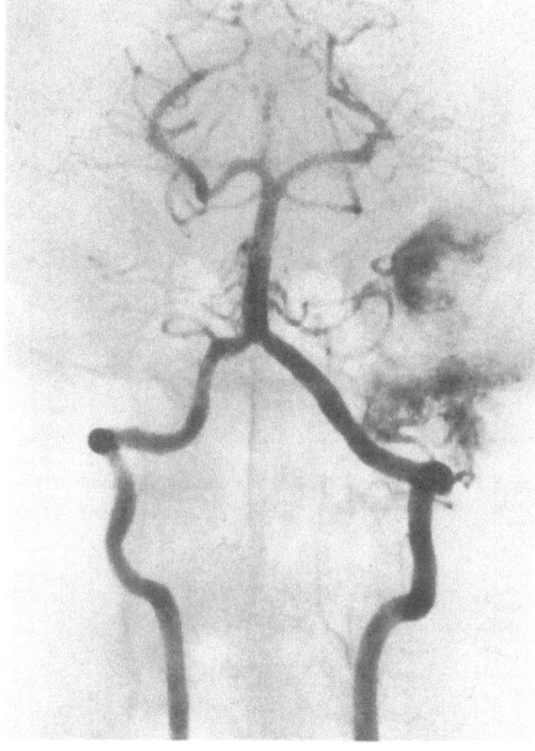

Fig. 8.17. Typical angiographic appearances of a small glomus jugulare tumour showing the tumour blush and the supply from the ascending pharyngeal branch of the external carotid. Common carotid injection.

Fig. 8.19. A larger glomus tumour may have an additional blood supply from the vertebral system in this case from the anterior inferior cerebellar artery (*AICA*) and muscular branches.

Fig. 8.18. External carotid injection showing a large glomus jugulare tumour.

▼

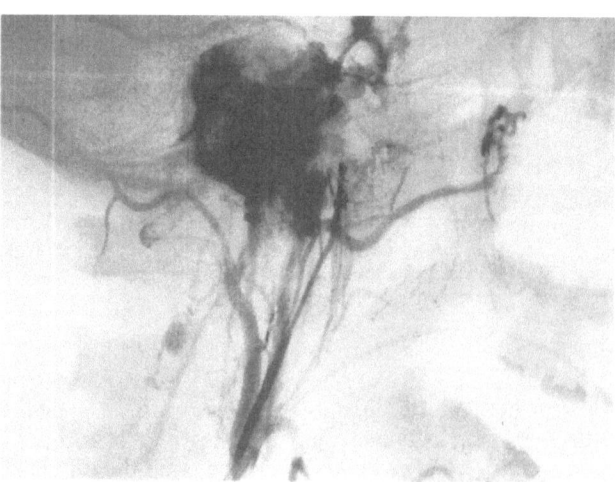

infancy, and has not yet been fully assessed. Tumours of both the jugulare and tympanicum types are shown in two recent textbooks by Swartz (1986) and Valavanis et al. (1987).

The soft tissue mass of the tumours is shown as mixed intensity on both T_1- and T_2-weighted images. Olsen et al. (1987) describe serpiginous areas of signal void in all tumours more than 2 cm

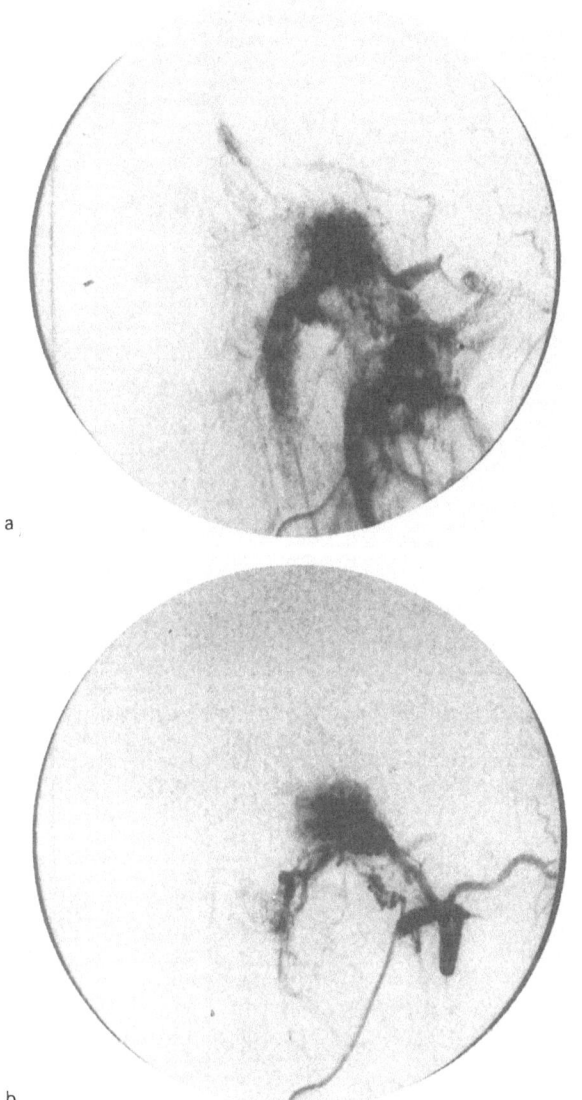

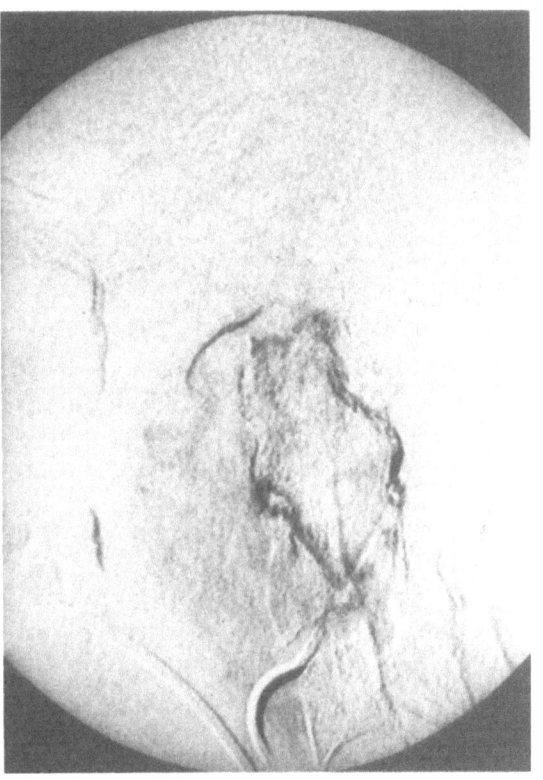

Fig. 8.20 a–c. Occipital angiogram, lateral projection. a Arterial; b venous phase. There is rich pathological circulation in the glomus jugulare tumour supplied by the petromastoid artery. The internal jugular vein is occluded: the tumour drains to the petrosal sinuses and cervical vertebral venous plexus. c Angiogram after embolisation with PVA particles. The catheter tip has been advanced into the petromastoid artery. Some PVA particles are outlined by contrast medium within the vessel. The tumour vessels have been occluded. (Courtesy of Dr. Brian Kendall, National Hospital, London.)

in diameter. These areas represent fast flowing blood in pools, and fair-sized tumour vessels, and are, in fact, a feature of all vascular tumours, including juvenile nasopharyngeal angiofibromas (Lloyd and Phelps 1986). In the petromastoid, they are almost diagnostic of a glomus tumour (Fig. 8.22).

Intracranial extension is as well shown by MRI as by CT and extension downwards into the neck is better shown than by CT (Fig. 8.23). The multiplanar imaging possibility is of considerable advantage in this latter area in particular. The growth of the tumour into the jugular vein and sigmoid sinus can be assessed in a way that was possible pre-viously only by the contrast studies of arteriography and retrograde jugulography.

We have used Gadolinium-DTPA enhancement for glomus jugulare and glomus tympanicum tumours. All tumours showed some degree of enhancement, especially on the inversion recovery sequences (Fig. 8.24). Small tumours in the middle ear became far more apparent (Fig. 8.25) and their boundaries were defined more clearly, especially at points of intracranial extension. A significant advantage was to show the tumour clearly different from fluid in the middle ear cleft and mastoid (Fig. 8.26).

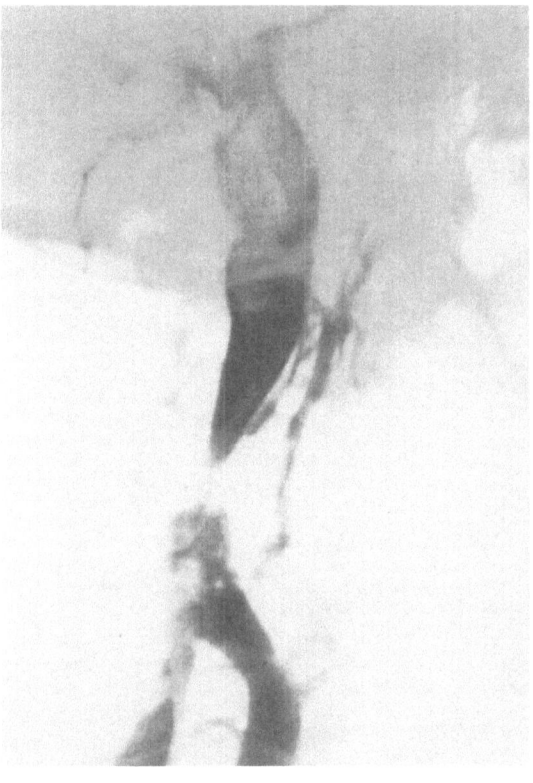

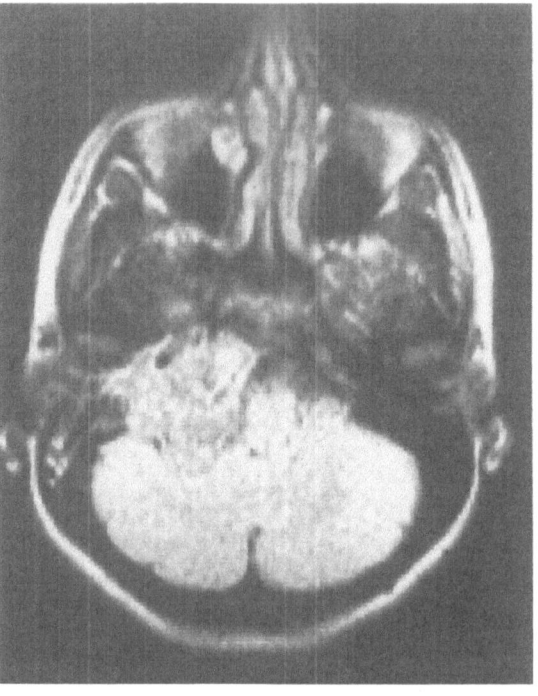

Fig. 8.21. Retrograde jugular venogram of a glomus jugulare tumour. (Courtesy of Dr. SR Srivatsa.)

Fig. 8.22. Base T_1-weighted MR scan showing the typical appearances of a large glomus tumour eroding the skull base and extending into the posterior cranial fossa. Note the non-homogeneous appearance and serpiginous streaks of signal void representing blood vessels.

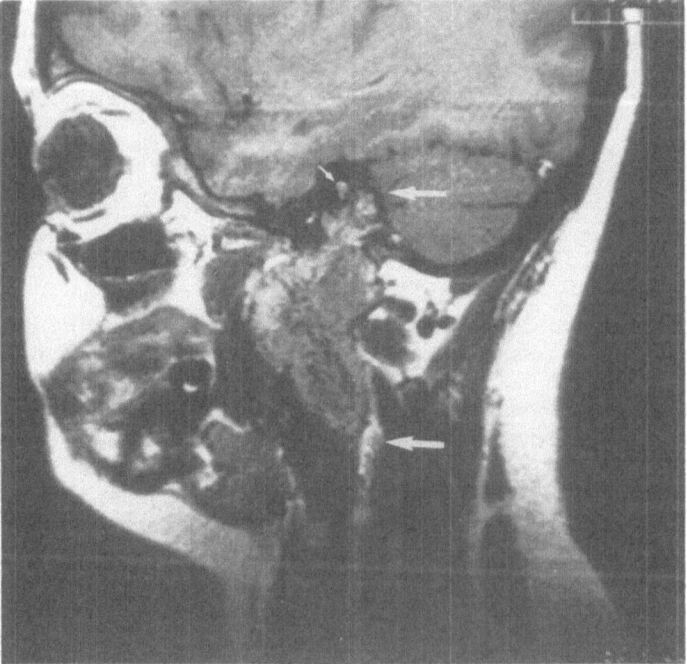

Fig. 8.23.

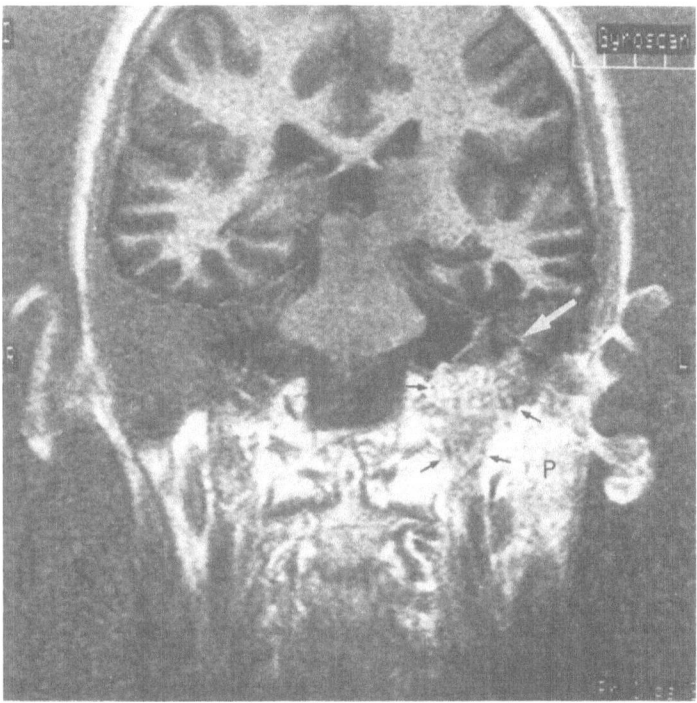

Fig. 8.24. Coronal GdMR section of the same glomus jugulare tumour showing intense enhancement especially when compared with the pre-contrast scan. Unfortunately, the tumour (*arrows*) thereby becomes *less* distinguishable from the surrounding fat and nearby parotid gland (*P*) IR 1400/400/30.

It would, therefore, seem that MRI offers great prospects as the investigation of choice for jugulo-tympanic glomus tumours but, at present, it presents two major problems. The first is its inability to define bony landmarks, a fact which means that parallel imaging by CT or tomography is essential. The second problem is in regard to the differentiation of soft tissue densities shown by CT, which give a strong signal on various MRI protocols. The most important of these are marrowfat (T_1) and serous otitis media, secondary to the presence of glomus tumour (T_2). Inflammatory reactions in the mastoid present as homogeneous zones of high signal intensity, which may be differentiated from tumour, especially on T_2-weighted sequences. However, an exact delineation between the tumour and inflammatory tissue cannot regularly be

◄——————————————————————————

Fig. 8.23. Lateral (sagittal) Gadolinium-enhanced MR scan (SE 450/30) of a large glomus jugulare extending from the jugular fossa down to the level of the angle of the mandible (*arrows*). Note the non-homogeneous appearance with variable Gd enhancement and black streaks of blood vessels. The *small arrow* points to the IAM.

obtained (Koenig et al. 1986). As bone and air in the middle ear cleft give essentially no signal, the margins of the cleft cannot be identified on an MR scan. To a certain extent, these important disadvantages can be overcome in two ways: 1) by using the clearly identifiable VIIth and VIIIth cranial nerves and the fluid in the membraneous labyrinth, and 2) by correlation with the accompanying CT scan, which is always necessary to show the important bone erosion. Fig. 8.27 shows how the normal structures and relevant anatomical features are represented on two base MR scans of the petromasoid.

A large glomus tumour surrounding the internal carotid artery in the infra-temporal region can be well demonstrated by MRI (Fig. 8.28). The relationship of the tumour to the intrapetrous carotid is much more difficult due to the marrowfat, which is invariably, but irregularly, present in the petrous apex. Bone marrow is like fat in the orbits and subcutaneous tissue, having a strong signal on T_1-weighted sequences (Table 8.1). A special fat-suppressing inversion recovery sequence, the so-called STIR, may be used, as in the orbit, to eliminate the marrowfat but, despite this, the arterial phase of the

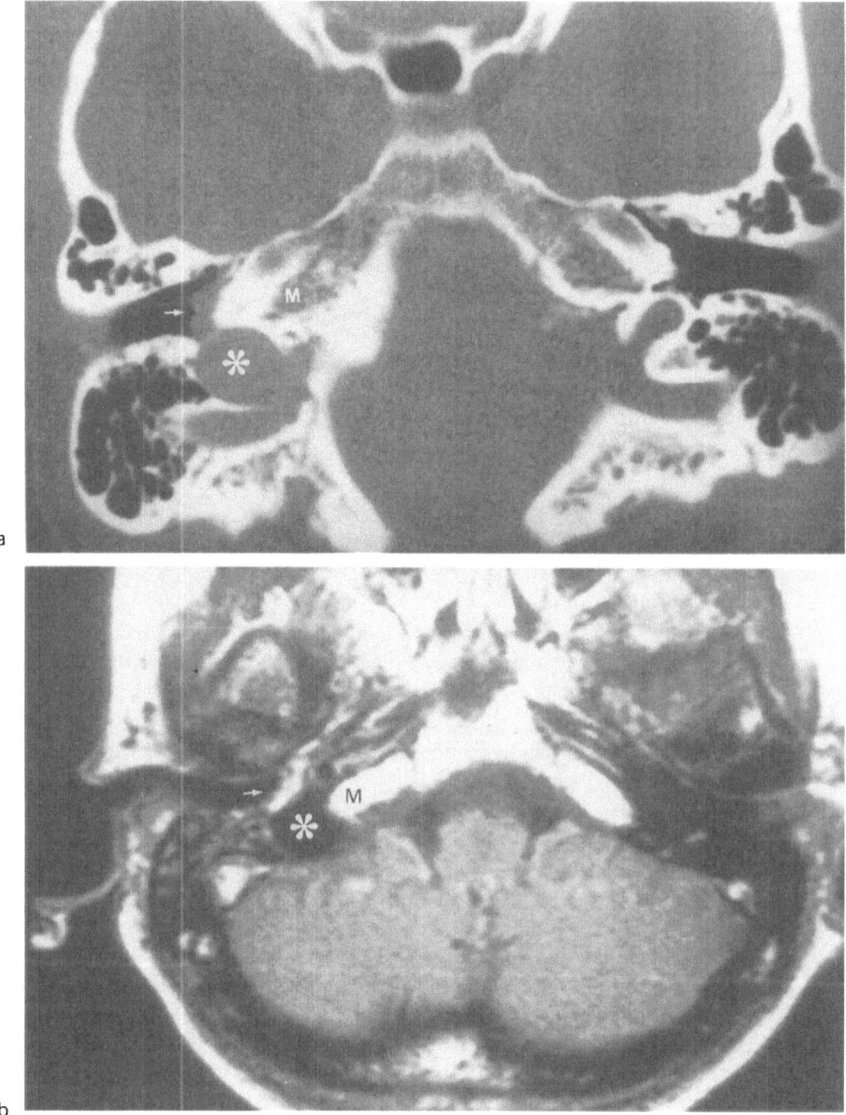

Fig. 8.25 a, b. Vascular mass behind the eardrum. (a) Base CT shows a soft tissue mass (*arrow*) in the middle ear, not clearly separate from the smoothly outlined jugular fossa (*asterisk*) which is larger than the contralateral fossa. *M*, bone marrow in the petrous apex. (b) Equivalent GdMRI shows the mass quite distinct from the jugular bulb. In both sections the arrow points to the glomus tympanicum tumour and the asterisk is in the middle of the jugular bulb. (From Phelps and Stansbie 1988.)

common carotid arteriogram will probably continue to give the best demonstration of the relationship of the tumour to the intrapetrous carotid. Extensive growth of what may appear to be a small tumour down the internal jugular vein can be well demonstrated on coronal or sagittal MR scans (Fig. 8.29).

Extension into the posterior cranial fossa is particularly well shown by Gd-MR and this may mimic an acoustic neuroma, both clinically and radiologically (Fig. 8.30).

The above radiological principles have been applied to our series of patients and have, in most cases, provided adequate assessment of individual

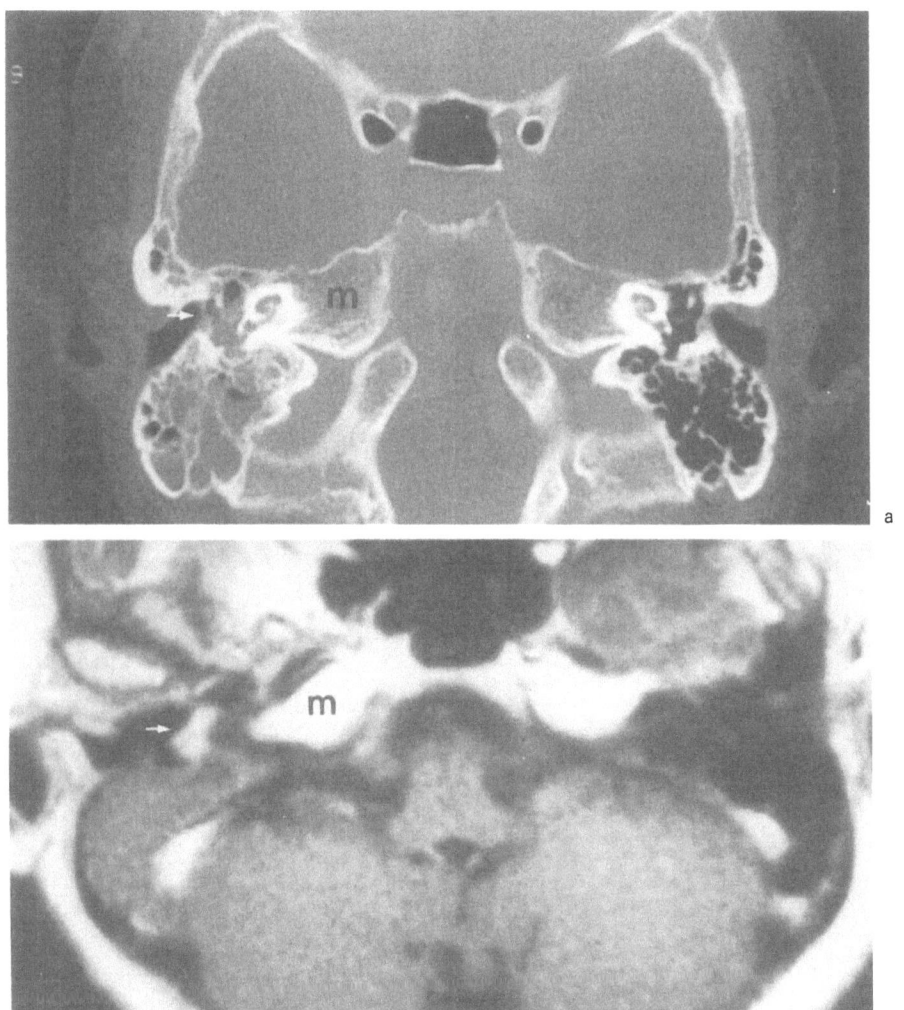

Fig. 8.26 a, b. A glomus tympanicum (*arrow*) can be distinguished clearly from fluid in the mastoid air cells on the GdMR scan (b)but not on the equivalent base CT section. (a). Note the strong MR signal from marrowfat (*m*) in the petrous apex.

cases. However, increasing experience has exposed problems, particularly in relation to the region of the dome of the jugular fossa, as exemplified by two cases which were initially assessed as glomus tympanicum but, at surgery, proved to be a glomus jugulare, with the main tumour mass in the middle ear.

These two cases examined on older CT scanners must be considered as diagnostic failures, as one suffered an extensive recurrence in the jugular fossa 6 years later and the other involved the surgeon in a more difficult operation than expected. It is interesting that Swartz (1986) also shows two cases of this type.

Such cases show no gross erosion of the jugular fossa and, therefore, extremely careful examination of good quality films is essential if minor erosions are to be detected. In addition, we believed formerly that an intact jugulo-carotid crest on lateral tomography excluded a jugulare tumour (Phelps and Lloyd 1986), but this is not necessarily so (Phelps and Stansbie 1988), where the erosion of the fossa is away from this region. Such erosions may clearly be so small that in the individual case they are identified only with the hindsight of information from surgery, particularly if the real problems of variation in the thickness and contour of the bone of the wall of the bulb, partial volume averaging,

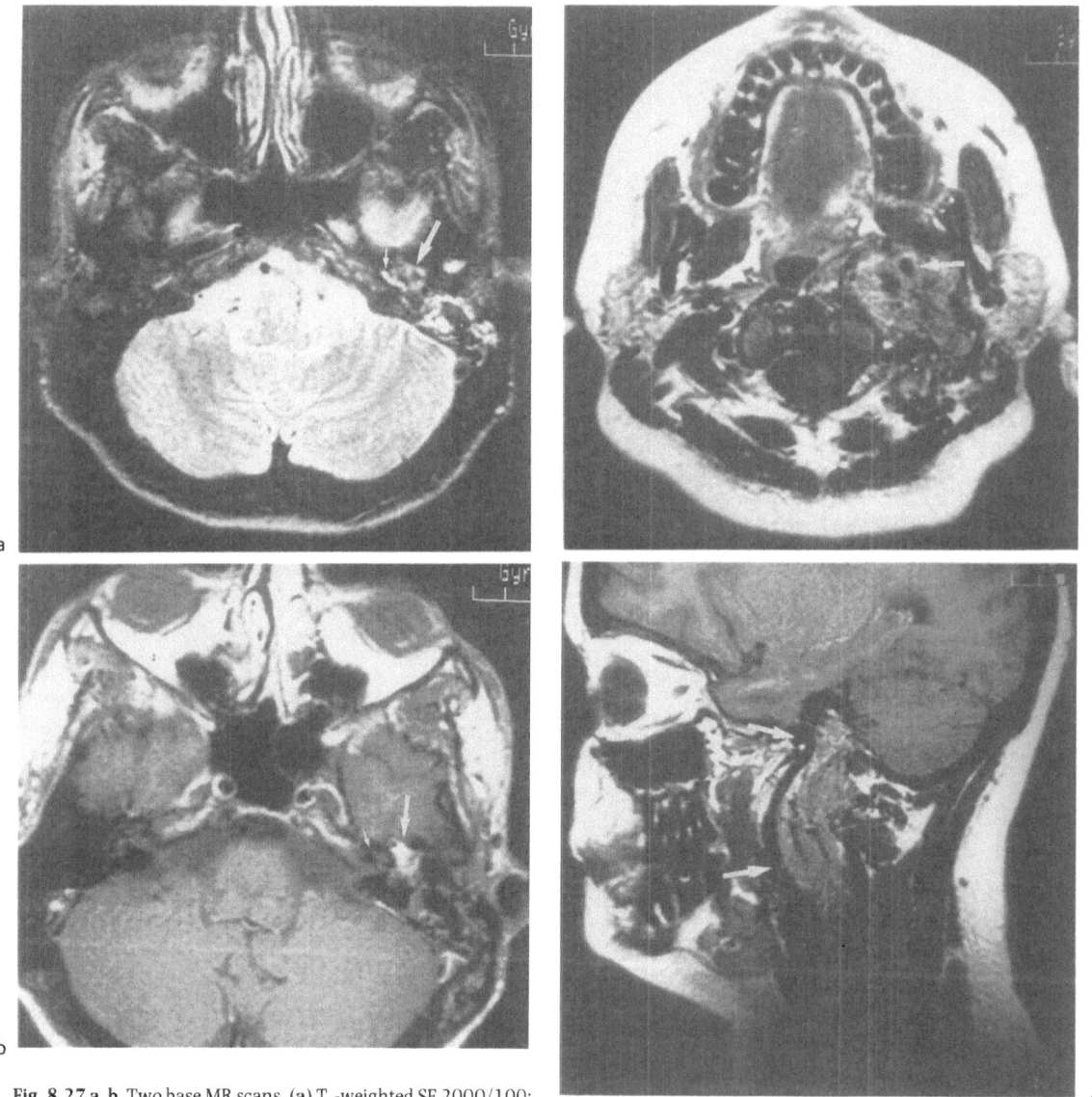

Fig. 8.27 a, b. Two base MR scans. (a) T_2-weighted SE 2000/100; (b) T_1-weighted Gd-enhanced (SE 450/30). The *large arrow* shows the tumour in the middle ear. The *small arrow* shows the cochlea. Note that in (a) the tumour is not as bright as the fluid in labyrinth and mastoid air cells, the reverse of section (b).

Fig. 8.28 a, b. Base (a) and (b) MR with Gd (SE 450/30). The carotid artery is displaced anteriorly and surrounded by tumour but again distinction from surroundings is poor.

and soft tissue silhouetting, have also to be taken into consideration (Table 8.2).

The crucial question from the surgeon's point of view has proved to be not only whether the bone of the jugular fossa is eroded, but whether the vein in the fossa is significantly involved by the lesion. This focusses attention in the borderline cases on the soft tissues of the region, and, in particular, on their demonstration by vascular studies and MR.

Angiography is of most use in assessing the arterial supply of tumour, especially if embolisation is planned, but it will not assess adequately the critical area of the jugular bulb. Digital vascular imaging may, in the venous phase, show minor soft tissue indentation of the jugular bulb, as may retrograde jugulography, but more hope now lies in MRI, despite the fact that, like the vascular studies, it has to be interpreted in the presence of inadequately

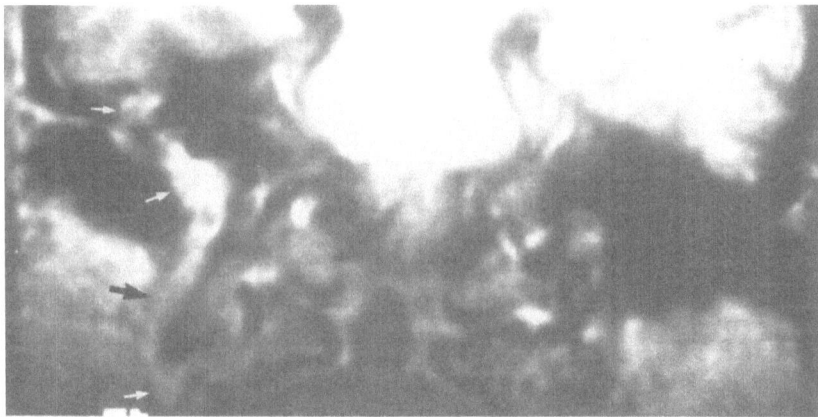

Fig. 8.29. Coronal GdMR scan (SE 450/30) showing extension of a small glomus tumour of the jugular bulb down the internal jugular vein (*arrows*).

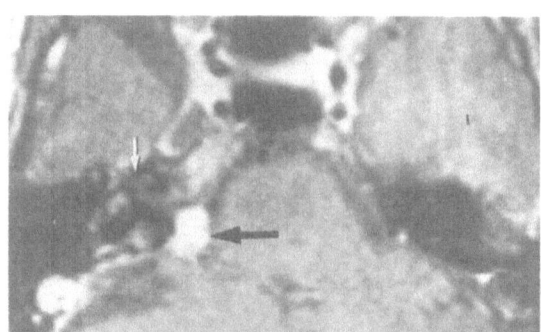

a

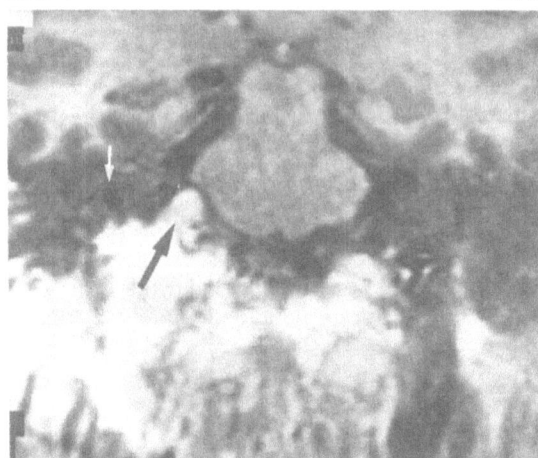

b

Fig. 8.30 a, b. A large glomus jugulare extending up into the cerebello-pontine angle and presenting with sensorineural deafness and other clinical features suggesting an acoustic neuroma. (a) Base GdMR scan (SE 500/20) shows the enhancing mass in the cerebello-pontine angle (*arrow*). The *small arrow* indicates the cochlea. (b) Coronal GdMR scan (IR 3200/30/800). The mass displaces the brainstem slightly (*arrow*) but is difficult to distinguish from fat below the skull base. The *small arrow* points to the vestibule.

imaged bony landmarks. Its advantages lie in its multi-planar potential, its clear demonstration of the jugular bulb as a dark void, so long as blood within it is flowing, and particularly in its ability to demonstrate Gadolinium-DTPA enhancement of the tumour in relation to the dark void (Fig. 8.31).

Differential Diagnosis of Middle Ear Masses Mimicking a Glomus Tumour

When the otolaryngologist sees a vascular mass in the middle ear behind an intact tympanic membrane, he usually diagnoses the lesion as a glomus tumour. There are two vascular anomalies and one inflammatory condition which lie behind an intact tympanic membrane and which may mimic a glomus tumour. The vascular anomalies are a high jugular bulb, and an ectopic intra-tympanic internal carotid artery. The inflammatory lesion is a solitary area of cholesterol granuloma, which may lie on the promontory behind an intact tympanic membrane or which may be located in the tympanic membrane itself. It is essential to differentiate a high jugular bulb and an ectopic internal carotid artery from a glomus tumour because biopsy is necessary to confirm the diagnosis of glomus tumour and cholesterol granuloma, while attempts to biopsy a jugular vein or carotid artery may lead to disastrous consequences.

Protrusion of the jugular bulb into the middle ear can be differentiated from glomus tumour tomographically by the lack of erosive changes. An intact bony spur will be present between the carotid canal and jugular fossa on lateral tomograms (see Chap.

Table 8.2 Imaging glomus tumours

	Bone erosion	Soft tissue mass	Vascularity	Diagnostic features
Conventional imaging (Jugular foramen view and lateral tomography)	+ +	−	−	Eroded margins of jugular fossa
Computerised tomography	+ +	+ +	−	Bone erosion and soft tissue mass in middle ear
Magnetic resonance	+	+ +	+	Serpiginous areas in non-homogeneous mass
Digital vascular imaging	−	+	+ +	Tumour blush
Carotid arteriography	−	+	+ +	Pathological circulation
Retrograde jugulography	−	+ +	−	Filling defect in bulb

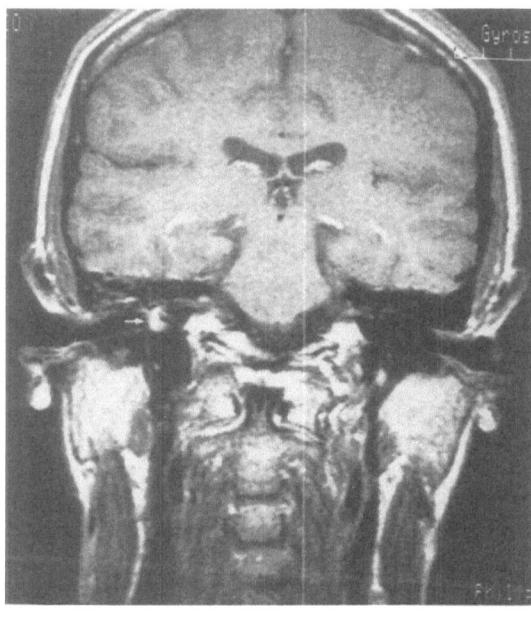

Fig. 8.31. Coronal GdMR section at the level of the oval window. The *arrow* points to a glomus tympanicum tumour. The signal void of the normal jugular bulb can be seen below it.

2 and Fig. 1.19). If necessary, the diagnosis may be confirmed by MR.

An ectopic position in the middle ear of the intratemporal portion of the internal carotid artery is extremely rare. The ectopic carotid enters the middle ear posteriorly, passes through the entire length of it and regains the normal position in the petrous apex. Sectional imaging shows a rounded soft-tissue mass throughout the entire length of the inferior portion of the middle ear cavity. There is an absence of the normal proximal portion of the carotid artery canal. This canal in the normal ear is always well visualised underneath the cochlea in coronal sections.

Neuromas

Neuromas, more correctly called schwannomas, may arise from any of the cranial nerves but have a peculiar tendency to occur in the vestibular components of the VIIIth nerve within the IAM. These so-called acoustic neuromas will be considered in detail in Chap. 9. Six cases of surgically proven intralabyrinthine schwannomas, presumably of the VIIIth nerve, have been reported (DeLozier et al. 1979). Five out of the six patients had a preoperative diagnosis of Ménière's disease and the radiographic examination was negative in all but one case.

Vth Cranial Nerve Neuromas

These usually grow into the middle cranial fossa, often with enlargement of the foramen ovale. If the neuroma is sufficiently large, erosion of the petrous apex occurs (Phelps et al. 1970; (Fig. 8.32). As well as bone erosion, trigeminal neuromas almost always enhance on CT and MR of the skull base although this enhancement may be homogeneous, non-homogeneous or ring-like due to cystic changes within the tumour (Valavanis et al. 1987). They may be an incidental finding in patients with neurofibromastosis (Fig. 8.33).

VIIth Nerve Neuroma

These are slow growing, uncommon but not rare tumours. A study of 600 human temporal bones revealed five undiagnosed facial nerve neuromas: an incidence of 0.8% (Saito and Baxter 1972). Pulec (1972) reported 14 cases and gave a thorough review of all previous reports, which at that time amounted to 98 cases. Since then, other reports have stressed the importance of radiology for this

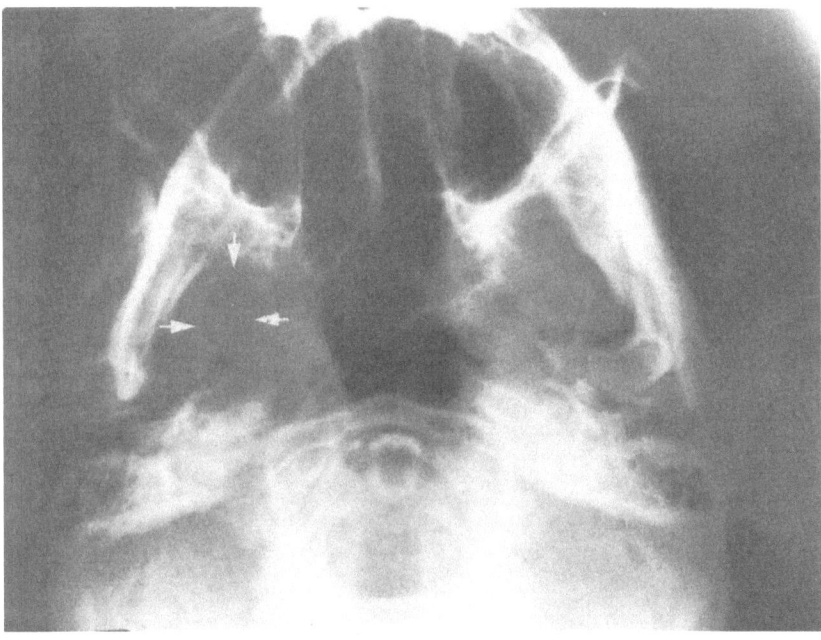

Fig. 8.32. Enlargement of the foramen ovale by a trigeminal neuroma (*arrow*) which has also eroded the apex of the right petrous bone.

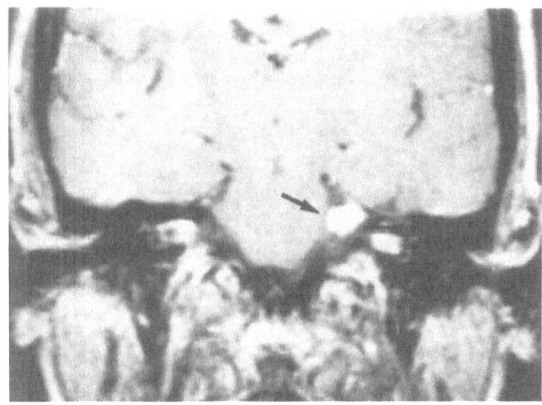

Fig. 8.33. Coronal T₁-weighted GdMR scan of a case of neuro-fibromatosis showing bilateral intrameatal acoustic neuromas as well as a trigeminal neuroma (*arrow*).

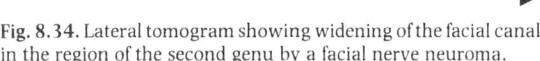

Fig. 8.34. Lateral tomogram showing widening of the facial canal in the region of the second genu by a facial nerve neuroma.

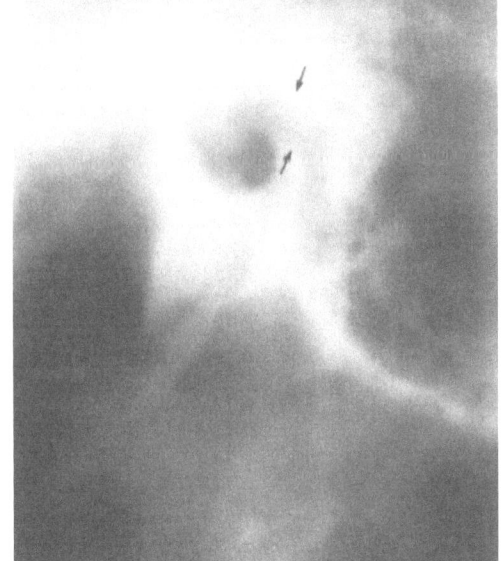

difficult diagnosis and for assessing the extent of the lesion (Latack et al. 1983; Wiet et al. 1983). These tumours can occur in any part of the intratemporal course of the facial nerve. Occurrence and pro-gression of the symptoms depend on the site of origin of the tumour and are those of facial tic or paralysis, hearing loss or vertigo. Steady pro-gression of the facial palsy is the usual feature but

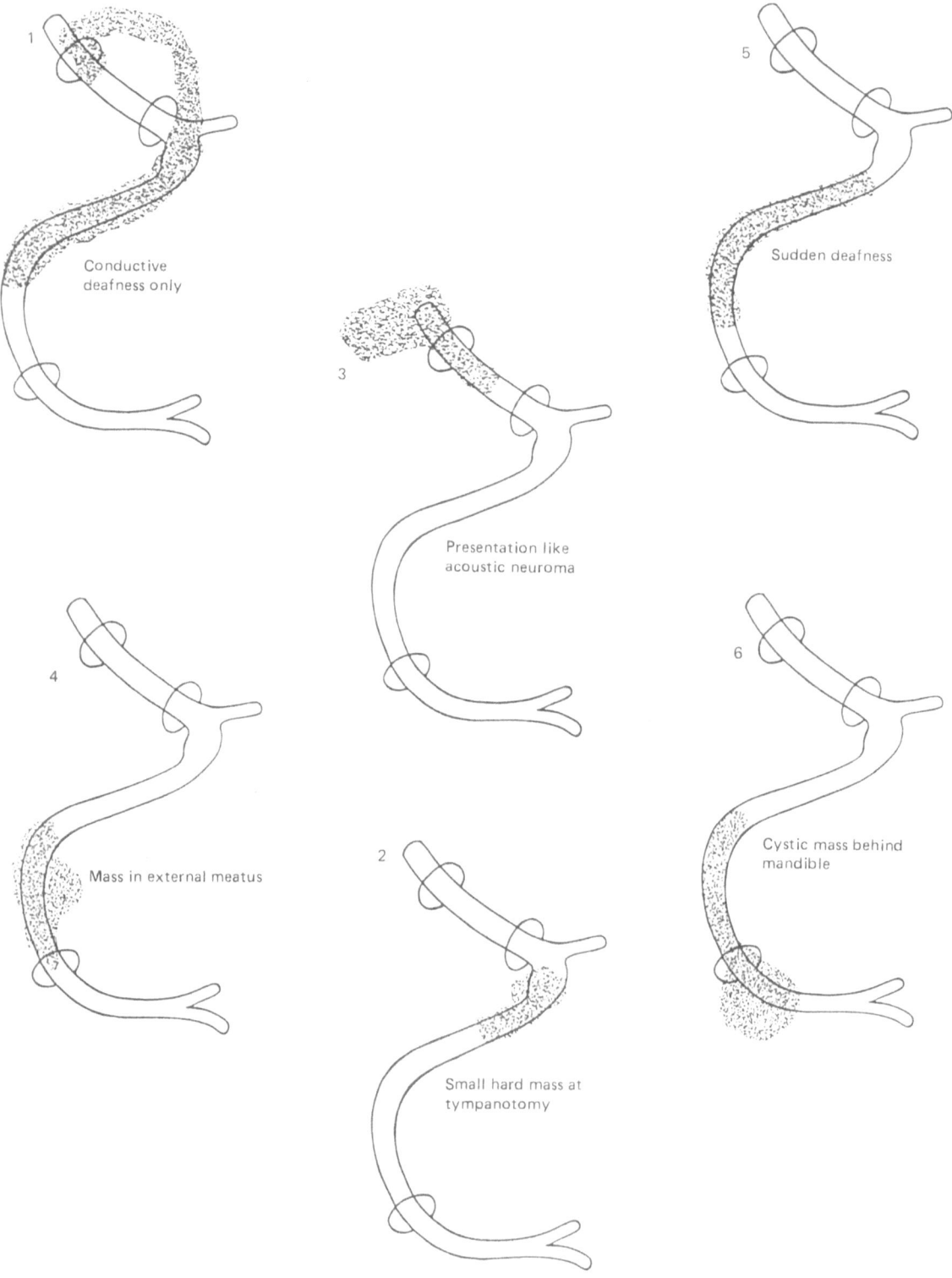

Fig. 8.35. Diagrams depicting the positions of tumours on the facial nerve in 11 patients, with a brief note on the mode of presentation which was very variable.

Fig. 8.35 continued

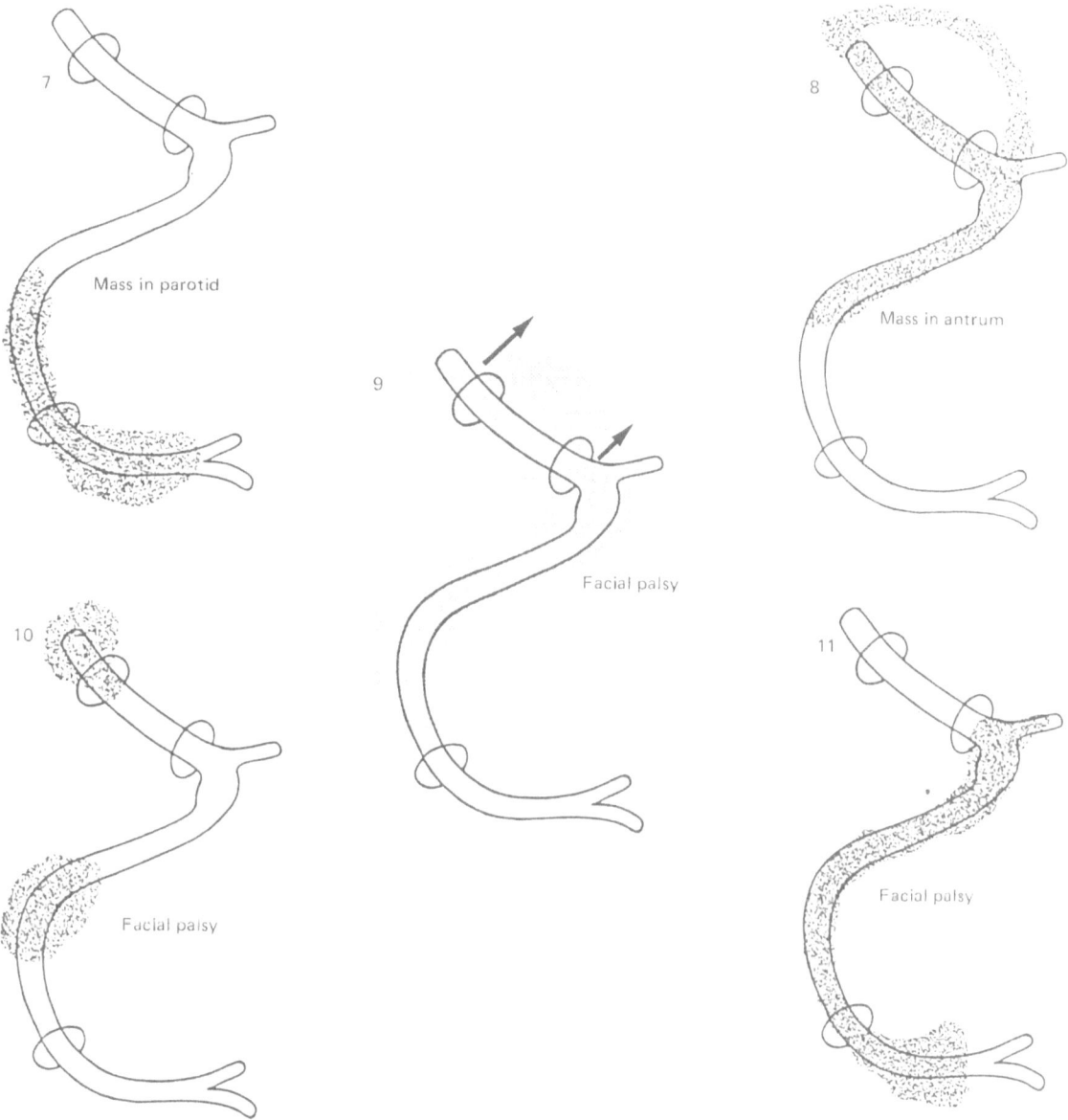

7

Mass in parotid

8

Mass in antrum

9

Facial palsy

10

Facial palsy

11

Facial palsy

cases occur with no paralysis or with paralysis of sudden onset. Initial facial paralysis may recover leading to a mistaken diagnosis of Bell's palsy. The tumour growth is in the direction of least resistance and often involves the intracranial cavity and air spaces such as the attic and mastoid. Extension proximally into the cerebello-pontine angle and distally into the parotid gland may occur.

Sectional imaging, formerly by polytomography but now largely replaced by high resolution CT, is necessary to show any widening or destruction of the intrapetrous facial nerve canal. We still prefer conventional tomography to demonstrate the canal in the lateral projection (Fig. 8.34). Computerised tomography will show the presence of a soft tissue mass in the middle ear cavity and an enhancing mass indistinguishable from an acoustic neuroma in the posterior cranial fossa. Magnetic resonance can demonstrate the whole length of the facial nerve and the situation of the neuroma, although correlation with the CT study is necessary. There have been a few MR reports and Mafee et al. (1988)

found an imaging of hypointensity to brain on T_1-weighted, isointensity in proton-weighted and hyperintensity in T_2-weighted scans.

We have studied 11 facial nerve neuromas by pluridirectional tomography, CT and MR. These are depicted in Fig. 8.35 and have a fairly even distribution over the intrapetrous course of the facial nerve. One case (3) was shown on CT as a large mass in the posterior cranial fossa. Although this was found at surgery to originate from the facial nerve, it was indistinguishable radiologically from an acoustic neuroma, except for some slight widening of the first part of the facial nerve canal shown on the tomograms. Two cases (1 and 8) had extension into the middle cranial fossa from the mass in the middle ear. Case 1 had a neuroma arising from the second (tympanic) part of the facial nerve. Clinically, there was no loss of cranial nerve function, and the presenting features were conductive deafness with a dark eardrum for which myringotomy was performed! Tomograms revealed erosion of the Fallopian canal of the facial nerve from the genicular ganglion to the second bend. However, the tumour had extended upwards and medially under the dura around the lip of the porus of the IAM. Extension under the middle fossa dura was also a feature in Case 8 who had had a previous partial removal of a neuroma in the middle ear cavity, but in this patient the tumour spread also along the proximal part of the facial nerve into the cerebello-pontine angle (Fig. 8.36).

The descending third part of the facial canal was affected predominantly in 5 patients. One presented with a visible mass projecting into the external auditory meatus and subsequently developed a facial palsy. Conventional tomography showed a destructive process interrupting the line of the descending part of the facial nerve canal. This was confirmed by high resolution CT, which showed the erosion of the facial canal in the coronal plane and a more anterior section showed the soft tissue mass of the tumour projecting into the external auditory meatus and encroaching on the middle ear cleft (Fig. 8.37). An axial section also showed the soft tissue mass in the external meatus and demonstrated erosion posteriorly into the posterior cranial fossa. In three cases, the tumour extended below the stylo-mastoid foramen.

Three facial neuromas have been assessed by MR. One was a massive well-defined tumour extending into the middle cranial fossa and showing a non-homogeneous appearance on the proton density and a low signal on T_1-weighted scans (Fig. 8.38). A longstanding facial nerve palsy with normal hearing was the presenting feature in a 28-year-old female with neurofibromatosis. The initial lateral tomograms demonstrated widening of the second bend of the facial canal, although a CT study was reported as normal. Magnetic resonance confirmed the soft tissue swelling in the region of the second tumour in the cerebello-pontine angle not apparent on the unenhanced MR (Fig. 8.39). The third patient (11) studied by MR was an 18-year-old male, also with a history of progressive facial palsy. This neuroma extended the whole length of the intrapetrous facial nerve and into the parotid gland. Magnetic resonance showed the tumour in cross-section in the descending facial canal but also on coronal sections revealed the proximal extension into the fundus of the IAM (Fig. 8.40).

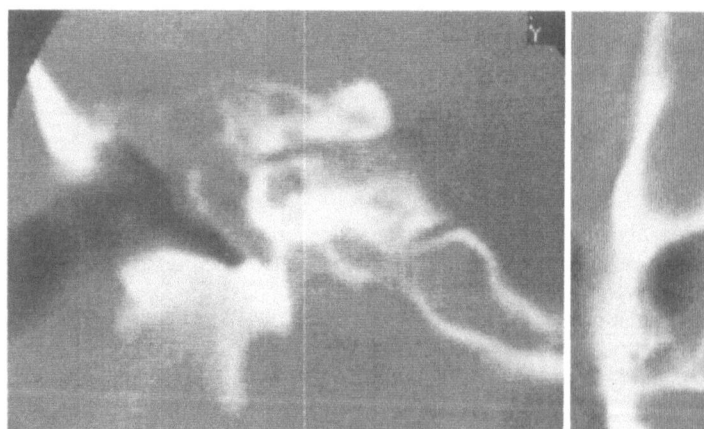
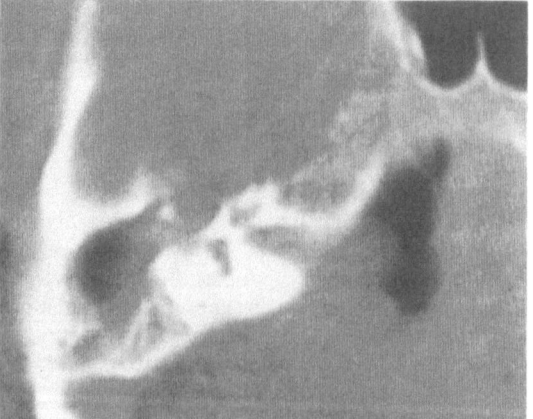

a   b

Fig. 8.36 a, b. Coronal (**a**) and base (**b**) air meatogram. CT study of a patient with a facial neuroma extending from the middle ear cavity over the top of the petrous pyramid as well as through the first part of the facial nerve canal and IAM to fill the cerebello-pontine angle.

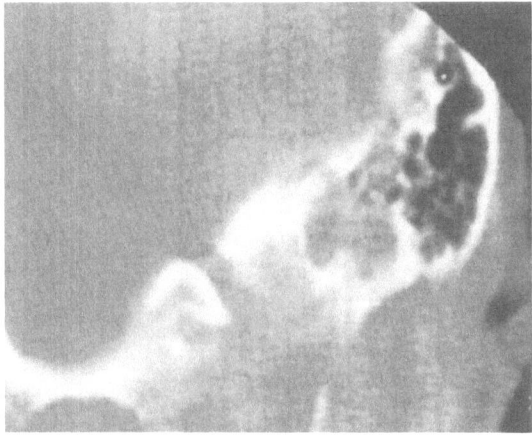
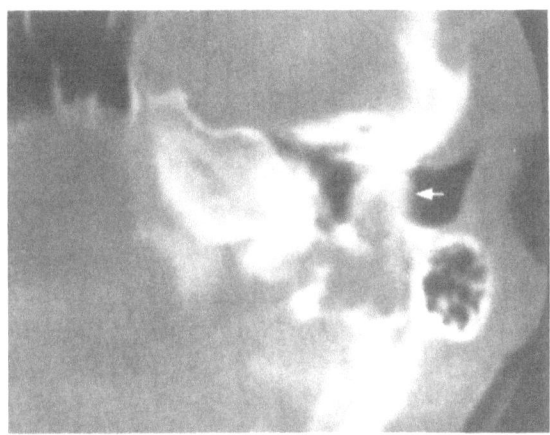

a

b

Fig. 8.37 a. Coronal CT scan, showing a facial nerve neuroma arising from the third part of the nerve. The intact lower part of the descending facial canal can be seen (*arrow*). (b) Base CT section, showing the facial neuroma in the external auditory meatus (*arrow*).

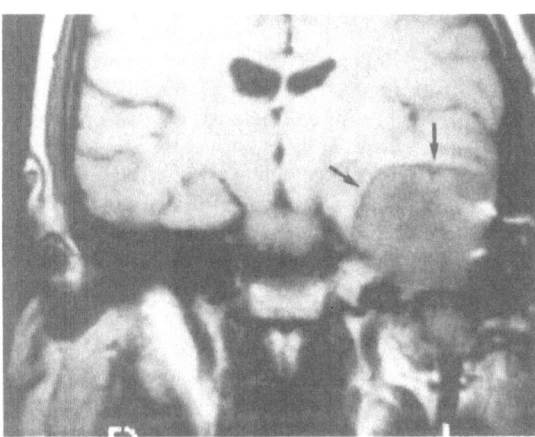

Fig. 8.38. A massive neuroma of the facial nerve extending up into the middle cranial fossa. Note the dark rim around the tumour, which is supposedly a feature of meningiomas (SE 600/27).

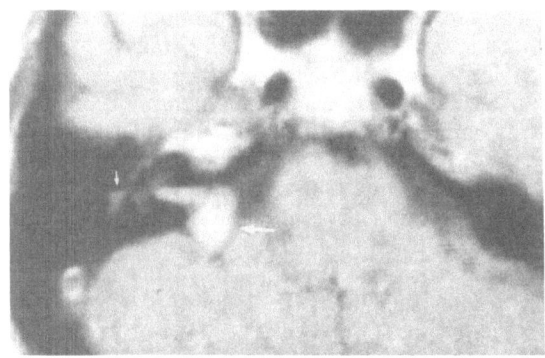

This latest case underlines the need for extensive and specialised surgery in many of these cases and, therefore, the necessity to image the limits of the tumour accurately, when long portions of the facial canal may be involved. Moreover, in three of our patients there was extension, mostly extradural, into the middle and posterior cranial fossae. This intracranial involvement was only shown satisfactorily by intrathecal contrast studies (Fig. 8.36) although MR would now appear to demonstrate any such intracranial component of the neuroma. The most satisfactory regime for imaging these tumors would, therefore, appear to be CT supported by pluridirectional tomography to show the facial nerve canal and a soft tissue mass in the middle ear. If polytomography is not available, reformatted CT sections in the sagittal plane can give an adequate demonstration of the descending facial canal (Fig. 8.41). Magnetic resonance should be used to show the whole length of the facial nerve and to demonstrate any proximal or distal extension of the neuroma beyond the facial nerve canal.

The differential diagnoses include meningiomas of the IAM or the first part of the facial canal, where haemangiomas may also give a similar radiological picture to neuroma. Perhaps the most important differentiation, however, is from a small cholesteatoma, either congenital or recurrent, which affects particularly the proximal segment of the

Fig. 8.39. Base GdMR scan shows a neuroma in the cerebello-pontine angle and IAM (*arrow*) and another at the second genu in the middle ear (*small arrow*).

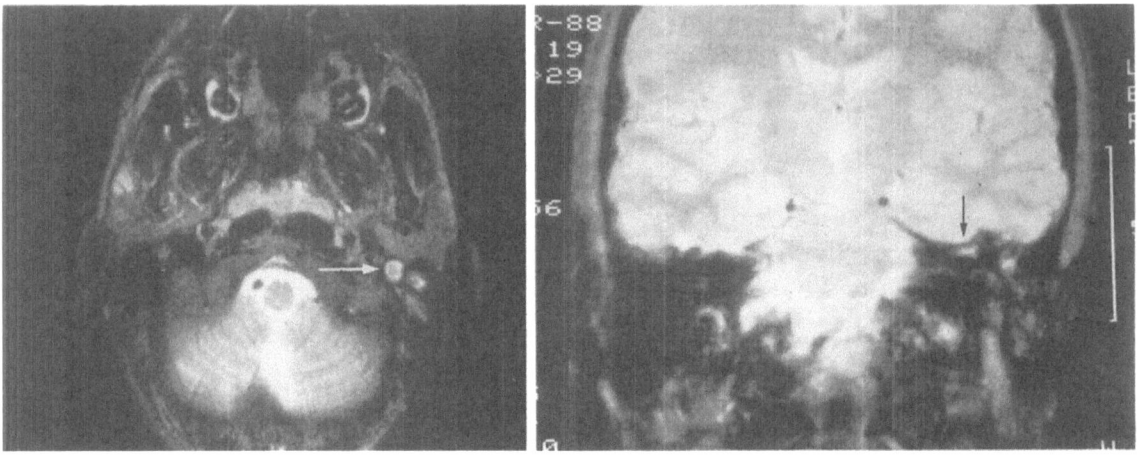

a   b

Fig. 8.40 a. Base (SE 320/90) and **(b)** coronal (SE 150/14) MR scans showing a facial nerve neuroma.

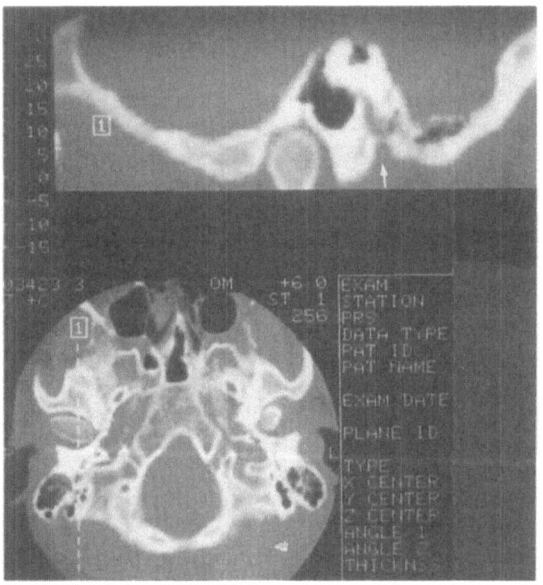

Fig. 8.41. Reformatted lateral CT of a neuroma of the descending facial nerve. The *arrow* indicates the stylomastoid foramen.

facial nerve in the region of the genicular ganglion (see Chap. 7).

IXth, Xth, XIth, XIIth Nerve Neuromas

Neuromas of the last four cranial nerves involve the jugular foramen and cause expansion. It is often impossible to determine the exact nerve of origin of these tumours at surgery, since the mass usually envelops them all. Clinically, they may present with a full jugular foramen syndrome, but some may be almost asymptomatic, and others may present in the cerebello-pontine angle, giving rise to symptoms suggesting an VIIIth nerve tumour. Arenberg and McCreary (1971) recorded two such cases in which large tumours presented with unilateral hearing loss, tinnitus and imbalance. An acoustic neuroma was suspected clinically in both cases and in neither was there any neurological deficit related to the nerves passing through the jugular foramen. Radiologically, therefore, these tumours of the lower cranial nerves need to be differentiated from both glomus jugulare tumours and from acoustic neuromas. They differ radiologically from glomus tumours in three respects (Valvassori 1974); the contour of the bone is smooth and well-defined with a neuroma, but poorly defined and irregular when the jugular fossa is expanded by a glomus tumour; neuromas do not usually erode into the middle ear; expansion of the hypoglossal canal is almost pathognomic of a neuroma of the XIIth cranial nerve.

An example of a neuroma arising from the glossopharyngeal nerve was found in a 44-year-old female who presented with a facial tic only and was observed to have an enlarged jugular fossa on routine skull X-ray. The tumour showed on CT as a contrast-enhancing mass in the cerebello-pontine angle, mimicking an acoustic neuroma, but there was obvious enlargement of the jugular fossa with a smooth, well demarcated margin, and no invasion of the hypotympanum or middle ear (Fig. 8.42). A high-resolution CT scan showed that, essentially, the tumour had eroded the posterior part of the petrous pyramid by upward extension. Radiologically, the differential diagnosis from an acoustic neuroma is made by the presence of an expanded jugular fossa and pressure erosion of the petrous

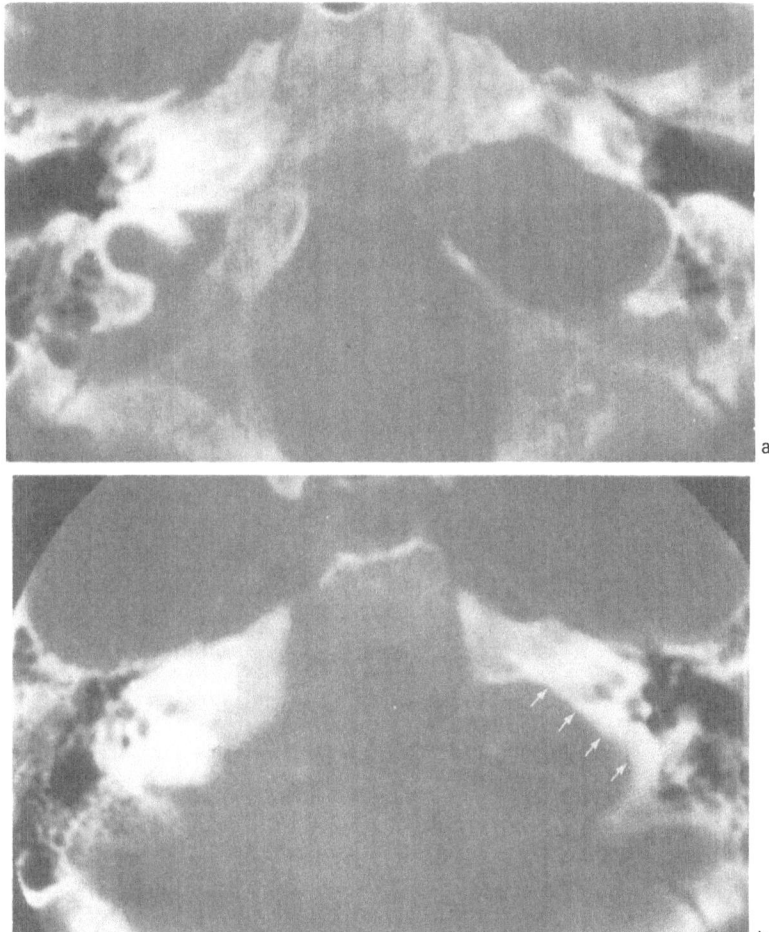

Fig. 8.42 a. Expansion of the left jugular fossa by a neuroma, shown by base CT. b. Smooth pressure erosion of the postero-medial surface of the petrous pyramid (*arrows*) by the same tumour.

pyramid posteriorly rather than the expansion of the IAM typical of an VIIIth nerve tumour. An even larger neuroma arising from the vagus nerve is shown extending into the middle ear cavity (Fig. 8.43). Once again, facial nerve dysfunction was the presenting feature. As with all neuromas, there was intense enhancement of the tumour with Gadolinium on a T_1-weighted MR scan (Fig. 8.44).

Meningioma

Meningiomas are thought to arise from "cap" cells or meningocytes located in clusters at the top of the arachnoid villi. Intracranial meningiomas take origin from the arachnoid granulations which are concentrated in the walls of the venous sinuses, while ectopic arachnoid cell rests are thought to be the origin of extradural meningiomas. Such cells are commonly located at the exit of cranial and spinal nerves from the skull and vertebrae and in the sheaths of the same nerves, both inside and outside the cranial cavity (Evard and Passy 1972).

Histopathological study of 200 temporal bones (Guzowski et al. 1976) has confirmed that the presence of arachnoid granulations within the ear is not a rare occurrence. Nevertheless, meningiomas localised within the middle ear space, which are entirely contained within the temporal bone and have no intracranial component, are very rarely encountered.

The jugular foramen, the IAM, the area of the genicular ganglion and the greater and lesser superficial petrosal nerves within the petrous pyramid,

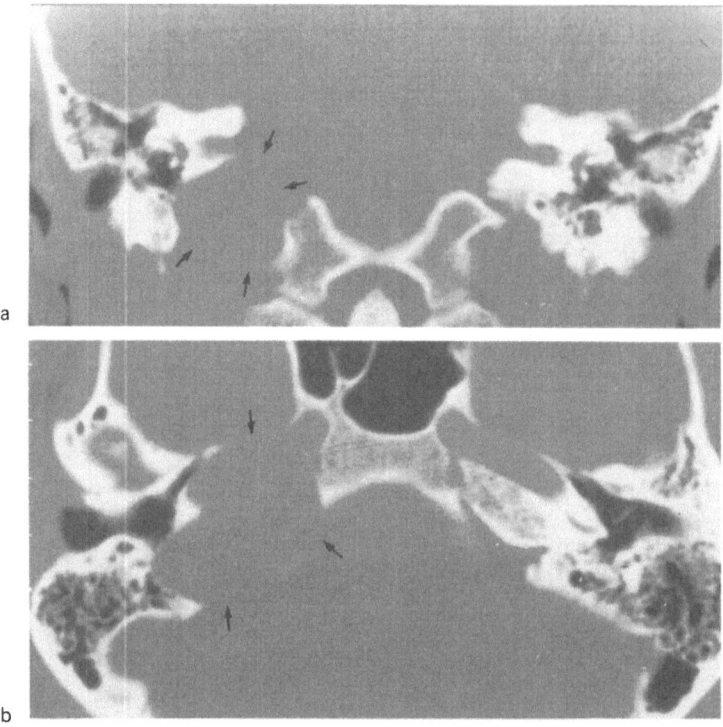

Fig. 8.43 a, b. Base (a) and coronal (b) scans of a large neuroma of the accessory nerve.

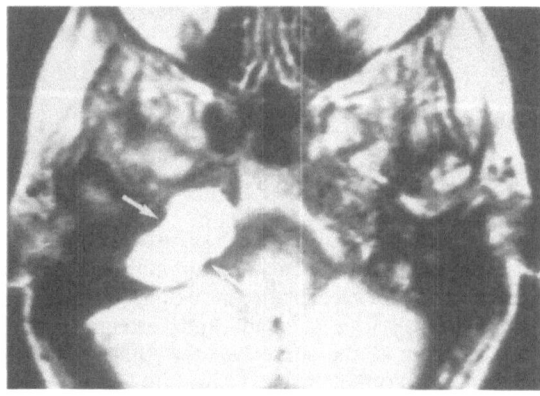

Fig. 8.44. Base GdMR (SE 300/18) showing the same tumour as Fig. 8.43. The patient had wasting of the sternomastoid muscle.

are sites of arachnoid cell clusters and can give rise to meningiomas involving the temporal bone. These tumours may be found in the middle ear, attic, hypotympanic region, jugular foramen mastoid and petrous portion of the temporal bone, including the IAM.

The type of clinical presentation depends to a large extent on the site of origin of the tumour. Nager (1967) reviewed the initial clinical signs in 30 patients with temporal bone meningiomas. The predominant symptoms in order of frequency were: progressive hearing loss, headaches, vertigo, tinnitus, otorrhoea, otalgia, and facial weakness or loss of sensation of taste.

In the cases reported, radiographic examination with mastoid projections and tomograms was not particularly helpful, being often normal or showing non-specific changes in the mastoid cell system. In only one case was there hyperostosis. All meningiomas are, however, well demonstrated by CT and this is now a mandatory investigation.

Secondary invasion of the temporal bone by a posterior fossa or middle fossa meningioma is more common than a tumour arising in the petrous temporal bone but it may be difficult or impossible to decide the point of origin. Parisier et al. (1978) reported three patients having meningiomas which were thought to be localised in the middle ear and which were treated by surgical excision; the patients were presumed to be cured of their disease. However, two to four years post-operatively these patients were examined using CT and all were found to have an adjacent large intracranial meningioma.

Much the commonest site of origin for a meningioma affecting the petrous temporal bone is the posterior surface, and meningiomas are second only to acoustic neuromas in frequency in the cerebello-

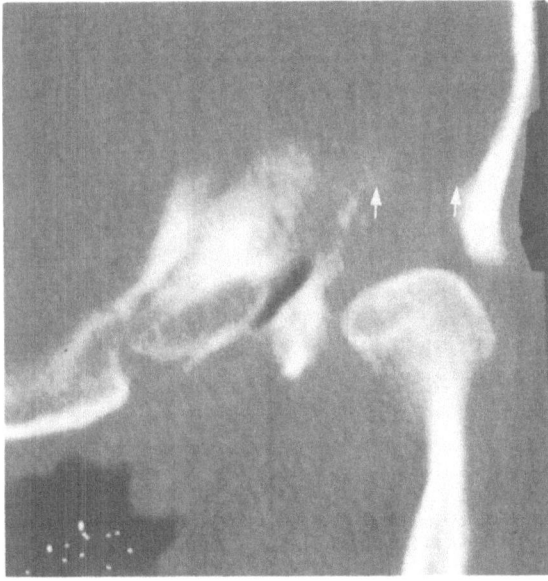

Fig. 8.45. Coronal CT scan showing erosion of the articular fossa of the temporo-mandibular joint by a meningioma (*arrows*). Note the air in the lower middle ear cavity and Eustachian tube.

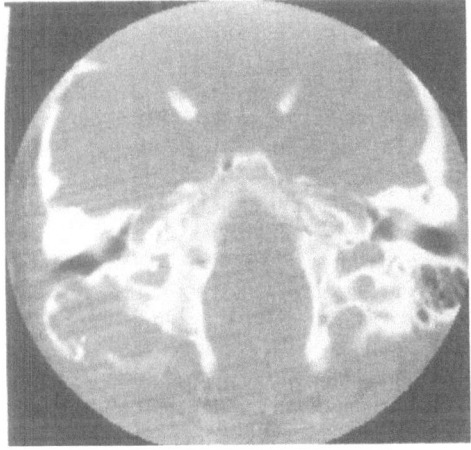

Fig. 8.46. A low grade extra dural meningioma expanding into the posterior cranial fossa.

pontine angle. The clinical presentation is similar. These posterior fossa tumours will be considered in Chapter 9.

We have seen six meningiomas which affected the petromastoid, but none appeared to have arisen in the middle ear cavity. One was a female patient of 56 years, who presented clinically with a mass protruding anteriorly into the external auditory meatus and a pulsating eardrum. Computerised tomography showed the mass projecting into the external auditory meatus. This was also shown in the middle ear and attic, spreading to the temporo-mandibular joint (Fig. 8.45). A coronal scan made at the level of the temporo-mandibular joint showed that the tumour had eroded through the tegmen. Findings at surgery appeared to confirm a meningioma en plaque of the floor of the middle cranial fossa, which had extended downwards and in front of the genicular ganglion.

Another patient presented with a facial tic followed by a complete right facial palsy. Plain skull views showed a large area of rarefaction in the mastoid region. Computerised tomography revealed a discreet mass with thin bony covering, which extended up into the posterior fossa (Fig. 8.46). A firm mass was removed through a suboccipital craniotomy. This was in an extradural situation, suggesting an origin from within the mastoid air cells, and appeared to have involved the descending portion of the intratemporal facial nerve.

Three cases presented as parapharyngeal masses. These large meningiomas probably arose in the jugular fossa and the diagnosis was indicated by CT, which showed hyperostosis of the temporal bone and calcification within the soft tissue mass (Fig. 8.47). Magnetic resonance was a useful complementary examination and in one case showed the tumour extending around the brainstem, thereby precluding any attempt at surgical resection. A positive biopsy was not obtained in two cases of severe hyperostosis of the temporal bone. One was a 15-year-old girl with neurofibromatosis meningiomas at other sites, and the other was a boy with progressive facial palsy and virtual obliteration of the IAM (Fig. 8.48). Air meatography was unsuccessful, presumably due to the presence of arachnoid adhesions from the meningioma en plaque.

In these few cases we found CT superior to magnetic resonance, which has been the experience of other authors (Mawhinney et al. 1986). Hyperostosis and calcification within the tumour are well shown by CT as well as enhancement by iodine-containing contrast agents. The often difficult MR differentiation of meningiomas from normal brain can be greatly improved by enhancement with GdDTPA (see Chap. 9).

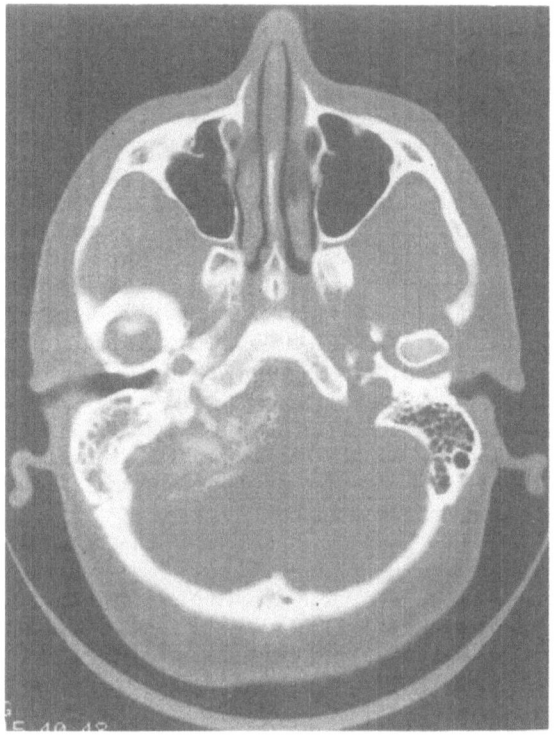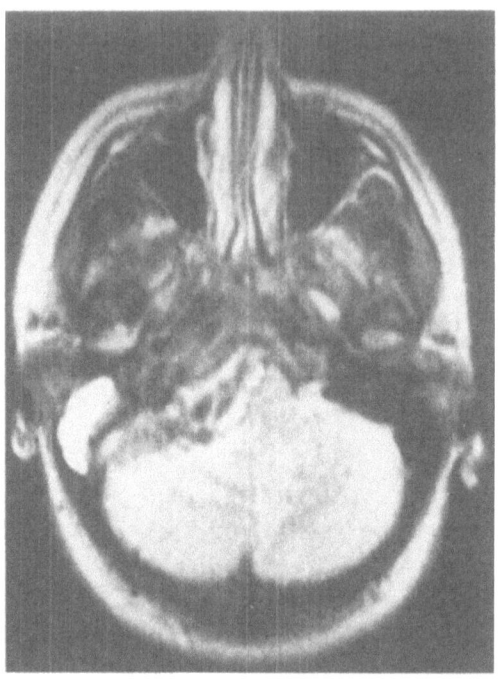

Fig. 8.47 a, b. Meningioma in the lower part of the posterior cranial fossa having probably arisen in the jugular fossa. There is both calcification in the tumour and hyperostosis of the adjacent skull base. This is better shown on the plain high resolution CT (**a**) than on the T_1-weighted base MR scan (**b**): the bright signal is from the retained fluid in the mastoid.

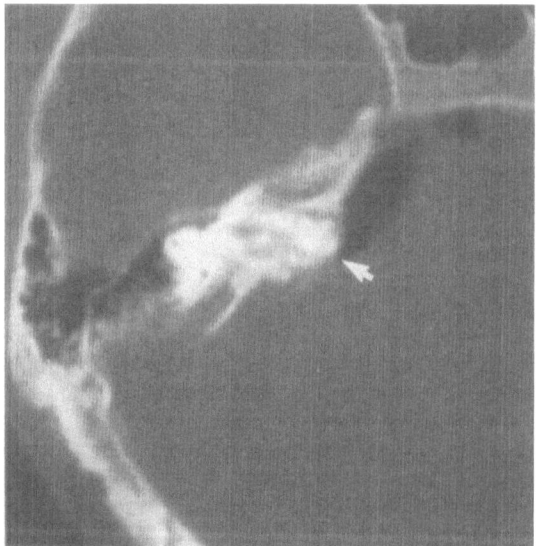

Fig. 8.48. Hyperostosis of the petrous pyramid from a presumed meningioma. The IAM was partly obliterated and air meatography was unsuccessful, presumably due to arachnoid adhesions.

Adenoma

These tumours arise from the middle ear mucosal epithelium and their clinical behaviour is that of a benign localised non-metastasising lesion. Hyams and Michaels (1976) described 20 examples of this condition. Their patients had an age range of 14 to 80 years, with the sexes evenly divided, and their chief symptom was a unilateral increasing hearing loss. No history of chronic middle ear disease was present in any of their patients and the preoperative diagnosis was usually that of a glomus tumour. In none of their patients was bone destruction recorded, either at surgery or on X-ray examination and the radiographic features are therefore confined to a soft tissue mass in the middle ear or mastoid antrum.

We have seen three patients with an adenoma of the middle ear. One patient presented with left otalgia and an aural polyp, subsequently developing a left facial palsy. At mastoid exploration, a soft tissue mass was found in the antrum and middle ear. It was enveloping the incus and was insep-

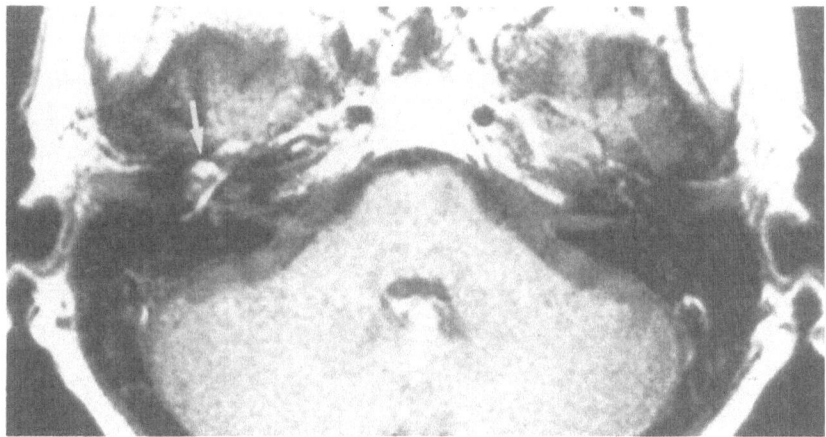

Fig. 8.49. Base GdMR scan showing a small adenoma in the anterior hypotympanum of the right middle ear (*arrow*). Note how well the second part of the facial nerve is demonstrated.

arable from the facial nerve. Biopsy showed the tumour to have the features of a benign adenoma. An example of a small adenoma in the anterior hypotympanum was poorly demonstrated by CT but became clearly apparent with Gadolinium-enhanced MR (Fig. 8.49).

Malignant Neoplasms

Carcinoma

Carcinoma of the ear arising in the external auditory meatus, middle ear cleft or in a mastoid cavity, is a rare but distressing disease, which is seldom diagnosed early. Lewis (1973) estimates an average period of time from initial symptoms to diagnosis of six months. Only about 10% of squamous carcinomas can be classified as early lesions, usually arising from the cartilaginous external auditory meatus. Lewis suggests that the classic features of bloody discharge and pain in fact indicate fairly advanced disease. The association of carcinoma of the ear with chronic suppurative otitis media is well recognised and variously estimated as occurring in 30–75% of cases (Maran and Jacobsen 1979; Phelps and Lloyd 1981). The presence of a cholesteatoma has been described in a few cases (Lewis 1973).

Carcinoma arising in the cartilaginous auditory meatus tends to spread into the parotid gland and the post-auricular sulcus, whereas a tumour arising from the deep bony meatus may perforate the eardrum at an early stage. It is, therefore, often impossible to assess the exact site of origin of the tumour or to decide whether it has arisen from the deep meatus or middle ear cleft. Treatment by various regimes of surgery and radiotherapy can give a 30% five-year-salvage rate, depending on the site of origin and extent of the disease.

Early diagnosis depends upon a high index of suspicion leading to biopsy of polyps or "granulation tissue" in the middle ear or external meatus. The diagnosis of carcinoma in the mastoid is usually made while performing a mastoidectomy in an effort to control presumed chronic mastoiditis (Clairmont and Conley 1977), since preceding middle ear infection is to be expected in at least 40% of patients (Phelps and Lloyd 1981). Sclerosis of the mastoid and clouding of the cells are, therefore, radiological signs of little value but the presence of ragged erosion, usually extensive or in an unusual site, suggests neoplastic change (Fig. 8.50). An important sign on the lateral mastoid view is erosion of the articular fossa of the temporo-mandibular joint. This was present on the initial radiographs in 30% of cases. Much better demonstration of the bony external auditory meatus and back of the temporo-mandibular joint was given by lateral tomograms (Fig. 8.51) and the authors consider this to be an obligatory investigation when a carcinoma of the ear is suspected. Minor erosions will indicate the site for further exploration and biopsy if the initial biopsies prove negative.

Almost all malignant epithelial tumours of the middle ear are squamous in type, although very rarely adenoid cystic and adenocarcinomas, presumably arising from glandular epithelium lining the middle ear cleft, have been reported. An exten-

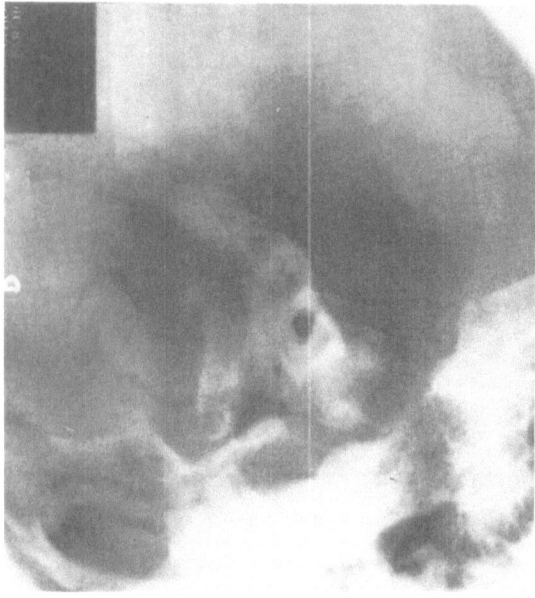

Fig. 8.50. Extensive ragged erosion of the squamous temporal bone; lateral oblique view showing the preservation of the labyrinthine capsule.

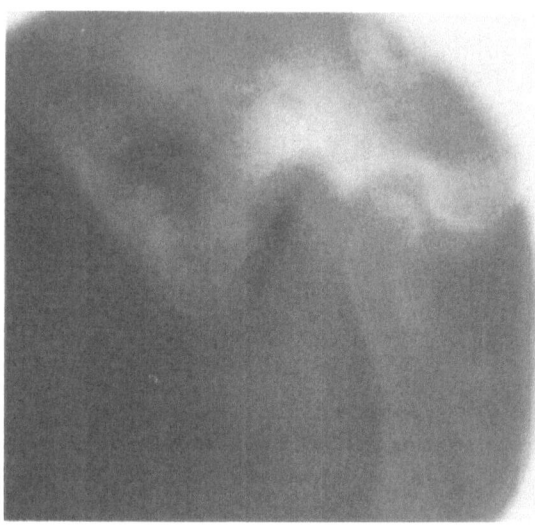

Fig. 8.51. Lateral tomogram showing soft-tissue swelling in the external auditory meatus with erosion of the anterior and inferior walls and extension into the temporomandibular joint. Note the well-pneumatised mastoid process.

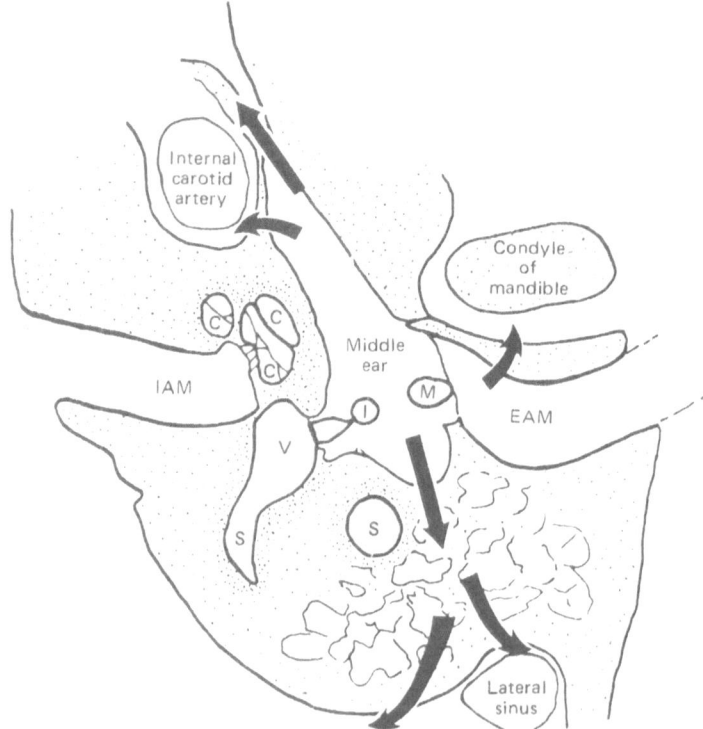

Fig. 8.52. Diagram based on axial histological and tomographic sections of the petrous temporal bone. The *arrows* indicate the usual directions of spread of carcinoma of the middle ear and bony external auditory meatus. *C*, cochlea; *V*, vestibule; *S*, semicircular canal; I, incus; M, malleus. The top of the diagram is anterior.

sive review of carcinoma of the external auditory meatus and middle ear and its management is given by Stell (1984).

Diseases which may have similar radiological appearance to squamous-cell carcinoma of the ear, are tuberculous otitis media, where there may be extensive bone destruction, and malignant otitis externa, a non-neoplastic condition which almost always occurs in elderly diabetics. Endarteritis and superadded infection lead to extensive destruction of the external auditory meatus, temporo-mandibular joint and middle ear, making radiological differentiation from carcinoma difficult. Symmetrical expanding erosion around the external auditory meatus is suggestive of infective, rather than neoplastic, disease (see Chap. 6). Glomus tumours also cause ragged erosion of the skull base but the involvement of the margins of the jugular fossa, a late feature with carcinoma or malignant otitis, will suggest the correct diagnosis.

The hard avascular bone of the labyrinthine capsule is relatively unaffected by carcinoma of the ear and erosion of the capsule with direct invasion of the inner ear is a late radiological feature only present with extensive surrounding bone destruction. Michaels and Wells (1980) have shown by means of serially sectioned temporal bones, that there are two important modes of spread of carcinoma of the middle ear (Fig. 8.52). The tumour first extends anteriorly and penetrates the bony septum separating the middle ear cavity from the carotid artery. It then spreads around the artery and extends down around the Eustachian tube towards the postnasal space. Erosion of the carotid septum (Fig. 8.53), margins of the bony Eustachian tube and even soft tissue extension of the tumour anteriorly can be demonstrated by CT. Secondly, the tumour may spread upwards, through the tegmen tympani and backwards through the mastoid air cells, then through the thin plate forming the posterior wall of the petrous pyramid and underlying the lateral sinus (Fig. 8.54). Erosion of these thin bony structures may also be demonstrated radiologically. Once inside the cranial cavity, infiltration along the dura occurs and when this is breached, death soon follows.

The CT findings in ten primary malignant neoplasms of the ear were described by Bird et al. (1983). They stressed the improved prognosis when a normal air-containing middle ear is demonstrated, and the importance of contrast-enhanced scans for showing extension into parotid, infratemporal fossa and intracranially. However, they had two false negative results in evaluating intracranial extension: at surgery both patients were found to have a thin layer of tumour along the dura, but no adjacent

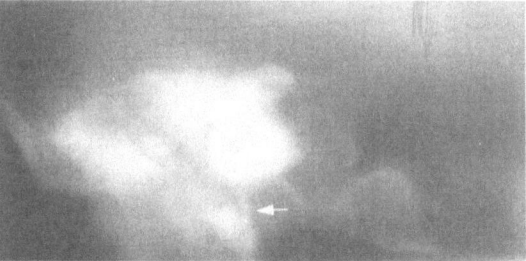
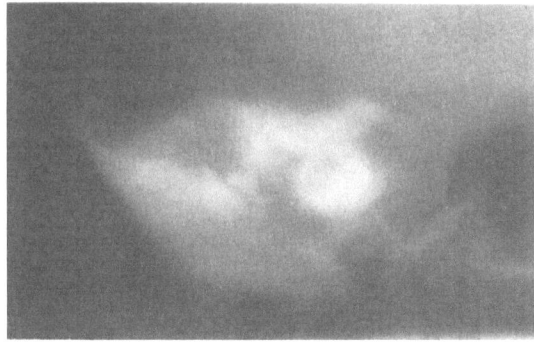

Fig. 8.53. Two equivalent coronal sections at the level of the cochlea, taken five months apart. The upper print shows an intact carotid septum (*arrow*), which can no longer be demonstrated on the later section. Extension of disease beyond the carotid canal was subsequently confirmed at surgery.

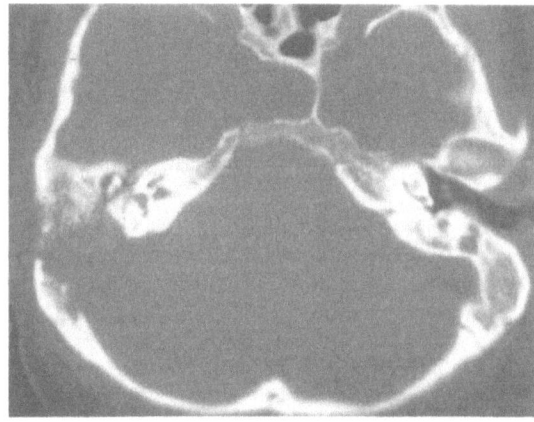

Fig. 8.54. Base CT showing ragged erosion of the posterior part of the petromastoid by a squamous cell carcinoma of the ear.

bone destruction or abnormal enhancement were noted on CT.

Magnetic resonance has been little used for carcinoma of the ear. A non-homogeneous mass may be shown and a better assessment of its extent when correlated with CT especially for spread beyond the temporal bone (Fig. 8.55).

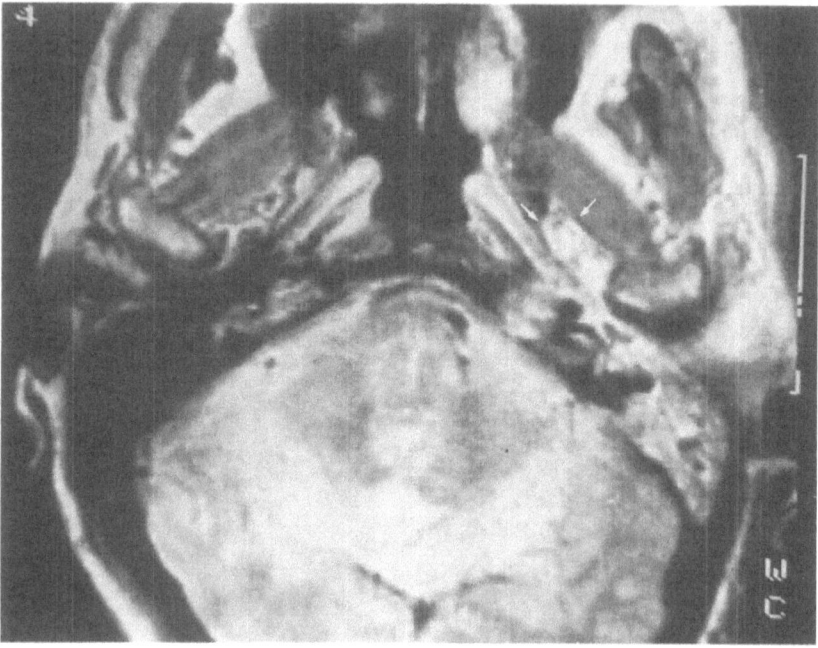

Fig. 8.55. Base MR (SE 320/30) shows a squamous cell carcinoma of the middle ear extending forwards into the infratemporal fossa (*arrows*).

Sarcoma

The most common sarcoma of tne middle ear, excluding systemic disorders, is the embryonal rhabdomyosarcoma of children. Osteogenic sarcoma, fibrosarcoma, chondrosarcoma and primary malignant melanoma of the temporal bone are extremely rare tumours, which usually produce rapidly expanding osteolytic lesions. Lymphomas and leukaemias infiltrate into the temporal bone, the middle ear and mastoid. The authors have seen a lymphoma causing destruction of the external auditory meatus entirely similar to that produced by a carcinoma.

Rhabdomyosarcoma

This is a rare tumour of mesenchymal tissue. The origin in the middle ear cleft is almost exclusively seen in young patients. Earlier reviews judged this tumour to be uniformly fatal and the results of treatment in middle ear sarcoma were disappointing. In the last few years, however, reports have shown that mastoidectomy or even simple biopsy followed by radiation therapy and multiple drug systemic chemotherapy, have given several long-term survivals (Goepfert et al. 1979).

Harwood-Nash (1971) has described the radiological features of rhabdomyosarcoma of the middle ear with intracranial extension in children. In the three cases described, more destruction of the petrous bone was demonstrated by tomography than by conventional mastoid radiographs. Ragged erosion of the petrous pyramid and mastoid region occurs but the labyrinth is usually not involved and in fact may be "skeletonised". The tegmen is usually destroyed with extension into the middle fossa. Recently, Proops and Mann (1984) have described the presenting features of rhabdomyosarcoma of the petrous temporal bone. These usually include a fleshy polyp in the external ear canal, conductive deafness and facial palsy. Early and adequate biopsy is vital, but CT can show the bone destruction and soft-tissue mass often extending into the infratemporal fossa.

Metastatic Tumours

Metastatic tumours of the temporal bone are considered uncommon. However, Jahn et al. (1979), who examined 19 temporal bones from 11 patients with metastatic temporal bone disease from a distant primary, noted the high incidence of occult

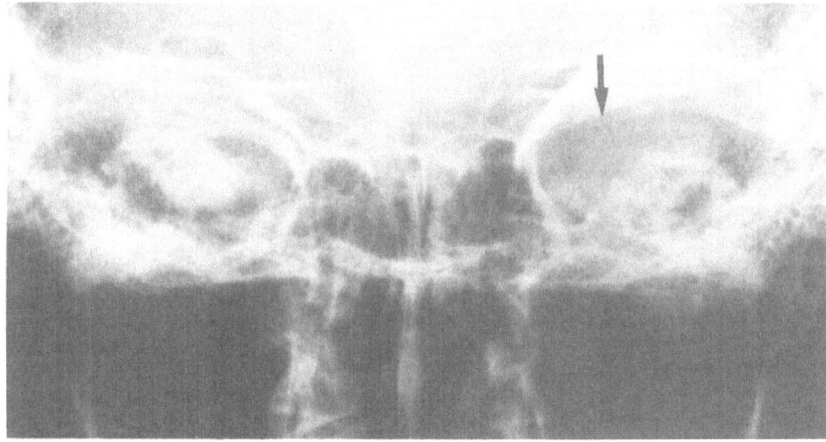

a

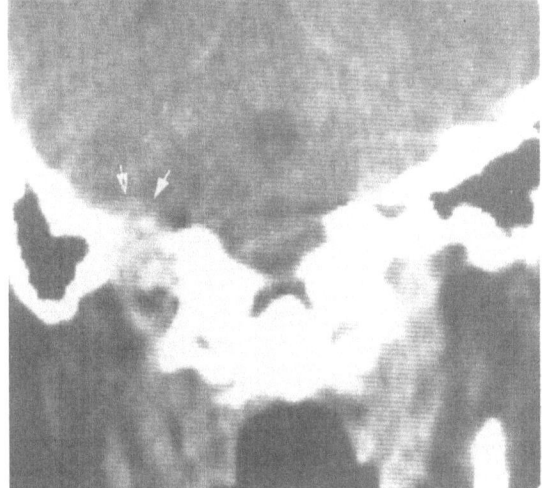

b

Fig. 8.56 a. Perorbital view shows ragged erosion of the petrous apex from a secondary deposit from carcinoma of the breast. (b) The same deposit is shown on this coronal CT section. There is only slight intracranial extension (*arrow*). The patient presented with acute vertigo from labyrinthine involvement.

temporal bone involvement as well as the considerable incidence of melanoma. A comprehensive literature survey by Hill and Kohut (1976) revealed 103 cases of metastatic temporal bone malignancies, to which they added one original case. This paper identified tumours with the greatest proclivity for spread to the temporal bone. They are cancers of the breast, lung, kidney and stomach in that order.

A ragged osteolytic lesion of the petrous pyramid and, particularly, the petrous apex, is the almost invariable radiological finding (Fig. 8.56). The labyrinthine capsule seems relatively resistant to invasion, perhaps because of its limited vascularity.

Facial palsy from invasion of the facial nerve canal is, however, a very common feature. CT may be used to assess the degree of intracranial extension of the deposit.

Extension from Adjacent Sites

Tumours for parotid and nasopharynx in particular can affect the petrous temporal bone by direct extension and be shown by bone erosion (Fig. 8.57) or directly by CT or MRI (Fig. 8.58).

Myeloma

Myeloma of the skull base is rare and fewer than 30 cases have been reported. Presentation as a solitary lesion or plasmacytoma and involvement of the temporal bone are even rarer, there having been few documented cases. Toland and Phelps (1971) described a patient who presented with mixed deafness and serous otitis media. Radiographs showed an extensive destructive lesion in the base of the skull, including the undersurface of the petrous bone. Biopsy showed sheets of plasma cells. There was subsequently further erosion of the occiput and basisphenoid without any sign of systemic disease.

Histiocytosis X

This is a disease of unknown aetiology, characterised by one or more proliferative granulomatous lesions of histiocytes with accumulations of lipid, giant cells and eosinophils.

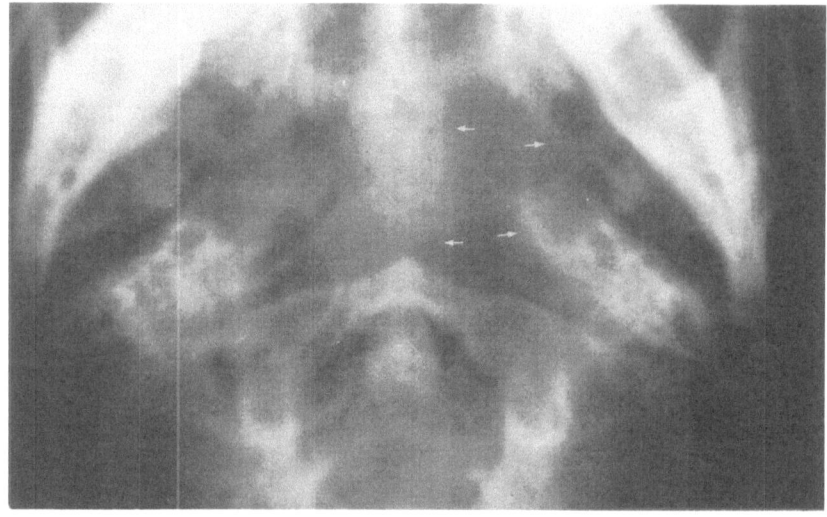

Fig. 8.57. Erosion of the petrous apex and region of the foramen lacerum by a nasopharyngeal carcinoma (*arrows*). Plain SMV view.

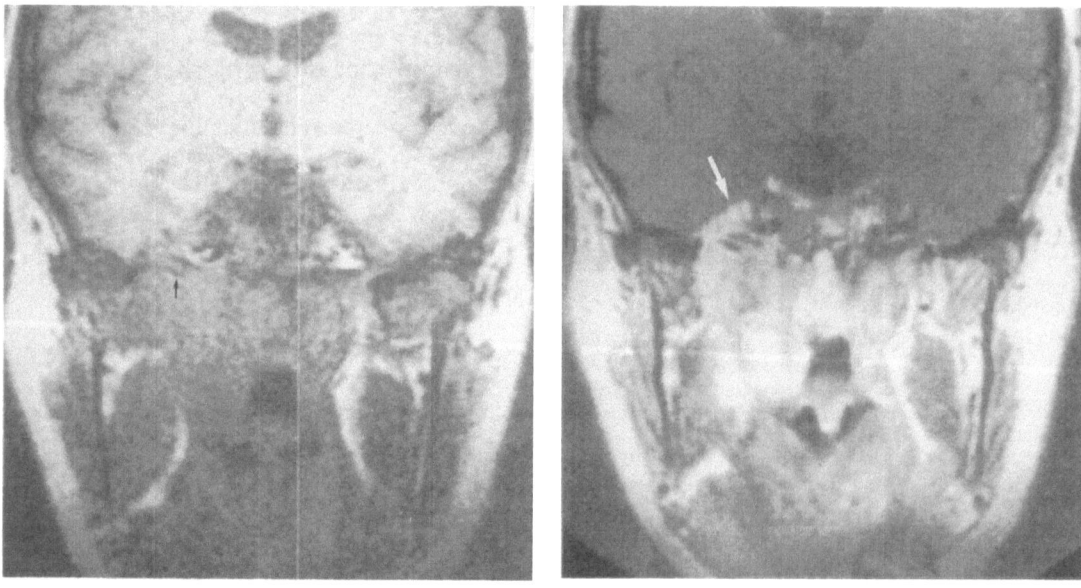

a

b

Fig. 8.58 a, b. An adenoid cystic carcinoma of the parotid which spread upwards through the floor of the middle cranial fossa (*arrow*). T_1-weighted coronal MR scans (a) unenhanced; (b) after Gd. The *small arrow* points to the IAM.

Three variants of histiocytosis X are described which have related manifestations but are symptomatically and prognostically different.

1. Letterer–Siwe disease is usually rapidly fatal and occurs most frequently in children below the age of three years

2. Hand–Schuller–Christian disease was originally described as a triad syndrome manifested by skull destruction, exophthalmos and diabetes insipidus. The latter two components are the result of destructive involvement of the sphenoid bone. In present-day descriptions, the exo-

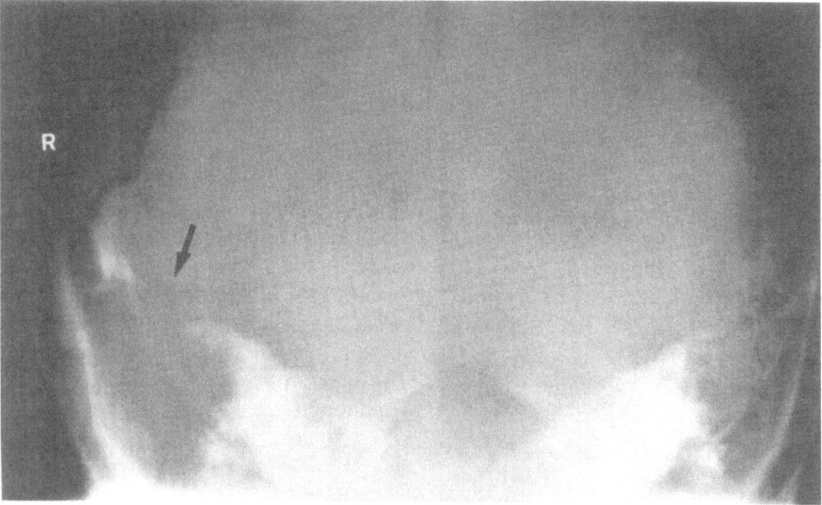

Fig. 8.59. Towne's view showing extensive destruction of the right mastoid from Hand–Schuller–Christian disease in a child.

phthalmos and diabetes insipidus need not occur

3. Eosinophilic granuloma occurs as single or multiple lesion of bone destruction. It is seen more commonly in children or young adults, although it may be found at all ages

Kirtane et al. (1978) described three cases of eosinophilic granuloma who presented with post-auricular swellings. One had a facial palsy, and mastoid radiographs showed osteolytic lesions in all three. Tos (1966) reviewed a total of 500 cases of Hand–Schuller–Christian disease described in the world literature. He found that 61% of these had aural and temporal bone manifestations and that the initial symptoms were from the ear and temporal bone in 16% of cases. He classified these cases into four groups:

1. Temporal bone defects without aural discharge or polyp
2. Aural discharge with temporal bone defects
3. Aural discharge with polyp in the external auditory canal and temporal bone defects
4. Aural discharge without temporal bone defects or polyp

Radiographic changes were varied, with blurring of the mastoid cells, destruction of the septa and defects in the mastoid process or in the petrous pyramid. Only 64 cases had radiological changes without perforation to the surface. In these instances, the destructions usually affected the pyramid and were small. In the great majority of cases, the granuloma primarily involved the mastoid process or the petrous portion, from which it became disseminated to the temporal squama or base of the skull.

There is frequently considerable destruction of the temporal bone, with or without perforation to the surface but without any aural discharge or otitis. Often, the disease is bilateral. Characteristically, the lesions are "punched out" (Fig. 8.59) but the appearances are by no means as diagnostic as they are when deposits of histiocytosis occur in the skull vault.

A mistaken diagnosis of mastoiditis with abscess formation or cholesteatoma is frequently made and even biopsy of an aural polyp may be inconclusive. The prognosis of eosinophil granuloma, with treatment by steroids, surgery and radiotherapy, is more optimistic than with other two variants of histiocytosis (Kirtane et al. 1978).

Xanthoma

Xanthoma are soft tissue tumours composed of lipid-laden, "foamy" histiocytes associated with cholesterol clefts and inflammation. They are considered to be specialised granulomata rather than true neoplasms and are usually associated with disorders of lipid metabolism, most commonly one of the hyperlipoproteinaemia syndromes. A case of xanthoma involving the temporal bone and causing extensive destruction of the skull base was described by Jackler and Brackmann (1987). We have investigated two patients with xanthoma affecting the temporal bone associated with hyperlipidaemia; in one there was a familial association since the patient's mother also had hypercholesterolaemia.

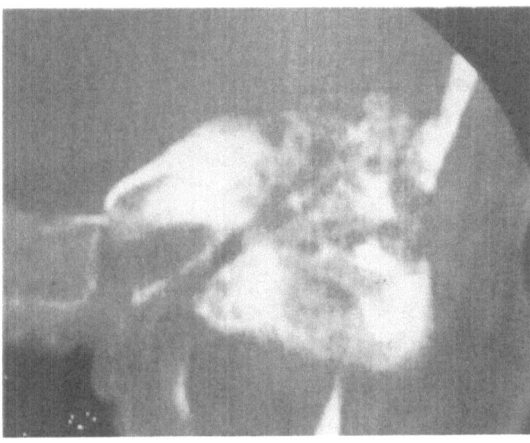

Fig. 8.60. Coronal CT section showing mixed osteolysis and new bone formation from a xanthoma of the petrous temporal bone.

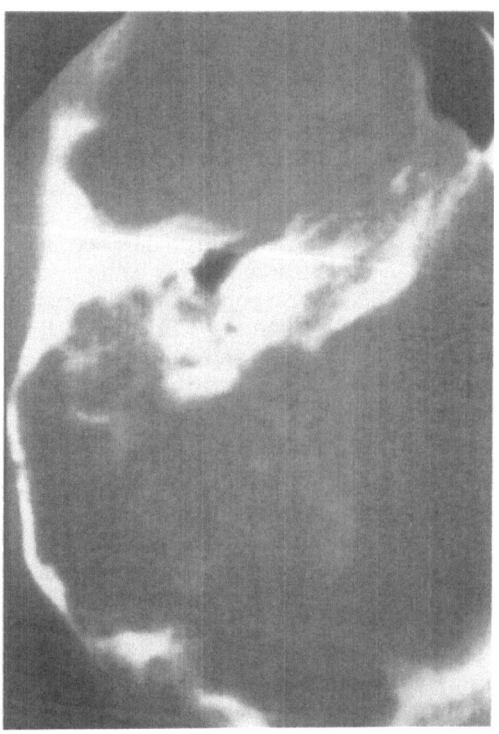

Fig. 8.61. Familial hyperlipidaemia with xanthoma: the base CT shows massive destruction of the petro-mastoid with a partially calcified soft tissue mass in the posterior fossa.

The first patient was a 67-year-old male who presented clinically with a 6-week history of a non-functioning ear and a bony hard mass in the external auditory canal. Conventional radiographs and CT demonstrated a mixture of new bone formation and osteolytic change in the petromastoid (Fig. 8.60). Biopsy revealed dense cortical bone mixed with firm yellowish soft tissue. Microscopy showed extensive xanthoma-cell deposition with cholesterol clefts: the lesion was diagnosed as hypercholesterolaemia xanthomatosis. A second case was seen in a 30-year-old male patient, who presented with a posterior fossa mass and gross destruction of the petromastoid (Fig. 8.61) due to a hyperlipidaemia xanthoma.

References

Arenberg IK, McCreary HS (1971) Neurilemmoma of the jugular foramen. Laryngoscope 81: 544–557

Beale DJ, Phelps PD (1987) Osteomas of the temporal bone: a report of three cases. Clin Radiol 38: 67–69

Bird CR, Hasso AN, Stewart CE, Hinshaw DB, Thompson JR (1983) Malignant primary neoplasms of the ear and temporal bone studied by high-resolution computed tomography. Radiology 149: 171–174

Clairmont AA, Conley JJ (1977) Primary carcinoma of the mastoid bone. Ann Otol Rhinol Laryngol 86: 306–309

Curtin HD (1986) The Facial Nerve Canal. In: Vignaud J, Jardin C, Rosen L (eds). The ear: diagnostic imaging. Masson, Paris, p 329

Dayal VS, Lafond G, Van Nostrand AW, Holgate RC (1983) Lesions simulating glomus tumours of the middle ear. J Otolaryngol 12: 175–179

Delozier HL, Gacek RR, Dana ST (1979) Intralabyrinthine schwannoma. Ann Otol Rhinol Laryngol 88: 187–191

Denia A, Perez F, Canalis R, Graham M (1979) Extracanalicular osteomas of the temporal bone. Arch Otolaryngol 105: 706–709

Evard N, Passy V (1972) Von Recklinghausen's disease with multiple meningiomas. Laryngoscope 82: 2222–2225

Fisch U (1982) Infratemporal fossa approach for glomus tumors of the temporal bone. Ann Otol Rhinol Laryngol 91: 474–479

Glasscock ME III, Jackson CG, Dickin JF et al (1978) Panel discussion: glomus jugulare tumors of the temporal bone. Laryngoscope 89: 1640–1653.

Goebel JA, Smith PG, Kemink JL, Graham MD (1987) Primary adenocarcinoma of the temporal bone mimicking paragangliomas: radiographic and clinical recognition. Otolaryngol Head Neck Surg 96: 231–238

Goepfert H, Langir A, Lindberg R, Ayala A (1979) Rhabdomyosarcoma of the temporal bone. Arch Otolaryngol 105: 310–313

Guzowski J, Paparella MM, Rao KN, Hoshino T (1976) Meningiomas of the temporal bone. Laryngoscope 86: 1141–1146

Harwood-Nash DC (1971) The radiology of rhabdomyosarcomas of the middle ear with intracranial extension in children. Clin Radiol 22: 321–329

Hesselink JR, Davis KR, Taveras JM (1981) Selective arteriography of glomus tympanicum and jugular tumours. AJR 2: 289–297

Hill BA, Kohut RJ (1976) Metastatic adenocarcinoma of the temporal bone. Arch Otolaryngol 102: 568–571

Hyams VJ, Michaels L (1976) Benign adenomatous neoplasms (adenoma) of the middle ear. Clin Otolaryngol 1: 17–26

Jackler RK, Brackmann DE (1987) Xanthoma of the temporal bone and skull base. Am J Otology 8: 111–114

Jahn AF, Farkashidy J, Berman JM (1979) Metastatic tumors of the temporal bone – a pathophysiologic study. J Otolaryngol 8: 85–96

Kirtane JM, Kirtane MV, Karnik PP (1978) Eosinophilic granuloma of the temporal bone. J Postgrad Med 24: 50–54

Koenig H, Lenz M, Sauter R (1986) Temporal bone region high resolution MR imaging using surface coils. Radiology 159: 191–194

Larson TC, Reese DF, Baker HL, McDonald TJ (1987) Glomus tympanicum chemodectomas: radiographic and clinical characteristics. Radiology 163: 801–806

Latack JT, Gabrielsen TO, Knake JE (1983) Facial nerve neuromas radiologic evaluation. Radiology 149: 731–739

Latchaw ER (1986) In: Lee Harker (ed) Otolaryngology Head and Neck Surgery, vol. 4. CV Mosby, St Louis, p 15

Lewis JS (1973) Squamous carcinoma of the ear. Arch Otolaryngol 97: 41–42

Livingstone PA (1974) Differential diagnosis of radiolucent lesions of the temporal bone. Radiol Clin North Am 12: 571–583

Lloyd GAS, Phelps PD (1986) Juvenile angiofibroma: imaging by magnetic resonance CT and conventional techniques. Clin Otolaryngol 11: 247–259

Mafee MF, Valvassori GE, Shugar MA, Yannas DA, Dobben GD (1983) High resolution and dynamic sequential computed tomography use in the evaluation of glomus complex tumors. Arch Otolaryngol 109: 691–696

Mafee MF, Valvassori GE, Kumar A (1988) Tumors and tumor-like conditions of the middle ear and mastoid: role of CT and MRI. Otolaryngol Clin North Am 21: 349–375

Maran AGD, Jacobsen I (1979) Tumours of the ear. In: Maran AGD, Stell PM (ed) Clinical Otolaryngology, Blackwells, Oxford pp 464–469

Mawhinney RR, Buckley JH, Holland IM, Worthington BS (1986) The value of magnetic resonance imaging in the diagnosis of intracranial meningiomas. Clin Radiol 37: 429–439

Mazzoni MD, Pareseki R, Calabrese MD (1988) Intratemporal vascular tumours. J Laryngol 102: 353–356

Michaels L, Wells M (1980) Squamous carcinoma of the middle ear. Clin Otolaryngol 5: 235–248

Moody DM, Ghatak NR, Kelly DL (1976) Extensive calcification in a tumor of the glomus jugulare. Neuroradiology 12: 131–135

Moyes PD, Bratty PJA, Dolman CL (1970) Osteoclastoma of the jugular foramen. J Neurosurg 32: 255–257

Nager GT (1967) Gliomas involving the temporal bone. Laryngoscope 77: 454–488

Olsen WL, Dillon WP, Kelly WM, Norman D, Brant-Zawadski M, Newton TH (1987) MR imaging of paragangliomas. AJNR 148:201–204

Parisier SC, Som PM, Shugar JMA, Marovitz MF (1978) The evaluation of middle ear meningiomas using computerised axial tomography. Laryngoscope 88: 1170–1177

Phelps PD, Lloyd GAS (1981) The radiology of carcinoma of the ear. Br J Radiol 54: 103–109

Phelps PD, Lloyd GAS (1986) Vascular masses in the middle ear. Clin Radiol 37: 359–364

Phelps PD, Stansbie JM (1988) Glomus jugulare and tympanicum. The role of CT and MR with Gadolinium DTPA. J Laryngol 102: 766–776

Phelps PD, Toland JA, Sheldon PWE (1970) Erosions of the petrous temporal bone. J Laryngol 84: 1205–1230

Proops DW, Mann JR (1984) The presentation of rhabdomyosarcomas of the head and neck in children. J Laryngol 98: 381–390

Pulec JL (1972) Facial nerve neuroma. Laryngoscope 82: 1160–1172

Rosenwasser H (1974) Glomus jugulare tumours. Proc R Soc Med 67: 259–264

Saito H, Baxter A (1972) Undiagnosed intratemporal facial nerve neurilemmomas. Arch Otolaryngol 95: 415–419

Stell PM (1984) Carcinoma of the external auditory meatus and middle ear. Clin Otolaryngol 9: 281–299

Swartz JD (1986): Imaging of the Temporal Bone, vol 9. Thieme Medical Publishers, New York

Toland JA, Phelps PD (1971) Plasmacytoma of the skull base. Clin Radiol 22: 39–43

Tos M (1966) A survey of Hand–Schuller–Christian's disease in otolaryngology. 62: 217–228

Valavanis A, Schubiger O, Naiditch TP (1987) Clinical Imaging of the Cerebello-pontine Angle, Springer-Verlag, Berlin, pp 100, 116, 170, 95.

Valvassori GE (1974) Benign tumors of the temporal bone. Radiol Clin North Am 3: 533–540

Wiet RJ, Lotan AN, Monsell EM, Shambaugh GE (1983) Tumour involvement of the facial nerve. Laryngoscope 93: 1301–1308

Wolfowitz BL, Schmaman A (1973) Giant cell lesions of the temporal bone. S Af Med J 47: 1397–1399

9 Lesions of the Internal Auditory Meatus and Posterior Cranial Fossa: the Investigation and Differential Diagnosis of Acoustic Neuroma

No aspect of imaging in ENT practice has changed so much in the last ten years as the investigations for acoustic neuroma. Yet despite the tremendous advances in imaging, there is still no simple, readily available, cheap, non-invasive test, either clinical or radiological, which will conclusively confirm or exclude the presence of a small tumour in the internal auditory meatus. Consequently, a great deal of time is spent investigating patients with unilateral signs and symptoms confined to the VIIIth nerve.

Internal Auditory Meatus (IAM)

The IAM is a bony sleeve surrounding four components of two cranial nerves and the vascular supply to the inner ear. It gradually assumes its definitive shape and position during fetal life, with development of the labyrinth, growth of the skull base and ossification of the petrous temporal bone. Various studies have been undertaken to assess the normal range of sizes and shapes of the IAM (Papangelou 1972; Valvassori and Pierce 1964). These authors stress the lack of variation between the two sides in normal cases (Fig. 9.1). The vertical diameter or "width" of the IAM is the most important measurement and 2–8 mm is usually accepted as the normal range, with only 1–2-mm variation

between the width of the porus, fundus or middle of the meatus. The length is less important and more variable, with an average length of floor and roof of approximately 12 mm. The length may depend partly on the degree of pneumatisation of the petrous apex. These figures should be used only as a guide; exceptions are found which have no

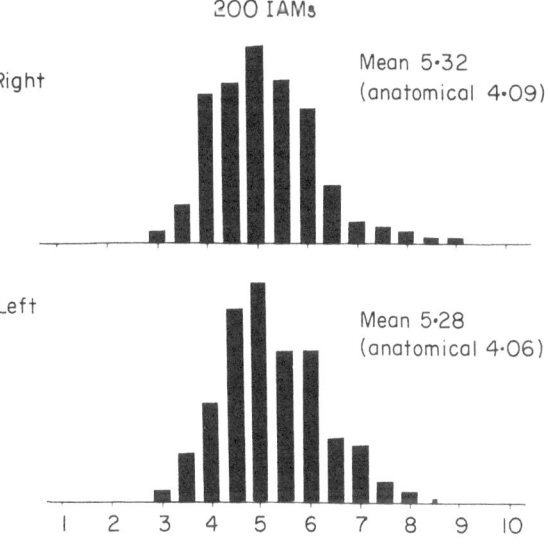

Fig. 9.1. The width of 200 normal IAMs based on measurements made on coronal section tomograms.

Fig. 9.2. Zonogram showing typical flaring of the IAM by an acoustic neuroma.

pathological significance. Dolan et al. (1978) provide a good review of the problem and report nine cases of unilateral enlargement of the IAM, as shown on tomography and subsequent free-filling of the large meatus with contrast medium.

Traditionally, studies of the bony margins of the IAM have always been the major investigation when looking for acoustic neuromas, especially when previously the definitive demonstration was only possible by the major invasive procedures of cerebral angiography and air encephalography. There is now a tendency to do all screening assessments on a clinical basis and then follow with imaging studies. We believe, however, that bone studies of the IAM by conventional techniques are still an integral part of the initial investigation and provide a quick and cheap screening procedure; hence the study of the IAMs will be fully described.

Towne's and Stenver's views may be used to show the IAMs on plain X-ray but the perorbital projection, particularly if a magnification technique is used, provides the best demonstration. This view will satisfactorily show expansion of the porus, especially if there is solid bone around the meatus, but if there is pneumatisation of the petrous pyramid, as in 30% of patients, the IAMs may not be adequately shown, with the danger of false positive or false negative evaluation. Plain radiographs do not, therefore, provide adequate bone studies, and zonograms are preferred. Using rotational zonography with 10–12° angulation of tube arc, exposures are made in a similar head position to the perorbital view, producing films which are in effect a superior version of this projection (see Chap. 1). When a large number of patients need to be screened to exclude an acoustic neuroma, zonography is a satisfactory method since only two or three zonograms are needed to show if the IAM's are normal (Fig. 9.2). When there is suspected abnormality, it may be useful to augment these coronal projections with lateral tomograms, which

will show when apparent expansion is, in fact, due to asymmetry and also give the best assessment of air cells around the meatus (Fig. 9.3). The bony margins of the IAM can also be studied by high resolution CT although, in our opinion, less satisfactorily. This, however, will result in excessive scan time especially if large numbers of patients with VIIIth nerve symptoms need to be screened and if the necessary views in two planes are obtained to exclude simple asymmetry of the IAMs (congenital aberrations have been considered in Chap. 3).

Acquired Disease

The IAM may be narrowed by bone dysplasias such as Paget's disease and fibrous dysplasia (Fig. 11.16) and in such rare congenital bone disorders as osteopetrosis. Subsequent mechanical pressure on the nerves in the IAM as a cause for the hearing loss seems doubtful, as the loss is mainly cochlear in type (Olivares and Schucknecht 1979). A more common abnormality is expansion by a space-occupying lesion, such as a tumour or cyst, and rarely a vascular anomaly of the posterior fossa. For acoustic neuroma, Valvassori (1969) gives the following criteria of abnormality in the IAM as shown by tomography:

1. Erosion of the cortical line surrounding the lumen of the canal seen in the lateral tomograms
2. Widening of 2 mm or more of any portion of the IAM when compared with the corresponding segment of the opposite canal
3. Shortening of the posterior wall of the canal by at least 3 mm in comparison with the opposite side
4. Demonstration of the crista falciformis running closer to the inferior than to the superior wall. The crista should normally be located at or

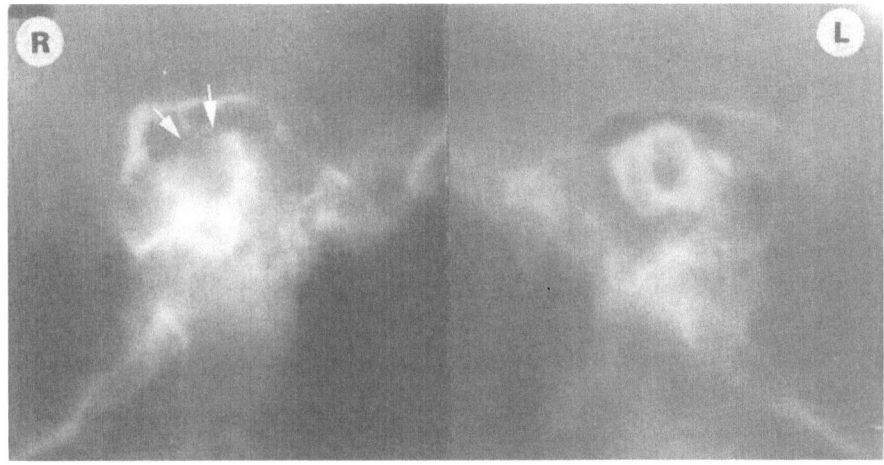

Fig. 9.3. Lateral tomograms of a patient with extensive bilateral pneumatisation of the petrous pyramid. Note the erosion of the roof of the IAM on the right (*arrow*), indicating the presence of an acoustic neuroma.

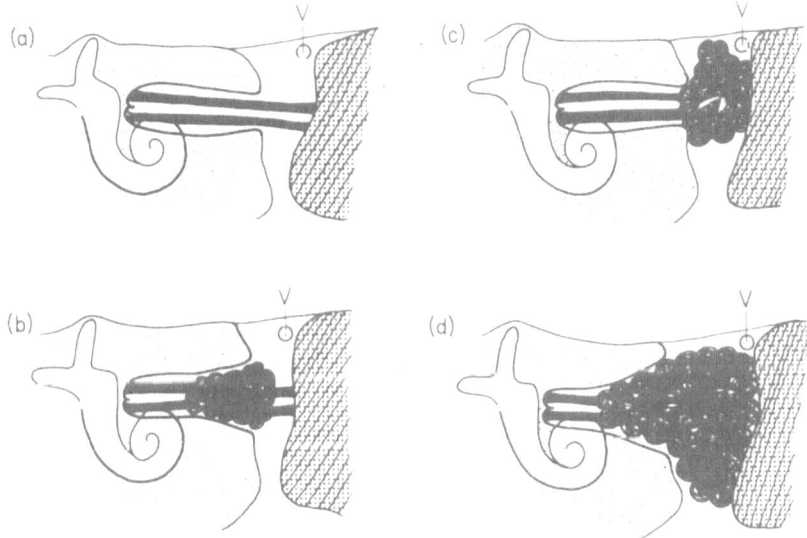

Fig. 9.4 a. Diagram based on coronal tomograms showing the nerves in the IAM passing from brainstem to labyrinth; **b** predominantly intrameatal; **c** extrameatal; **d** large acoustic neuromas. V, trigeminal nerve.

above the mid-point of the vertical diameter of the canal

The majority of acoustic neuromas arise within the IAM (Fig. 9.4). The tumour then grows medially into the cerebello-pontine angle and, as it does so, it produces expansion of the IAM at its medial end with erosion of the posterior wall. The typical appearance suggesting an acoustic neuroma is therefore a "funnel shaped" IAM (Fig. 9.2) and assessment of the state of the meatus at the porus or medial end is of the utmost importance.

A less common but more pathognomonic appearance of the IAM occurs when there is irregular and pronounced destruction of the walls of the meatus (Fig. 9.5). Why a minority of neuromas should produce this type of erosion, instead of the more usual expansion of the IAM, is unknown.

Other space-occupying lesions which may expand the IAM include facial nerve neuromas, arachnoid cysts, anomalies of the basilar artery (Rao and Woodlief 1979), often without hearing loss (Azar-Kia et al. 1976), and aneurysms. Eleven cases of aneurysm of the anterior inferior cerebellar

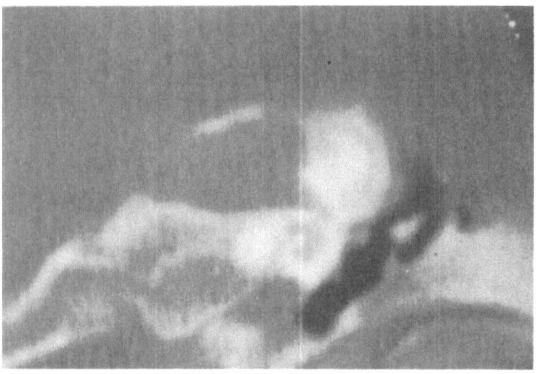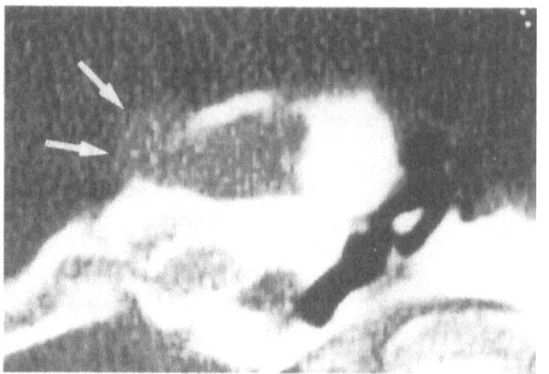

a   b

Fig. 9.5 a, b. High resolution CT. **a** Wide window setting shows the bone destruction around the IAM. **b** After contrast enhancement the neuroma can be seen protruding into the cerebello-pontine angle (*arrow*).

artery were reported by Johnson and Kline (1978). Ten of these had facial paralysis and four had enlargement of the IAM.

Cerebello-pontine Angle

The cerebello-pontine angle cistern is a triangular space limited medially and anteriorly by the pons and by the cerebellum posteriorly. The flocculus of the cerebellum often overhangs the angle. Laterally lies the medial wall of the petrous pyramid and the porus of the IAM which is just in front of the mid-

point of the posterior wall. The porus usually has an oval shape. The tentorium forms the roof of the cerebello-pontine angle and the jugular tubercle the floor.

Neurovascular Anatomy of the IAM and Cerebello-pontine Angle

The VIIIth cranial nerve, in close association with the VIIth, which lies anterior to it, passes from the brainstem across the cerebello-pontine angle to enter the porus of the IAM. An extension of the subarachnoid space from the angle surrounds the

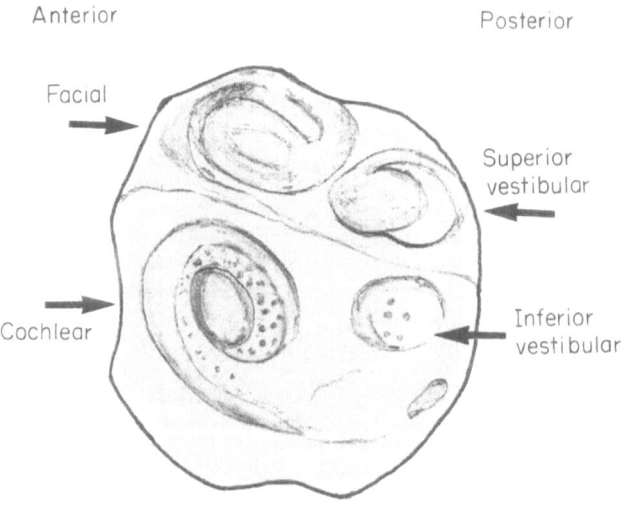

Anterior   Posterior

Facial

Superior
vestibular

Cochlear

Inferior
vestibular

Fig. 9.6. The lateral end of the IAM and the openings for the nerves in the lamina cribrosa.

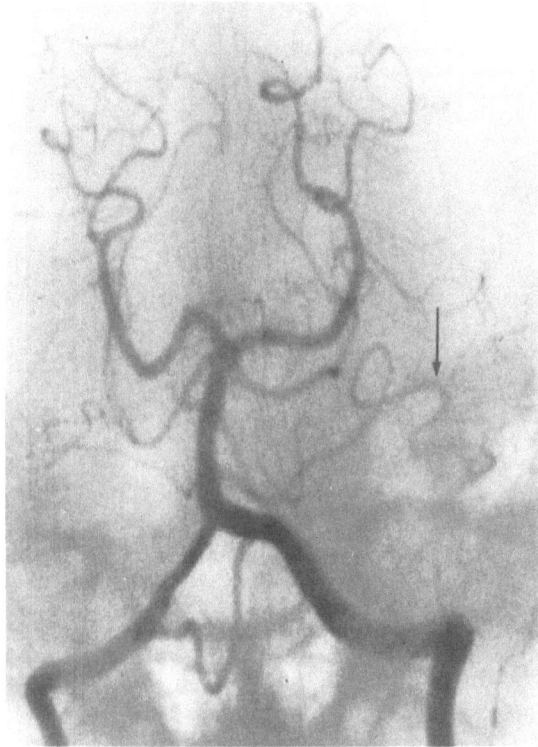

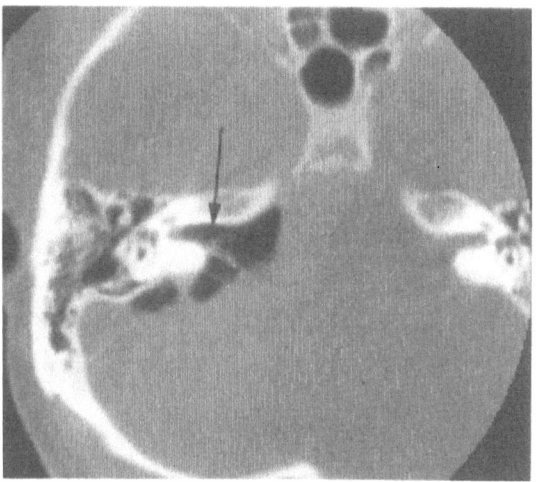

Fig. 9.8. The loop of the AICA extending into the porus of the IAM.

Fig. 9.7. Preoperative vertebral angiogram. The *arrow* points to the loop of the anterior inferior cerebellar artery, adjacent to the porus of the left IAM. On this side, the AICA is larger than the PICA, an unusual variant.

nerves in the meatus. The lateral end of the meatus can be divided into four quadrants for the components of these two cranial nerves, as shown in Fig. 9.6.

The principal blood supply of the inner ear is from the labyrinthine artery which almost always arises from the anterior inferior cerebellar artery (AICA). The AICA varies considerably in size and position and its distribution is usually in inverse proportion to the posterior inferior cerebellar artery (PICA) (Fig. 9.7). It forms a distinctive loop before supplying part of the pons and cerebellum. Mazzoni (1969), in a study of 100 human specimens, found the loop of the AICA to lie inside the IAM in 40% of cases, at the porus in 27% and in the cerebello-pontine angle in 33%. However, the loop extends to the lateral half of the IAM in only 5% of people. This loop can be shown by high-resolution air-CT meatography (Fig. 9.8; Phelps and Lloyd 1982). The AICA is usually pushed upwards by acoustic tumours (Fig. 9.9) and its recognition and preservation are very desirable when surgical exicision is undertaken.

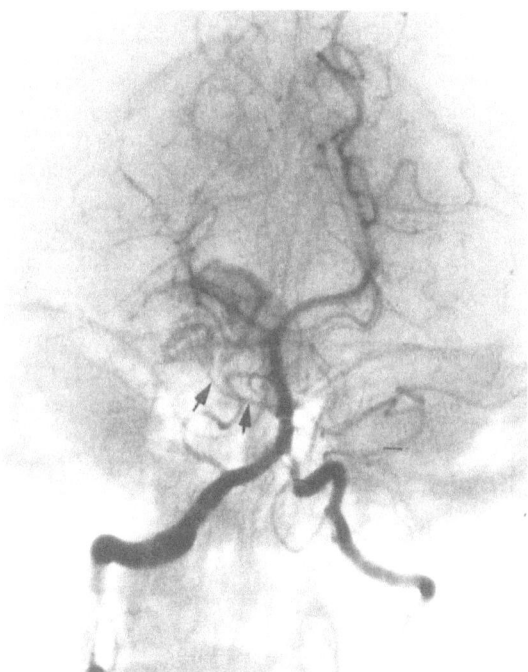

Fig. 9.9. A very vascular acoustic neuroma with a prominent pathological circulation. The *arrows* indicate elevation of the AICA.

This close association of the AICA with the VIIIth nerve suggests that the artery may be the cause of dysfunction of the nerves. Applebaum and Valvassori (1984) reported hearing loss in ten patients with prominent vascular loops in the ipsilateral IAM but not in the other ear. This deafness was of the

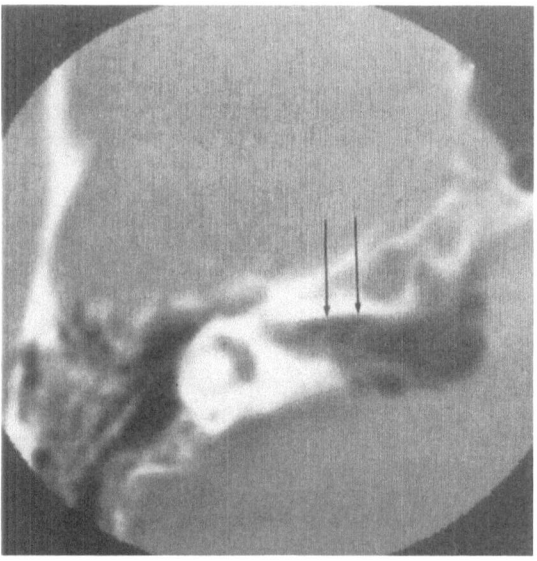

Fig. 9.10. A double loop of AICA (*arrows*).

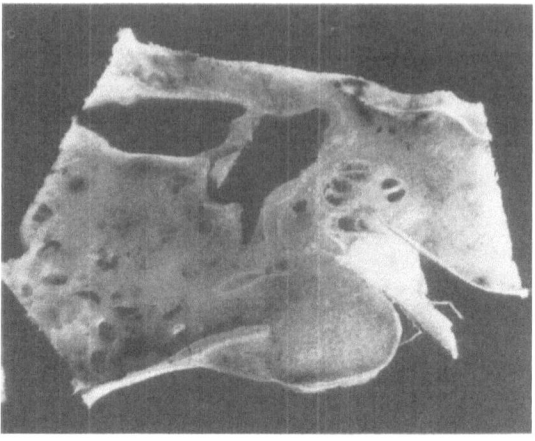

Fig. 9.11. Histological section of a temporal bone showing an acoustic neuroma arising within the IAM from one of the vestibular nerves. Note the compression of the cochlea nerve as it passes from the base of the modiolus of the cochlea. The neuroma was an incidental finding in a bone from the "temporal bone bank".

cochlear type with excellent speech discrimination and caloric tests were normal. On the other hand, McCabe and Harker (1983) considered that vascular loops surgically verified in close association with the nerves in the IAM were the cause of vertigo and severe motion intolerance. In each of their eight cases, a loop large enough to indent the nerve was present, and in one case a double loop was found, one loop on each side of the superior vestibular nerve flattening it visibly between the loops. We have also seen a double loop of AICA in a vertiginous patient (Fig. 9.10).

Acoustic Neuroma

Pathogenesis

Acoustic tumours are benign, well encapsulated lesions with a variable rate of growth. Duration of symptoms may vary from a few weeks to 40 years or more, and symptomless vestibular tumours, some within the labyrinth are occasionally found in sectioned temporal bones (Fig. 9.11). However, in a review of 214 patients with large acoustic neuromas treated at the Radcliffe Infirmary, Oxford, the average period between onset of symptoms and significant neurological deficit necessitating surgical relief was only 4.5 years (Ellis and Wright 1974). The majority of acoustic neuromas arise from the

vestibular part of the VIIIth nerve, usually the superior division.

There is much confusion over nomenclature of these tumours, resulting mainly from the uncertainty about the cell of origin. Electron microscope studies have shown that this is almost certainly the Schwann cell, and therefore, "schwannoma" would seem the correct term, although "neuroma" is the best known. The distal part of the VIIIth nerve is invested by Schwann cells and this presumably accounts for the majority of acoustic neuromas arising in the IAM, from which they characteristically extend medially into the cerebellopontine angle.

Vascularity of the tumours is variable, as is well shown by vertebral angiography (Fig. 9.7) and by the variable degree of contrast enhancement shown on CT scans. Necrosis and cystic change is usual in large tumours, accounting for the variable attenuation of the lesion on enhanced CT. Occasionally, acoustic neuromas may contain large cysts.

Bilateral tumours are rare (Fig. 9.12) and are usually associated with neurofibromatosis. In this disease, vestibular schwannomas occur in about 5% of reported cases and are nearly always bilateral (Schuknecht 1974). There may be one or multiple schwannomas involving an individual nerve or any of numerous nerves, as well as one or multiple meningiomas.

Microscopically, in most cases of neurofibromatosis, the acoustic neuroma is identical on H and E stain to any of the usual unilateral tumours.

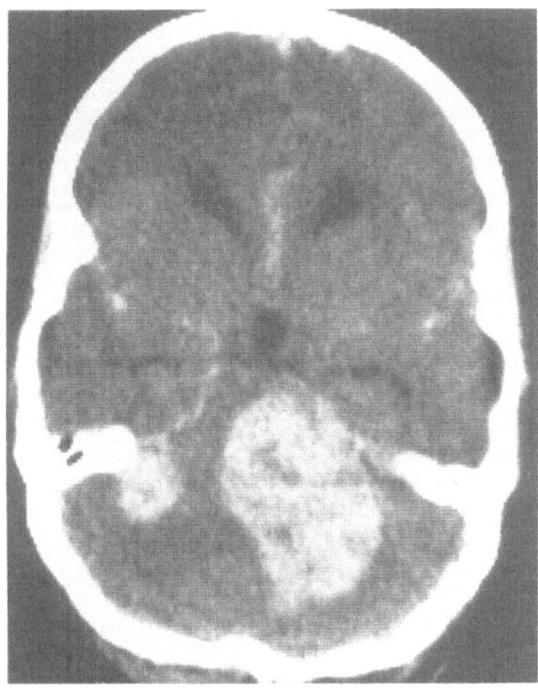

Fig. 9.12. Bilateral acoustic neuromas in a patient with neurofibromatosis. Note the areas of low attenuation in the larger tumour, presumably representing areas of necrosis.

Occasionally, the tumours in neurofibromatosis may show areas that appear to be intermediate in pattern between meningioma and schwannoma. Another feature of neurofibromatosis is the association with dura ectasia (Sarwar and Swischuk 1977). Just as widening of the spinal canal and foramina occurs without the presence of intraspinal tumour, so patulous IAMs may sometimes be filled with contrast medium when cisternomeatography is undertaken to exclude an acoustic neuroma.

Clinical Features

These are very variable and depend on the site of origin and rate of growth; a slow-growing tumour may reach a considerable size before it produces symptoms other than unilateral deafness. However, otologists see hundreds of patients with unilateral cochlear dysfunction, very few of whom have an acoustic neuroma. Careful radiological assessment is, therefore, necessary before proceeding to sophisticated and expensive radiological investigations, which will decide whether or not there is a neuroma present. Only a broad outline of these clinical features will be given here.

The first sign of involvement of the cochlear nerve is a loss of speech discrimination that is disproportionate to the pure tone threshold as shown on a standard audiogram. The patient may discover the loss when using the telephone. Speech audiometry is, therefore, an important test as is that for auditory adaptation (tone decay) which is usually present with an acoustic neuroma. Fluctuant or sudden hearing loss may occur due to interference with the blood supply or venous drainage of the inner ear and Morrison (1975) estimated that 17% of acoustic neuromas present with sudden deafness.

Although the majority of tumours arise from the vestibular nerve, vestibular symptoms are often minimal or absent because the vestibular system readily compensates for vestibular deficits. Attacks of vertigo are most unusual and the most common complaint is a feeling of unsteadiness. Impaired caloric response occurs in over 80% of cases and the authors believe that the caloric test should be performed before any radiological investigation.

Gross facial dysfunction is a most unusual feature of acoustic neuroma, except as a very late sign. This is because the facial nerve seems to be able to tolerate a considerable degree of stretching around the tumour, although sophisticated tests of the facial nerve function may show some impairment. In the authors' experience, a cerebello-pontine mass that presents with a facial palsy is almost always found to be another type of lesion such as a cholesteatoma. When the tumour fills the cerebellopontine angle, either from extension out of the meatus, or at an early stage in the 20% of cases where the origin is from the extrameatal portion of the VIIIth nerve, then the so-called neurological stage is reached. Pressure on the Vth nerve causes pain or altered sensation in the face and loss of the corneal reflex is an important sign. Brainstem and cerebellar signs, VIth nerve loss, headache and papilloedema, indicating raised intracranial pressure, are all features of very large tumours.

In recent years, sophisticated objective audiometric tests have been introduced which have shown a high success rate in predicting the presence of an acoustic neuroma. Impedance audiometry is accurate but can only be used if hearing is present.

The best screening audiometric test has in recent years proved to be brainstem-evoked response (BSER), otherwise known as auditory brainstem response (ABR). This is a simple procedure and a normal tracing almost excludes an acoustic neuroma. However, there is a high rate of false positives, especially in patients with Ménière's disease and the test is unsatisfactory if the hearing loss is greater than 75 dB. Thus claims of 98% success rate (Johnson and Selters 1987) are unrealistic if patients with poor hearing are first excluded. The Royal National series (Pfleiderer et al. 1988) showed that ABR provided positive diagnostic information in 54% and in 65% of those studied by electrocochleography. In combination, 92% of acoustic neuromas were correctly suspected on one of these tests. Electrocochleography can be done on the same machine as ABR but besides increasing the length of the examination, has the disadvantage of being invasive, albeit with an extremely low morbidity.

Screening assessments of vestibular function should always be obtained before computerised imaging is requested, despite their relatively high false positive and false negative rates. This should be by caloric testing with or without electronystagmography.

Computerised Tomography with Intravenous Contrast

Acoustic neuromas show variable attenuation. In about 50% this is similar to normal brain but may be more or less or mixed. However, almost all acoustic neuromas show some degree of contrast enhancement and should appear on the scan if they are of sufficient size (Fig. 9.13). Indirect signs, such as displacement of the brainstem and fourth ventricle, obliteration and widening of the cisterns and ventricular dilatation from obstructive hydrocephalus, indicate the presence of a space-occupying lesion.

Improvements in scanner technology have lessened the problem of posterior fossa artefacts caused by the dense bone of the petrous pyramids. Typically acoustic neuromas are round or lobulated (Fig. 9.14), often with non-homogeneous areas of enhancement. Areas of low attenuation may be due to cystic changes in the tumour.

Schubiger et al. (1978) have shown the advantages of thin overlapping sections for the diagnosis of small acoustic neuromas. Eight proven acoustic neuromas, 1 cm or less in diameter, were detected by these authors. Nevertheless, ordinary brain-scan techniques are at present unreliable for the detection of tumours less than 1.0 to 1.5 cm in size.

We perform a limited brain scan when an acoustic neuroma is suspected. One section 4-mm thick is obtained at the level of the IAMs. The chin of the patient is slightly depressed so that the section passes just above the orbits. Five 4-mm sections at 4-mm intervals are than obtained after intravenous contrast injection. These should cover the posterior fossa from the jugular tubercles to the petrous ridges above. One further section 2 cm higher, is then obtained to confirm that the ventricles are not dilated. It is important to exclude obstructive hydrocephalus and the danger of "coning" before proceeding to posterior fossa contrast studies. Sections in the coronal plane may help to assess the tumour size.

Air CT Meatography

To outline small tumours in the cerebello-pontine angle or confined to the meatus, it is necessary to introduce contrast into the subarachnoid space by

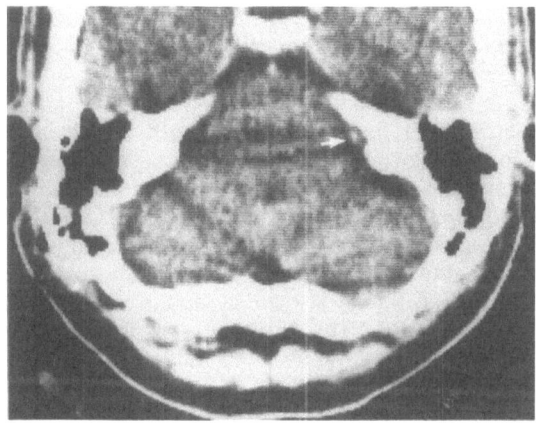 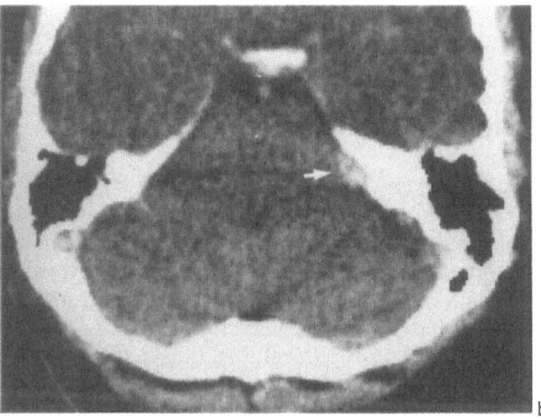

a   b

Fig. 9.13. Contrast-enhanced posterior fossa brain scan. The *arrow* shows a small acoustic neuroma in the cerebello-pontine angle. The two sections were taken 3 years apart and show the growth of the tumour. The patient refused operation (from Scott Brown's *Otolaryngology* Vol 3).

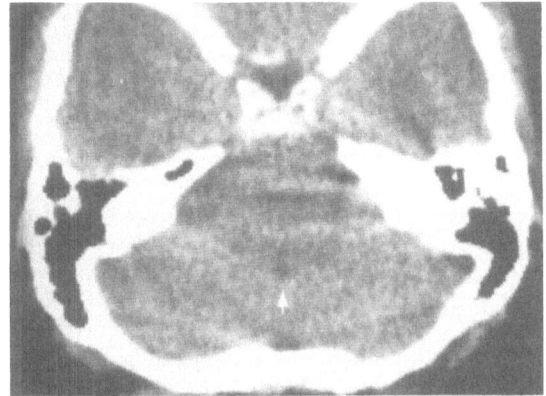

a

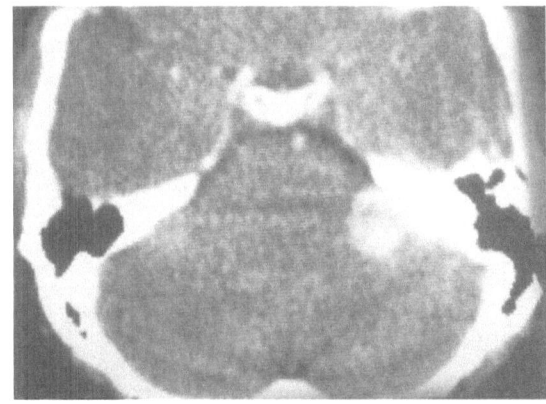

b

Fig. 9.14 a, b. Pre (a) and post-contrast (b) equivalent sections showing an acoustic neuroma. Note that the fourth ventricle is mid-line (*arrow*).

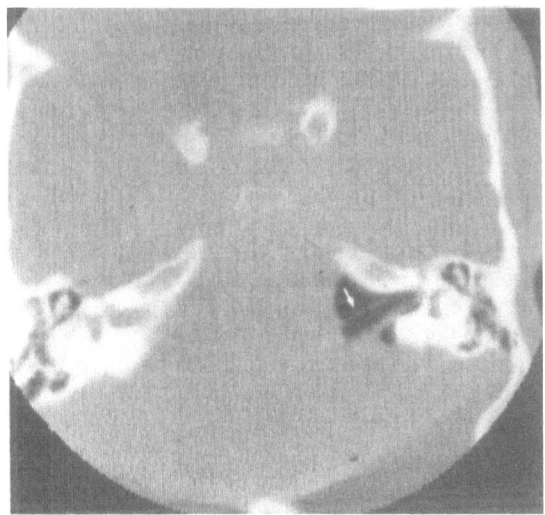

Fig. 9.15. A normal air meatogram showing VIIth (*arrow*) and thicker VIIIth cranial nerves in the IAM.

lumbar or cisternal puncture, and then manipulate it into the relevant part of the posterior cranial fossa. Air, oxygen, iophendylate (Myodil) and the water-soluble contrast medium Metrizamide, have all been used with fluoroscopy, plain views, tomography and computerised tomography. For complete exclusion of the presence of an acoustic neuroma, it is necessary to demonstrate the contrast within the IAM. This was previously only possible with iophendylate. We used very small quantities of the oily contrast with pluridirectional tomography. However, iophendylate is a known cause of arachnoiditis. Metrizamide is similarly not entirely free of complications, as well as being unsatisfactorily demonstrated within the IAM. Positive contrast studies have now been almost completely superseded by air CT meatography, a simple and safe procedure. The technique is described in detail below.

The patient lies on his side on the scanner table, with the ear to be examined uppermost. A lumbar puncture is performed and CSF sent for differential protein estimation. At a sufficient spinal gradient to allow it to pass up into the cervical region, 3 ml of air are introduced. After 2 minutes, the head is elevated momentarily to allow the air to pass through the foramen magnum and into the cerebello-pontine angle. This is the only time the head is displaced from the true lateral position during the examination. The first section is made at the level of the IAM and if air is demonstrated in the meatus, then the examination is ended. More air may need to be introduced if the cerebello-pontine angle has not been filled sufficiently. If air fails to fill the meatus and no definite space-occupying lesion has been shown, then the other ear should be examined. It is often possible to use the same 3 ml of air for this by turning the patient through the prone position onto his other side. The patient can usually feel the air enter the meatus.

Not only can air be demonstrated in the meatus by this technique, but various normal structures can also be recognised (Phelps and Lloyd 1982): in particular, the VIIIth nerve and often the VIIth nerve close to it (Fig. 9.15); but also the loop of the AICA, which may be in the angle, the porus of the IAM, or within the IAM (Fig. 9.8). Small acoustic neuromas may be shown protruding from the meatus (Fig. 9.16). If the tumour fills the angle, or alternatively is confined to the meatus, the demonstration may not be so definite. Non-filling of the IAM is not diagnostic of an intrameatal mass unless a definite convex border can be shown adjacent to the air (Fig. 9.17). In any doubtful case, where non-filling may be due to surface tension effects (the so-called "tomato ketchup" phenomenon), the

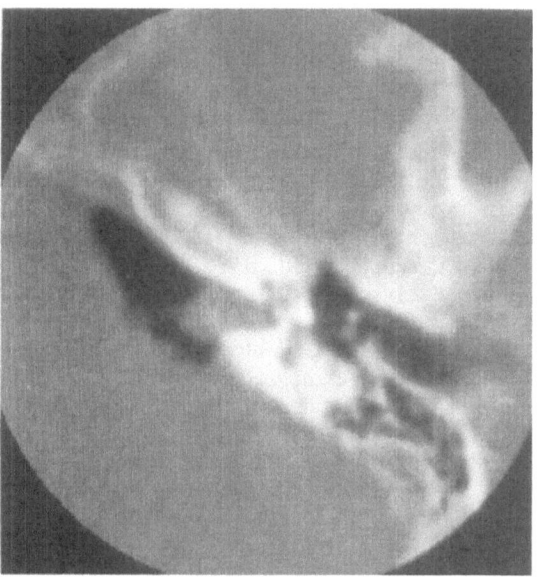

Fig. 9.16. Air meatogram. A small neuroma protrudes from the IAM. Note the coils of the cochlea.

patient's head should be shaken gently and then repositioned.

When first introduced, air CT meatography was thought to be an entirely innocuous procedure because of the small amount of air and the fine needles used. The patients were allowed to go home 1–2 hours afterwards. However, although no serious complications have been reported, it now appears that there is a significant level of morbidity in the form of headaches and general malaise occurring 1–2 days after the procedure (Greenberger et al. 1987). These authors recommend a return to 24-hour hospitalisation and recumbent posture. Our smaller series has shown similar results with two of 20 patients saying that they would not have the procedure repeated. It is not clear whether the ill-effects are due to the lumbar puncture, or the air but use of carbon dioxide or oxygen, which are more rapidly absorbed, might help. Our present policy is to allow patients to go home after 4–5 hours of lying flat as long as they have only a short car journey in a recumbent seat. Replacement of CT by magnetic resonance will obviate the problem.

Magnetic Resonance Imaging

Magnetic resonance is now better than CT for the investigation of lesions of the posterior fossa. Multiplanar imaging, lack of beam-hardening artefacts and improved density resolution, especially for lesions of the brainstem, are significant advantages. These make MR the investigation of choice for posterior fossa abnormalities, and MR has now been recommended as the primary imaging investigation when neurological examination indicates a retrocochlear lesion (Mafee 1987; Valvassori 1988).

The MR appearance of acoustic neuroma depends upon the pulse sequence used but at present, tissue specificity is limited (Stack et al 1988). The majority of acoustic neuromas appear on T_1-weighted images with a density similar to brain but appear brighter than the surrounding CSF (Fig. 9.18a). On T_2-weighted images, neuromas usually have a similar signal intensity to CSF but slightly greater than brain (Fig. 9.18b). However, they are often non-homogenous in intensity, especially if large. Small tumours may easily be missed on T_2-weighted images if there is no mass effect and the lesion is entirely or mostly confined to the IAM. It may also be confused with the usual bright signal from the normal nerves (Fig. 9.19). The use of surface coils can improve the anatomical demonstration of the structures in the petrous temporal bone but this is more than outweighed by the distinct dis-

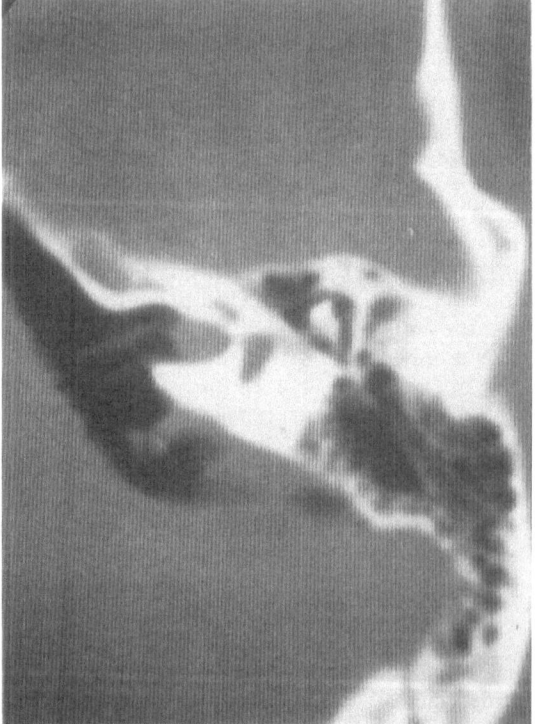

Fig. 9.17. Air meatogram. A smaller intrameatal neuroma. Note the convex outer margin.

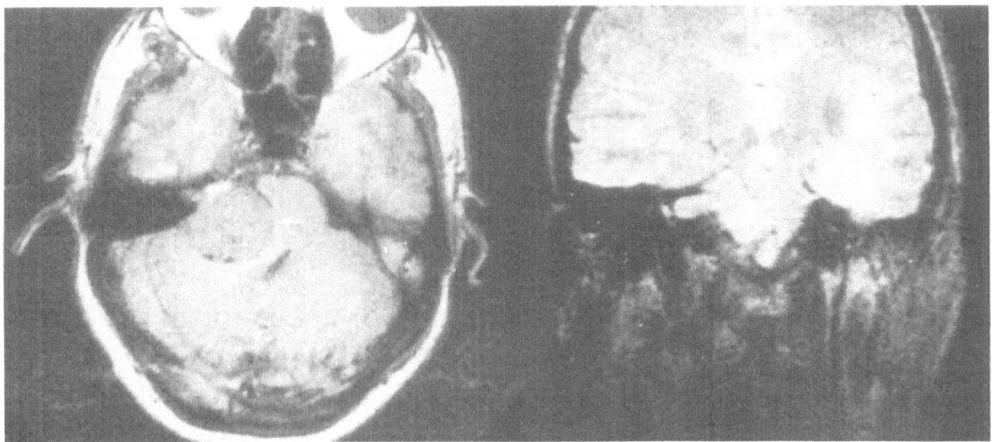

Fig. 9.18 a. T_1-weighted (SE 700/26) base MR section showing a large acoustic neuroma protruding from the IAM displacing the fourth ventricle and distorting the brainstem. (**b**). T_2-weighted (SE 1500/80) coronal MR section of the same neuroma with a bright signal similar to that from CSF. Note the non-homogeneous nature of the tumour.

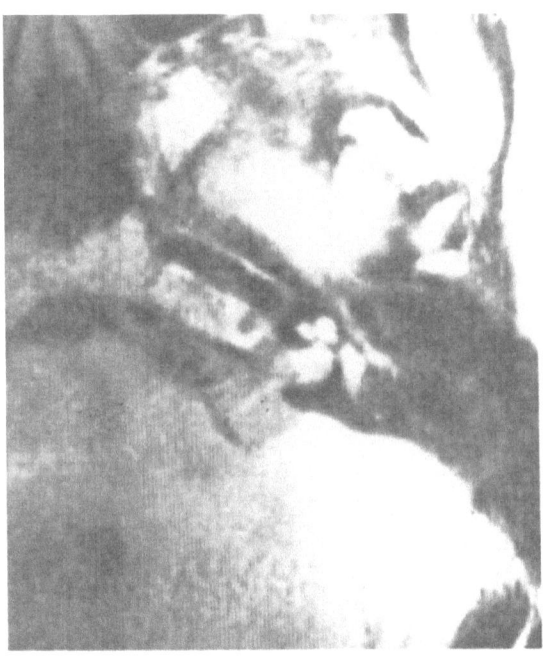

Fig. 9.19. A small (5 mm) surgically proven acoustic neuroma in the lateral end of the IAM. The tumour has equal signal intensity with the labyrinthine fluids and VIIth and VIIIth cranial nerves on this SE 1500/30 image with surface coil.

Magnetic Resonance with Enhancement by Gadolinium DTPA (GdMR)

Intense and homogeneous enhancement of all acoustic neuromas occurs after the intravenous administration of the paramagnetic contrast agent Gadolinium DTPA. Although GdDTPA has been shown to have no adverse side effects, it is only now being released for general use. Initial assessment showed that inversion recovery sequences (Fig. 9.20) give maximum enhancement followed by a short spin-echo protocol (Curati et al. 1986). Therefore, T_1-weighted sequences are required and a very accurate estimation of the tumour size, both in the IAM and the posterior cranial fossa, is provided (Fig. 9.21). Thus GdMR has replaced air meatography completely and moreover, has also been shown to be effective to demonstrate other masses in the posterior cranial fossa, both intra- and extra-axial (Stack et al. 1988). Some of these will be described subsequently.

Vertebral Angiography

With rare exceptions, vertebral angiography is no longer considered to be a diagnostic procedure for acoustic neuromas, but most neurosurgeons require it for preoperative assessment of the vascular anatomy in the region of the tumour. Angiography will also exclude the presence of an aneurysm or vascular anomaly mimicking a neoplasm. The vascularity of acoustic tumours varies greatly, most barely revealing their presence, others

advantages of being unable to compare the two sides. Surface coils are therefore not desirable for the detection of small acoustic neuromas. We would recommend initial T_2-and proton-density-weighted axial images such as TR 2000 and a double echo TE of 30 and 70 msec. This protocol is followed by T_1-weighted coronal sections (TR 500 TE 30).

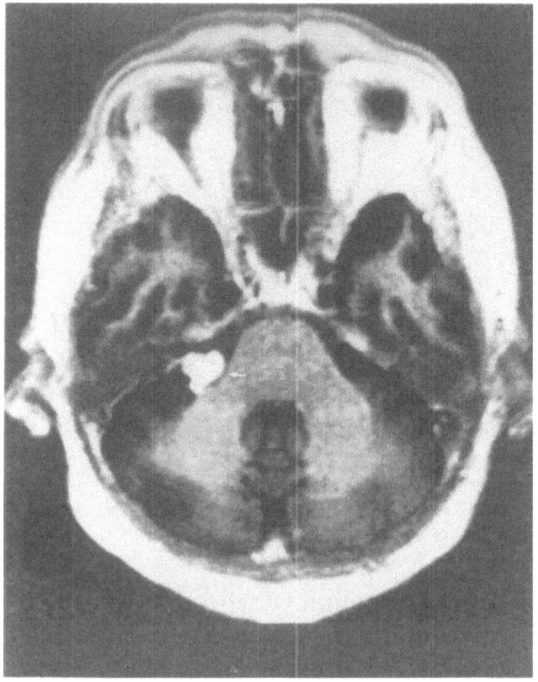

Fig. 9.20. A very bright signal from Gadolinium-enhanced acoustic neuroma in the cerebello-pontine angle on this inversion recovery sequence (IR 2800/600).

◀―――――――――――――――――――――――――――

showing extensive pathological circulation (Fig. 9.9).

Differential Diagnosis of Acoustic Neuroma

Acoustic neuromas account for 90% of tumours within the cerebello-pontine angle. The differential diagnosis of large tumours is primarily the differentiation of masses in the posterior cranial fossa and therefore outside the scope of this book.

Meningiomas are the next most common neoplasm that occur in the cerebello-pontine angle.

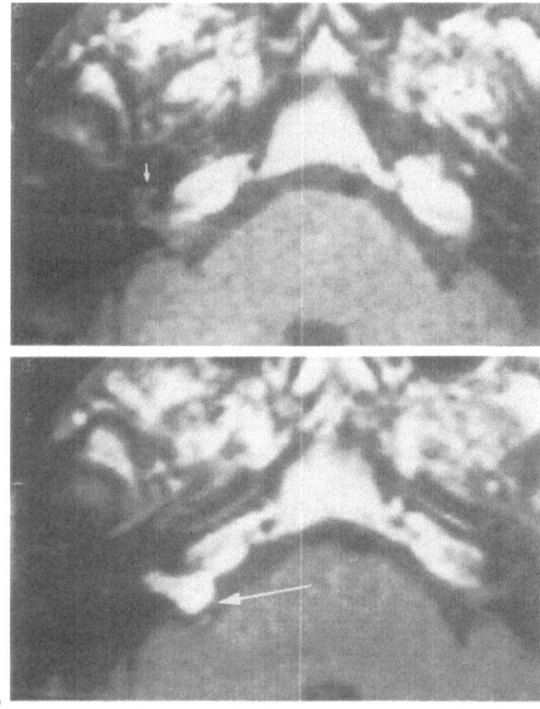

a

b

Fig. 9.21 a, b. Base T_1-weighted MR scan of a small acoustic neuroma in the IAM and cerebello-pontine angle shown before (a) and after (b) intravenous injection of GdDTPA (*arrow*). The *small arrow* points to the cochlea.

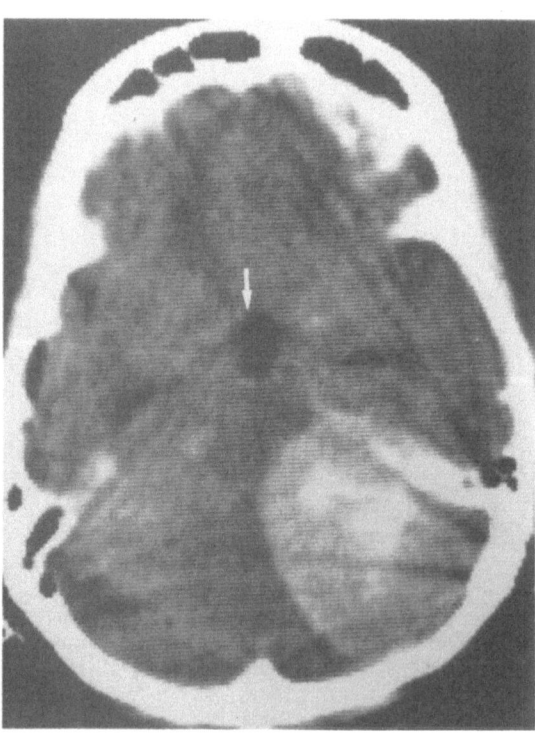

Fig. 9.22. Meningioma of the posterior cranial fossa: a smoothly outlined, homogeneously enhancing mass containing areas of calcification. The calcification was not shown on plain film or tomograms. Note the dilated third ventricle (*arrow*) indicating obstructive hydrocephalus. The patient had minimal symptoms and signs.

Several differentiating features have been described (Moller et al. 1978). Unlike the acoustic neuromas, the meningiomas often calcify. Both tumours may be large. Acoustic neuromas expand mainly posteriorly and medially and rarely have a broad attachment to the petrous bone. Meningiomas may be oval, which is unusual with acoustic tumours, and their long axis lies parallel to the petrous pyramid with an obtuse angle between the medial free tumour border and the bony surface (Valavanis et al. 1987). Changes in the IAM are rare with meningiomas and frequent with neuromas. Dense homogenous enhancement, a smooth outline (Fig. 9.22) and sometimes hyperostosis of the

petrous ridge are other features of a meningioma in the posterior fossa, although bony changes are less frequent than with sphenoidal ridge meningiomas. Occasionally, the hyperostosis of the petrous pyramid may result in narrowing of the IAM (Fig. 9.23) and a small exostosis at the base of the tumour can represent the hilum of the feeding vessels.

Magnetic resonance has not in general terms proved as satisfactory as CT for the demonstration of meningiomas (Mawhinney et al. 1986). The tumours often have a signal intensity similar to brain on both T_1 and T_2-weighted sequences and, unless there are secondary changes due to the mass effect, they may be missed. A peripheral rim of low intensity is thought to represent the tumour capsule (Fig. 9.24). Intense enhancement occurs after GdDTPA however (Stack et al. 1988), and this is obviously necessary for the best assessment for tumour extent.

Cholesteatoma (epidermoid) occurs in the angle or more anteriorly alongside the petrous apex (Phelps and Lloyd 1980). Non-enhancement of the lesion and low or even negative attenuation values are characteristic features (see Chap. 7), as is the irregular margin; a characteristic but, unfortunately, not

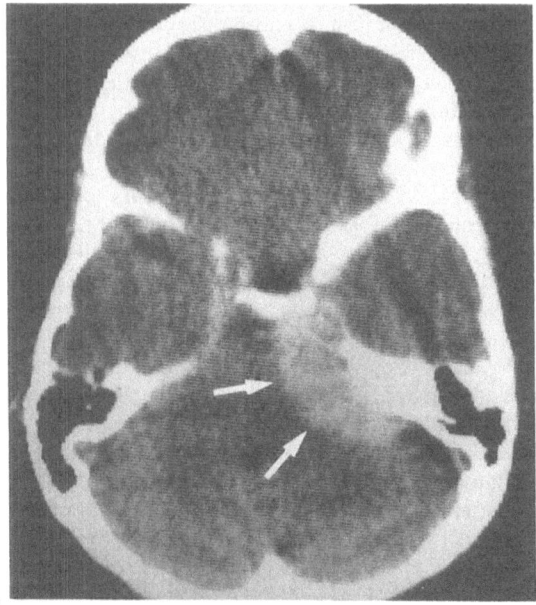

a

b

Fig. 9.23 a, b. A meningioma arising from the anterior petrous ridge. (a) Base CT showing the hyperostosis narrowing the porus of the IAM. (b) After contrast enhancement, showing the extent of the tumour.

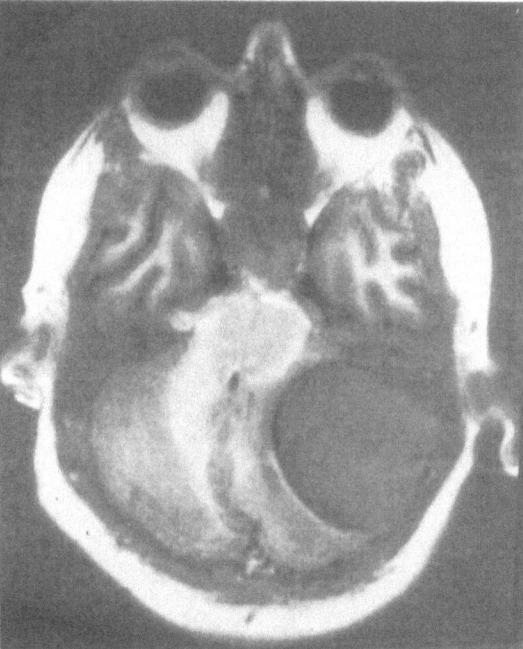

Fig. 9.24. Meningioma of the posterior cranial fossa well shown on inversion recovery MR sequence (IR 3200/800). Note the characteristic low signal rim probably representing the venous capsule around the tumour.

a constant feature which serves to distinguish epidermoids from arachnoid cysts.

Arachnoid Cysts

Approximately 0.5% of tumours of the cerebello-pontine angle are found at surgery to be arachnoid cysts but it is probable that there are many more small cysts of the IAM that produce minimal or no symptoms (Schuknecht and Gao 1983). These authors reported three cases of arachnoid cysts of the IAM in a histological study. The cysts had caused compression atrophy of the nerves in the IAM and severe VIIth and VIIIth nerve deficiencies in vivo. Other cases have been reported of marked expansion of the IAM, especially the mid portion, by an arachnoid cyst (Thyssen et al. 1976). Such space-occupying lesions in the IAM can be differentiated reliably from acoustic neuromas pre-operatively but the more common arachnoid cyst of the posterior cranial fossa will appear as a hypo-intense mass on enhanced CT, with a smooth outline which helps to differentiate it from the cauliflower appearance of an epidermoid. The cyst may cause pressure erosion of the posterior surface of

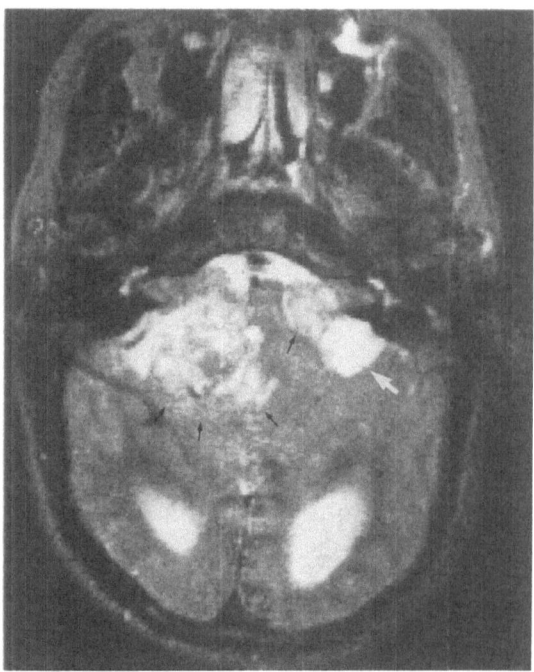

Fig. 9.25. Bilateral acoustic neuromas (*black arrows*) rather poorly demonstrated on this T$_2$-weighted base MR scan (SE 3200/90). There is a stronger signal from an arachnoid cyst associated with the smaller of the two neuromas (*white arrow*).

the petrous bone. The MR appearances show similar features, but with signal characteristics equivalent to CSF on the various protocols used (Fig. 9.25). The association of arachnoid cysts with acoustic neuromas is a common feature of large tumours.

Lipomas

Intracranial lipomas are extremely rare but have been found in the IAM (Olson et al. 1978) where they cause clinical features similar to acoustic neuromas.

Gliomas

Gliomas (Fig. 9.26) or large glomus jugulare tumours from below may appear as enhancing masses in the region of the cerebello-pontine angle. The pattern of bone erosion of the petrous pyramid will, however, suggest an extrinsic mass. Neuromas arising from the IXth, Xth and XIth nerves in the jugular fossa, may also extend up into the cerebello-pontine angle (See Chap. 8).

Neurofibromatosis

There are two distinct forms of this autosomal dominant disorder, which was described in Chap. 4 with other congenital syndromes. Central neuro-fibromatosis is the defined form of the disease, which presents typically with bilateral acoustic neuromas, but other tumours of the central nervous system, both axial and extra-axial, and particularly meningiomas, are found. There have recently been accounts of large numbers of patients affected by neurofibromatosis examined by magnetic resonance (Braffman et al. 1988; Bognano et al. 1988). These authors recommend a screening MR study in this population because of the large number of asymptomatic lesions detected.

Recent experience with GdMR in the assessment of a young patient with neurofibromatosis has convinced us of the need to use enhanced MR for this condition. This patient's only complaint was severe bilateral hearing loss, and a previous plain MR examination suggested only the acoustic neuromas. Gd MRI revealed a large trigeminal neuroma; and multiple meningiomas including several "en-plaque" lesions. However, the most relevant lesion was a tumour in the cervical spinal cord (Fig. 9.27). This case demonstrates the advantages of the use of Gadolinium, not only for neuromas, but for detecting meningiomas and intraspinal tumours.

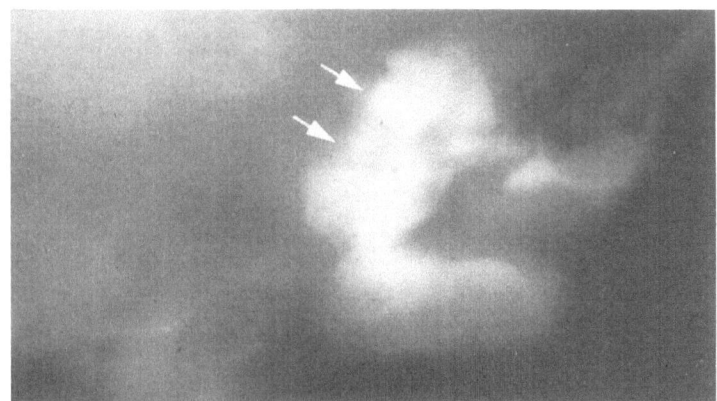

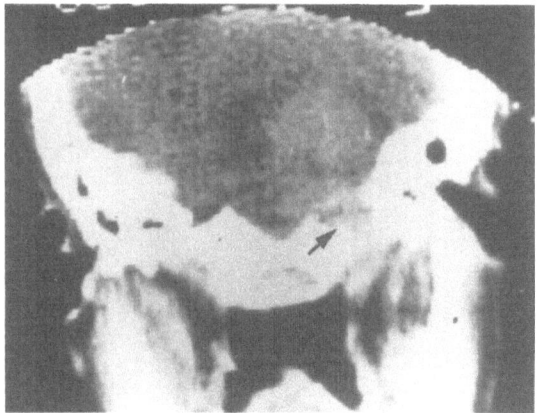

Fig. 9.26 a, b. An astrocytoma arising in the cranial cavity has here eroded the posterior surface of the petrous pyramid of the jugular fossa. (a) Coronal tomogram showing erosion of the posterior surface of the petrous bone. (b) Coronal CT showing the soft tissue mass as well as the eroded jugular fossa (*arrow*).

Conclusion

The variable and often insidious nature of presentation of small acoustic neuromas results from their differing rates of growth and points of origin on the VIIIth cranial nerve. Imaging provides not only the definitive demonstration of the tumour and its size and situation, but we believe has a most important role in screening the large numbers of patients with minimal signs and symptoms confined to the VIIIth nerve who are seen by the otologist. Approximately 1% of patients referred with sensorineural hearing loss and a suspected acoustic neuroma will eventually be shown to have a tumour (Pfleiderer et al. 1988). Only a minority require the full imaging investigation. There is, therefore, a need for an initial screening examination, which includes bone studies by conventional tomography, evoked response audiometry and caloric testing, before employing the definitive investigation of gadolinium-enhanced magnetic resonance. This regime is quick, cheap

and totally non-invasive and if two out of three of these tests are positive (Terkildsen and Thomsen 1983) there is a clear indication to proceed to GdMR without using CT.

An alternative screening protocol using ABR and contrast-enhanced CT has been advocated (Barrs et al. 1985) but cannot be considered totally non-invasive since contrast reactions, although rare, do occur with the iodine-containing compounds. It is possible to use CT for all stages of the imaging investigation for acoustic neuroma, but this involves two injections, one intravenous and one intrathecal, and is not to be recommended. Air meatography has a significant morbidity, as described above, and is not suitable for large acoustic neuromas or other masses in the posterior fossa, which first need to be excluded by brain-scan techniques. Magnetic resonance is the primary investigation of choice for pathology of the posterior cranial fossa, which can be less satisfactorily demonstrated by enhanced CT if MR is not available. These lesions are mostly outside the scope of this work, but some which may present to the neur-

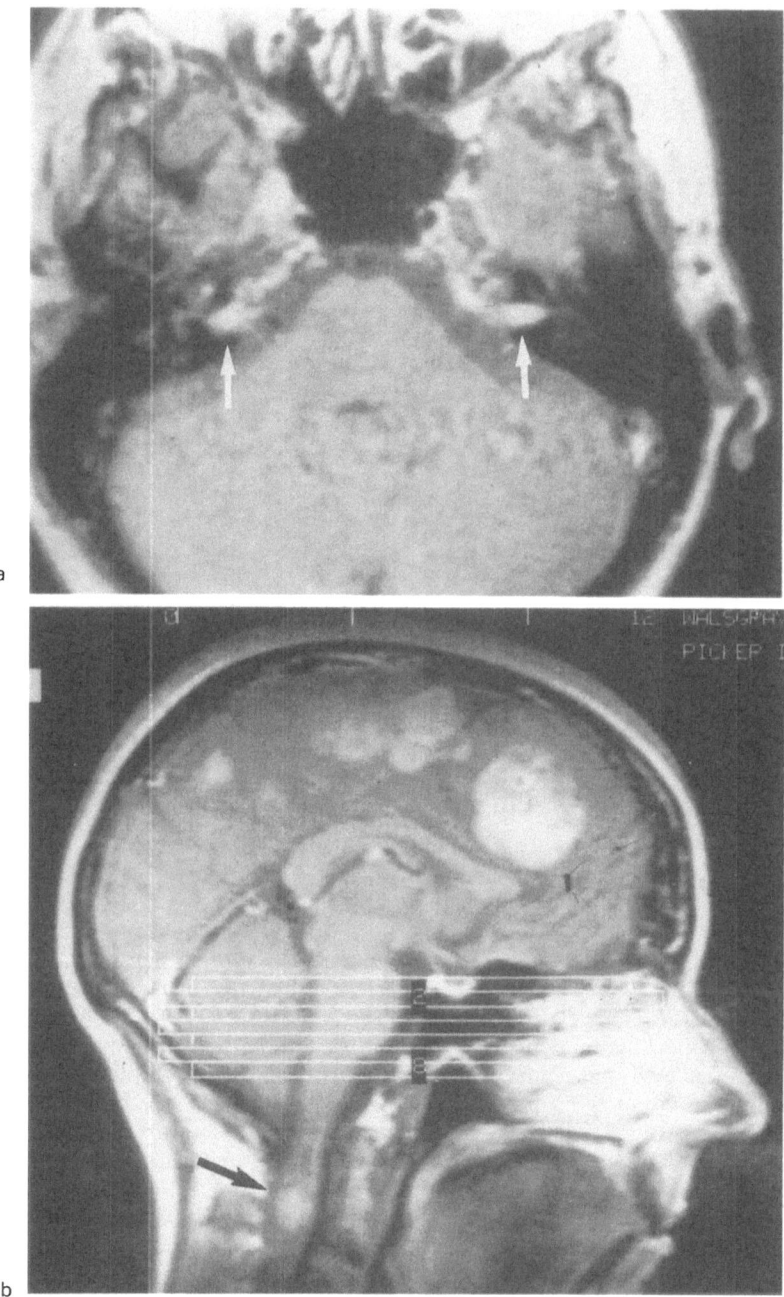

Fig. 9.27 a, b. Neurofibromatosis. (a) Base GdMR scan shows bilateral intrameatal acoustic neuromas (*arrows*). See also Fig. 8.33. (b) Lateral GdMR scout view revealed not only multiple intracranial meningiomas and neuromas, but also a tumour in the cervical cord (*black arrow*).

Fig. 9.28. Equivalent sections of air meatograms done 6 months apart showing considerable growth of the acoustic neuroma and prompting surgical intervention despite the age (67 years) of the patient. Note that in each section, the signet ring sign of the vestibule and lateral semicircular canal can be identified. (From Phelps and Lloyd 1987).

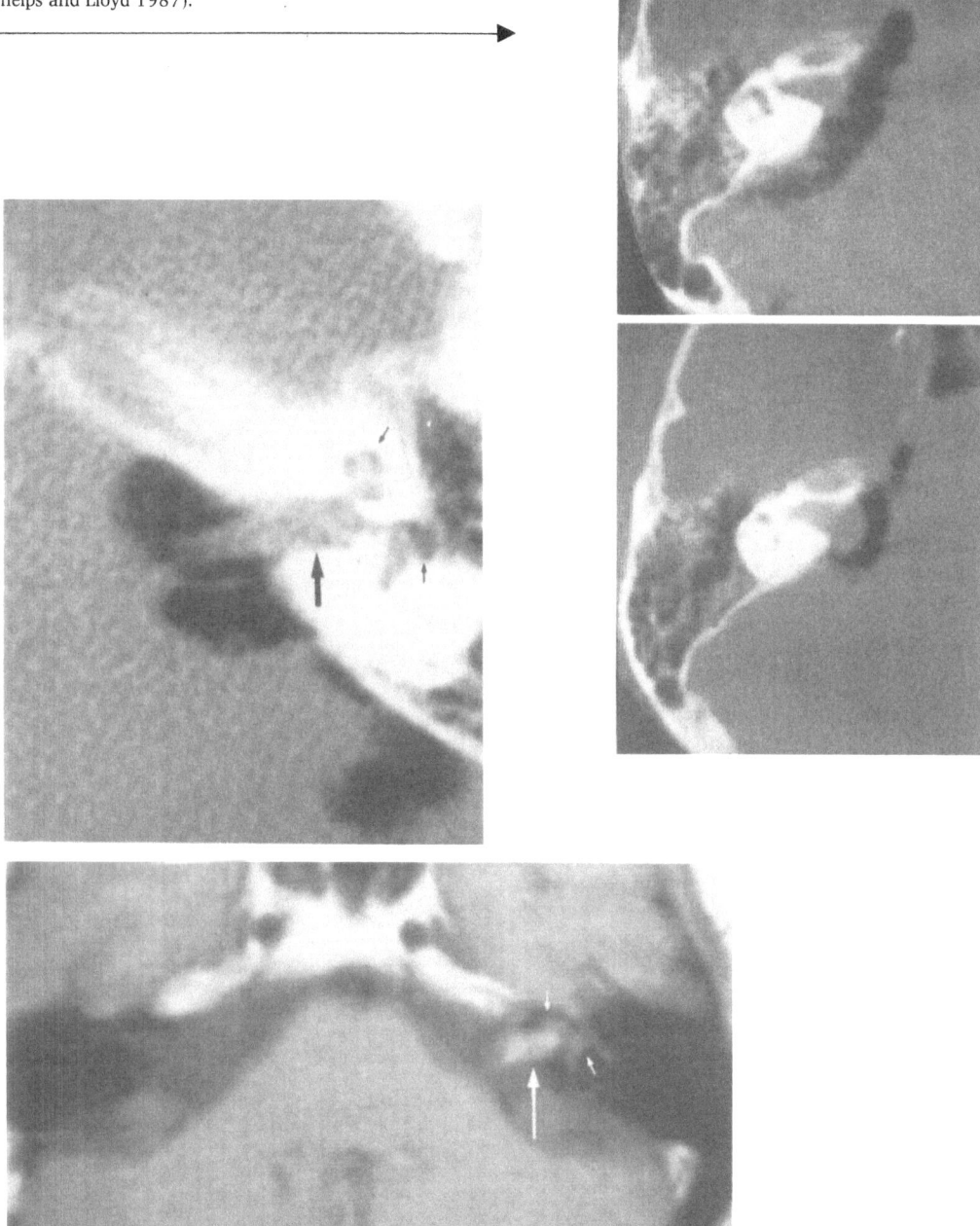

a

b

Fig. 9.29 a. Air meatogram showing an intrameatal acoustic neuroma (*large arrow*). The *small arrows* point to the cochlea in front and vestibule. (**b**) GdMR scan at the same level and showing the same features rather better. It is most important not to confuse the bright signal from the marrowfat in the petrous apex on these short spin echo, T_1–weighted images. This is especially important if no precontrast MR scans are obtained. A sound knowledge of MR petrous temporal bone anatomy is obviously important.

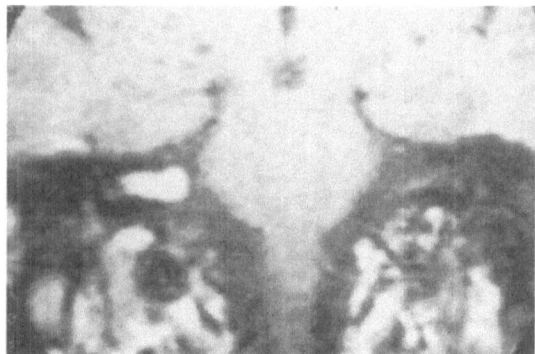 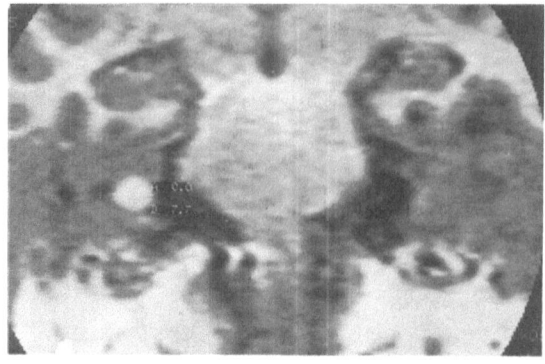

a   b

Fig. 9.30 a, b. Coronal MR scans of small acoustic neuromas. (**a**) A small neuroma fills the IAM and extends out into the cerebello-pontine angle (SE 500/26). (**b**) An even smaller tumour with a measured size of 7.7 mm is very well shown in the IAM on this inversion recovery sequence (IR 2000/400).

otologist, largely because of central vertigo, will be considered in the next chapter.

Small acoustic neuromas, wholly or largely confined to the IAM, can be demonstrated by magnetic resonance but not as reliably as by air meatography. This is unfortunate, because surgery for small tumours needs careful consideration and will depend mainly on two factors:

1. The age of the patient
2. The rate of growth of the tumour

The latter can only be partially assessed on the basis of deteriorating clinical features and really needs serial imaging studies (Fig. 9.28) (Phelps and Lloyd 1987). Gadolinium-enhanced MR will overcome these problems and rapid scans, with intravenous GdDTPA given before the patient goes into the scanner, will enable all acoustic neuromas to be demonstrated with an accurate estimation of their size, extent and position (Fig. 9.29). We would advocate short spin-echo T_1-weighted images in base and coronal planes with inversion recovery sequences if a better demonstration is required (Fig. 9.30).

References

Applebaum EL, Valvassori GE (1984) Auditory and vestibular system findings in patients with vascular loops in the internal auditory canal. Ann Otol Rhinol Laryngol (Suppl) 112: 63–70

Azar-Kia B, Palavos E, Spak M (1976) The megadolichobasilar artery anomaly and expansion of the internal auditory meatus. Neuroradiology 11: 109–111

Barrs DM, Brackmann DE, Olson JE, House WF (1985) Changing concept of acoustic neuroma diagnosis. Arch Otolaryngol 111: 17–21

Bognano JR, Edwards MK, Lee TA, Dann DW, Roos KL, Klatte EC (1988) Clinical MR imaging in neurofibromatosis. AJR 151: 381–388

Braffman BH, Bilanuik LT, Zimmerman RA (1988) The central nervous system manifestations of the phakomatoses on MR. Rad Clin North Am 26: 773–800

Curati WL, Graif M, Kingsley DPE, Neindorf HP, Young IR (1986) Acoustic Neuromas: Gd DTPA enhancement in MR imaging. Radiology 158: 447–451

Dolan KD, Babib RW, Jacoby CG (1978) Asymmetry of the internal auditory canals without acoustic neuroma. Ann Otol Rhinol Laryngol 87: 817–822

Ellis PDM, Wright JLW (1974) Acoustic neuroma – a plea for early diagnosis and treatment. J Laryngol Otol 11: 1095–1100

Greenberger R, Khangure MS, Chakera TMH (1987) The morbidity of CT air meatography: a follow-up of 84 patients. Clin Radiol 38: 535–536

Johnson EW, Selters WA (1987): In Handbook of Neurotological Diagnosis, eds. House JW and O'Connor, AF Marcel Dekker Inc., New York, p 76

Johnson JH, Kline DG (1978) Anterior inferior cerebellar artery aneurysms. J Neurosurg 48: 455–460

McCabe BF, Harker LE (1983) Vascular loop as a cause of vertigo. Ann Otol Rhinol Laryngol 92: 542–543

Mafee MF (1987) Acoustic neuroma and other acoustic nerve disorders. Role of MRI and CT: an analysis of 238 cases. Semin Ultrasound CT MR 3: 256–283

Mawhinney RR, Buckley JH, Holland IM, Worthington RS (1986) The value of magnetic resonance imaging in the diagnosis of intracranial meningiomas. Radiol 37: 429–438

Mazzoni A (1969) Internal auditory canal arterial relations at the porus acousticus. Ann Otol Rhinol Laryngol 78: 797–814

Moller A, Hatam A, Olwerona H (1978) The differential diagnosis of pontine angle meningioma and acoustic neuroma with computed tomography. Neuroradiology 17: 21–23

Morrison AW (1975) Management of Sensorineural Deafness. Butterworth, London, p 180

Olivares FP, Schuknecht HF (1979) Width of the internal auditory canal. A histological study. Ann Otol Rhinol Laryngol 88: 316–323

Olson JE, Glasscock ME, Hill Britton B (1978) Lipomas of the internal auditory canal. Arch Otolaryngol 104: 431–436

Papangelou L (1972) Study of the human internal auditory canal. Laryngoscope 82: 617–622

Pfleiderer AG, Evans KL, Grace ARH, Lloyd GAS (1988) A screening protocol used for the detection of acoustic neuromas: a clinical evaluation. Clin Otolaryngol 13: 145–151

Phelps PD, Lloyd GAS (1980) The radiology of cholesteatoma. Clin Radiol 31: 501–512

Phelps PD, Lloyd GAS (1982) High resolution air CT meatography. Br J Radiol 55: 19–22

Phelps PD, Lloyd GAS (1987) Which small acoustic neuromas need surgery? The influence of magnetic resonance and on air CT meatograms. Clin Otolaryngol 12: 191–196

Rao KG, Woodlief RM (1979) CT simulation of cerebellopontine angle tumour by tortuous vertebrobasilar artery. AJR 132: 672–673

Sarwar M, Swischuk LE (1977) Bilateral internal auditory canal enlargement due to dural ectasia in neurofibromatosis. Am J Roentgenol 129: 935–936

Schubiger O, Valavanis A, Menges H (1978) Computed tomography for small acoustic neuromas. Neuroradiology 15: 287–290

Schuknecht HF (1974) Pathology of the Ear. Harvard University Press, Cambridge, Mass p 415

Schuknecht HF, Gao YZ (1983) Arachnoid cyst of the internal auditory canal. Ann Otol Rhinol Laryngol 92: 535–541

Stack JP, Antoun NM, Jenkins JRR, Metcalfe R, Isherwood I (1988) Gadolinium DTPA as a contrast agent in magnetic resonance of the brain. Neuroradiology 30: 145–154

Terkildsen K, Thomsen J (1983) Editorial: Diagnostic screening for acoustic neuromas. Clin Otolaryngol 8: 295–296

Thyssen Hom, Marres EHM, Slooff JL (1976) Arachnoid cyst simulating acoustic neuroma. Neuroradiology 11: 205–207

Valavanis A, Schubiger O, Naidich TP (1987) Clinical imaging of the cerebello-pontine angle. Springer Verlag, Berlin, p 63

Valvassori GE (1969) The normal internal auditory canal. The diagnosis of acoustic neuroma. Radiology 92: 449–459

Valvassori GE (1988) Diagnosis of retrocochlear and central vestibular disease by magnetic resonance imaging. Ann Otol Rhinol Laryngol 97: 19–22

Valvassori GE, Pierce RH (1964) The normal internal auditory canal. Am J Roentgenol 92: 1232–1241

10   Radiology of Vertigo

Vertigo is an hallucination of movement and a symptom of a disturbed vestibular system. This system comprises the end organs in the temporal bone, the vestibular components of the VIIIth nerve and the central connections in the brainstem. The end organs are the cristae of the three semicircular canals which respond to movement of the head and the macula of the utricle, situated in the vestibule, which records the position of the head. The semicircular canals and utricle therefore record dynamic and static function.

A careful history is necessary to assess the duration and nature of the attacks, to rule out cardiovascular, cerebral and other problems and to assess "dizziness" and "unsteadiness' which may be due to a lesion of the VIIIth nerve or its central connections rather than the labyrinth. Complete, partial or temporary loss of labyrinthine function of rapid onset results in true vertigo. Mild vertigo is accompanied by nystagmus, involuntary jerky movements of the eyes, as well as nausea and vomiting. Failure of the end organ is referred to as peripheral vertigo. Central vertigo is caused by epilepsy, demyelinating disease, migraine, posterior fossa tumours – both axial and extra-axial – and vascular accidents and insufficiency affecting the brainstem and VIIIth nerve.

The ramifications of the vestibular system in the brain are more complex and extensive than the central auditory pathways and hence the central type is more common (Valvassori 1988). Montandon and Hausler (1984) in a retrospective study of 1000 cases, attributed the dizziness to a peripheral disorder in 25% and a CNS disorder in 46% of the patients.

Radiology may aid the diagnosis and indicate the site of the lesion in the conditions described below.

Peripheral Vertigo

Radiology is mostly concerned with demonstrating disease processes which affect the vestibular system by secondary extension. It is not of value in primary vestibular disorders such as vestibular neuronitis, streptomycin ototoxicity or benign positional vertigo.

Ménière's Disease

The medical history of Ménière's disease is usually quite typical. Severe episodic vertigo is accompanied by tinnitus, fluctuating hearing loss and a feeling of fullness in the affected ear or ears. Ménière's disease is a failure of the mechanism regulating the production and disposal of endolymph, resulting in recurrent attacks of endolymphatic hydrops. There is now strong evidence that the endolymphatic duct and sac are the site of resorption of endolymph, and therefore play a notable role in the pathogenesis of endolymphatic hydrops.   The success of various drainage type operations on the endolymphatic sac strengthens this point of view and has led to a great interest in the tomographic demonstration of the vestibular aqueduct – the fine bony canal in which the endolymphatic duct and sac lie.

There have been comprehensive descriptions of the radiographic anatomy of the vestibular aqueduct, particularly by the Uppsala School (Wilbrand et al. 1978). The vestibular aqueduct extends from the medial wall of the vestibule to the outer opening in the posterior surface of the petrous pyramid and has the shape of an inverted "J". The proximal segment of the aqueduct, formed by the short limb of

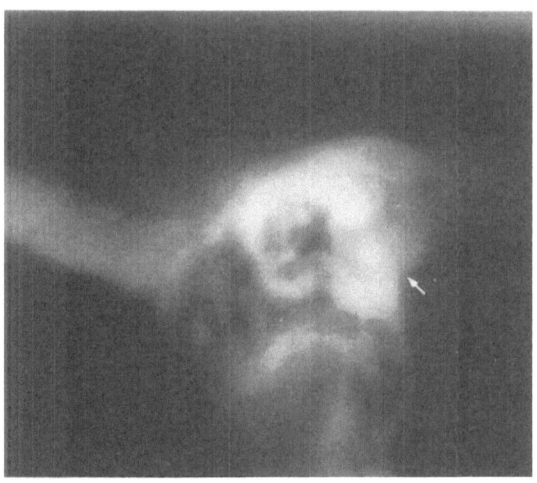

Fig. 10.1. Lateral tomogram showing the vestibular aqueduct (*arrow*). The aqueduct is short and curved (Wilbrand, Type 3).

erated anatomically. The Uppsala school were able to demonstrate the vestibular aqueduct in 100% of healthy ears, but in only 50%–60% of the diseased ears of the patients with Ménière's disease. They consider that non-visualisation of the aqueduct, and hence the relationship to the disease process, depends on the degree and type of periaqueductal pneumatisation and the length of the vestibular aqueduct. Three different types of periaqueductal pneumatisation were identified in their investigations (Fig. 10.2):

Type 1 – with large cell pneumatisation

Type 2 – with small air cells or bone marrow spaces (which cannot be differentiated from each other by tomography)

Type 3 – showing a complete absence of air cells (Stahle and Wilbrand 1974)

These different types of peri and infralabyrinthine air cell formation, together with varying sizes and positions of the jugular fossa, seem to have an influence upon both the appearance and shape of the vestibular aqueduct and its course through the pyramid.

The vestibular aqueduct is longer and its external aperture wider in a Type 1 pyramid and it exhibits a tomographically readily identifiable bend of about 80° between its proximal and peripheral portions. In a Type 3 pyramid, the aqueduct is shorter; it also shows a narrow external aperture and both its proximal and peripheral portions are curved without any clearly identifiable angulation between them. The Type 1 pneumatisation which is common in healthy individuals, was found in only a few patients with Ménière's disease at an early phase, but 74% of ears affected by Ménière's disease were of Type 3 without pneumatisation in the vicinity of the vestibular aqueduct. In Type 3 temporal bones, the course of the peripheral portion of the aqueduct through the pyramid may be curvilinear. Such digression from a straight course creates difficulties in exact tomographic positioning, is usually the reason for failure to reproduce the aqueduct, and probably explains the high frequency of non-visible aqueducts reported in Ménière's disease. In a smaller series, but with an added correlation between the X-ray appearances and histological section of 32 randomly selected temporal bones, we broadly confirmed the Swedish findings (Emery et al. 1983).

This evidence is refuted by Kraus and Dubois (1979) who, in a study of 190 ears, found that the tomographic appearance of the vestibular aqueduct was abnormal, either filiform or non-visualised, in

the "J", extends upwards medially and posteriorly, close to the crus commune, and then turns to run downwards posteriorly and medially to form the long limb of the "J" (Valvassori 1969). Generally, the best projection for demonstrating the aqueduct is the lateral, although variations in its course may mean that slight modifications of the lateral position should be tried, usually by turning the face as for the axial-pyramidal projection. The proximal segment and the bend or isthmus are very narrow and not satisfactorily demonstrated on the tomograms (Fig. 10.1).

Much controversy surrounds the significance of the tomographic findings. There is strong evidence that failure to visualise the aqueduct correlates to some extent with the occurrence of Ménière's disease. Valvassori and Clemis (1978) reviewed 3000 consecutive cases referred for tomographic studies of the vestibular aqueduct because of cochleo-vestibular disorders. A normal visualisation of both vestibular aqueducts was obtained in 57%. One or both vestibular aqueducts were abnormal in 43%. When the clinical findings were correlated to the radiological features, it was found that the vestibular aqueduct was normal in most of the cases referred for sudden hearing loss or mild paroxysms of positional vertigo. In contrast, a very high incidence of correlation was observed between radiographic non-visualisation of filiform aqueducts and clinical disturbances of the inner ear, of the type seen in Ménière's disease with abnormal audiometric and/or vestibular findings.

Tomographic non-visualisation does not necessarily mean that the vestibular aqueduct is oblit-

Type I

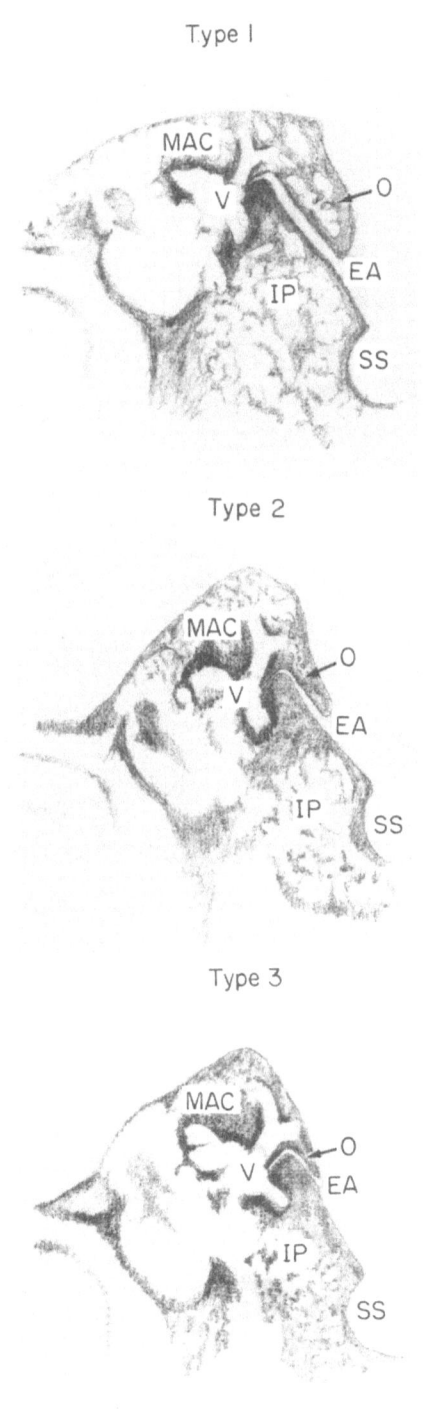

Type 2

Type 3

Fig. 10.2. The three types of vestibular aqueduct and surrounding pneumatisation (based on lateral tomograms). V, vestibule; SS, sigmoid sinus; EA, external aperture of the vestibular aqueduct; O, opercula; IP, inferior pneumatisation. (Courtesy Dr. HF Wilbrand.)

approximately the same percentage of patients with Ménière's disease as in patients with other diseases, no ear disease and normal ears. Similar negative findings were recorded by Hall et al. (1983), but the low rate of demonstration of the vestibular aqueduct may well be due to a limited tomographic examination.

The assessment of the vestibular aqueduct by multidirectional tomography or CT imaging or by histology of the temporal bones post mortem must be a study of sections in a predetermined plane. This is why the considerable variations between individual aqueducts as well as their small size causes such difficulties. The uncertainty of the role of the vestibular aqueduct and its morphology in the dizzy patient caused much discussion in the 1970s; little progress has been made in the present decade to solve this dilemma. Multidirectional tomography has now been replaced almost completely by CT, but CT is unsatisfactory for the study of the vestibular aqueduct, which is best demonstrated in the sagittal projection or, if necessary, by sections in the arc between the sagittal and axial-pyramidal planes. These projections are easy to reproduce by tomography but very difficult to achieve by CT and only the Utrecht school recommend this type of direct CT imaging (De Groot and Huizing 1987). Arenberg et al. (1984) advocate the reformatting technique to demonstrate the vestibular aqueduct. This is a convenient method and the plane of the vestibular aqueduct can be plotted on the base sections by a line joining the external aperture of the vestibular aqueduct with the crus commune. Unfortunately, 20–25 sections are necessary, which is likely to give a large radiation dose to the eyes, and the images are still suboptimal even if the patient remains motionless (for the reasons explained in Chap. 1).

Three recent works, one histological and two radiological, seem to confirm the abnormal aspects of the vestibular aqueduct in Ménière's disease. Sando and Ikeda (1984) measured the area, length, width, angle, position and external aperture of the vestibular aqueduct in 27 temporal bones of patients who had had Ménière's disease. These measurements were compared with measurements of the parameters in 88 normal temporal bones. A medial graphic reconstruction method was used to give a truer indication of the size of the vestibular aqueduct by volume rather than by measuring the length or width. It was found that small vestibular aqueducts were observed more often in the temporal bones of patients with Ménière's disease than in temporal bones from individuals without this disorder. Stimulated by these histological findings, Valvassori and Dobben (1984) extended their imaging study with an additional 400 cases of clinically diagnosed Ménière's disease. The cases were examined by multidirectional tomography, and CT. Once again, there was a statistically significant difference in size between the Ménière's and control groups. DeGroot and Huizing (1987) have recorded the only comprehensive CT study of the vestibular aqueduct in two planes perpendicular to each other. They used the standard base (transverse) plane and axial-pyramidal (axial petrosal) projections and measured the length from isthmus to external aperture. In the affected ears in patients with Ménière's disease this distal portion of the vestibular aqueduct was significantly shorter than in normal ears. These authors also pointed out that partial volume averaging effects (see Chap. 1) do not permit distinction between bony and soft tissue narrowing or obliteration.

In conclusion, therefore, the weight of evidence confirms that there is a statistically significant difference between the vestibular aqueduct in normal persons and in patients with Ménière's disease. The vestibular aqueduct in the Ménière's group is more likely to be short, hypoplastic, harder to demonstrate by tomography or CT, and with less periaqueductal pneumatisation. However, the obvious fact that a "Ménière's type" vestibular aqueduct occurs in normal persons and a normal vestibular aqueduct in patients with clinical Ménière's disease means that other, more direct causative factors need to be found and imaging has no place in the routine diagnosis of Ménière's disease, other than the exclusion of acoustic neuromas or other organic causes of vertigo. When surgery to the endolymphatic sac is planned, however, imaging contributes valuable preoperative information about variation in the location of the sac and the position of the external aperture particularly in relation to the jugular bulb. There is evidence that a diverticulum from a high jugular bulb can very rarely obstruct the endolymphatic duct (see Chap. 2). We believe that lateral tomography is the best means of demonstrating these relationships, although there is now considerable doubt about the efficacy of saccus drainage procedures (Fig. 10.3).

Large Vestibular Aqueduct Syndrome

A vestibular aqueduct that has a diameter of 1.5 mm or more measured at the mid point of the distal limb, is a very rare but definite congenital abnormality associated with fluctuant and progressive hearing loss. It has been described in Chapter 3 and is easily demonstrable on thin section high resolution axial CT (Fig. 3.24).

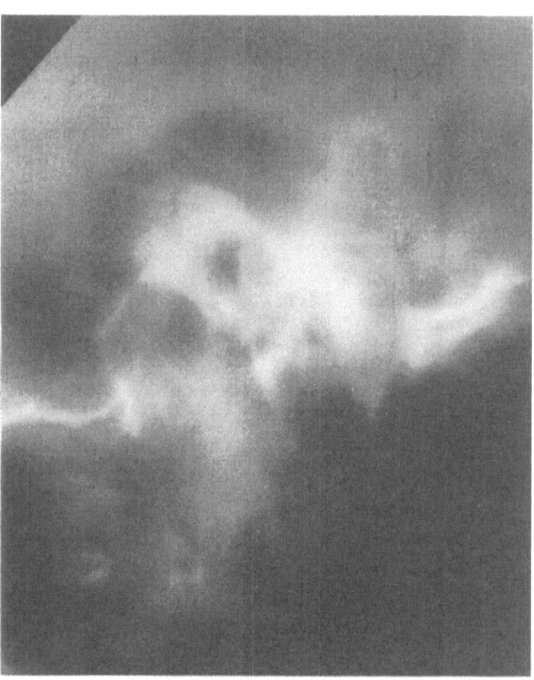

Fig. 10.3. The vestibular aqueduct is closely associated with a large jugular fossa.

Vertigo as a Complication of Otitis Media

Labyrinthitis may complicate an attack of acute otitis media. Radiology is of little value except to demonstrate accompanying mastoiditis (see Chap. 6). Imaging may show subsequent new bone formation totally or partially occluding the lumen of the affected labyrinth, but by this stage the damage has been done. This is known as labyrinthitis obliterans and a similar sequence of events may occur with a labyrinthitis secondary to meningitis. Chronic otitis media is a less common cause of vertigo except with cholesteatoma.

Cholesteatoma

Cholesteatoma may erode the capsule of the inner ear and invade the labyrinth. Before this occurs, i.e., in the pre-invasive phase, the patient may experience attacks of vertigo and it is at this stage that the "fistula sign", provocative of vertigo by variations in air pressure via a Seigal's speculum, is usually but not always positive. Immediate surgery is necessary to preserve labyrinthine function, and although radiology is of limited value in a straightforward case with obvious cholesteatoma and a positive fistula sign, it may nevertheless usefully demonstrate attico-antral erosion (see Chap. 7). The site of the fistula is usually the lateral semicircular canal where this bulges into the attico-antral space. Congenital cholesteatoma arising within the petrous pyramid may erode the labyrinth at any site depending on the location of the lesion.

Tumours in the Petrous Bone

Various benign or malignant tumours in the pyramid, such as glomus tumours, carcinomas of the middle ear or metastatic disease, may directly involve the labyrinth but usually vertigo caused by secondary deposits from carcinoma of the breast or bronchus has a central origin.

Imaging should demonstrate a radiolucent defect in the petrous pyramid, with ragged margins (Fig. 8.56) which will suggest a neoplastic lesion.

Trauma

A transverse fracture of the petrous bone destroys auditory and vestibular function and initially the patient has severe vertigo from the action of the opposite, unopposed labyrinth. Readjustment occurs after a few weeks. In less severe injuries and in fractures of the longitudinal type, there may be mild dizziness due to labyrinthine concussion.

Imaging in such a case may fail to show a fracture and if one is present it may not appear to involve the labyrinthine capsule (see Chap. 5).

Otosclerosis and Stapedectomy

Otosclerosis is an unusual cause of vertigo and tomographic recognition of involvement of the semicircular canals is usually limited to the lateral canal, and bone around the vestibule (Fig. 10.4).

Vertigo, although usually transient, may be a complication of the stapedectomy operation. Postoperative imaging may be of value, for example in demonstrating a prosthesis that protrudes too far into the vestibule (Fig. 10.5).

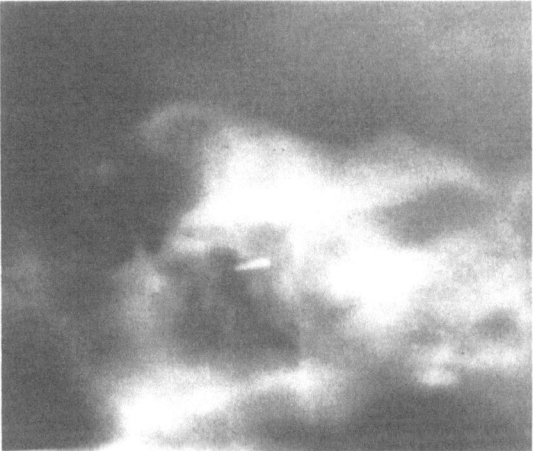

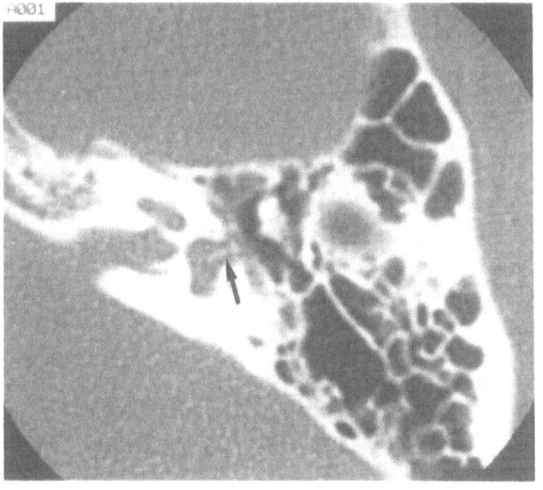

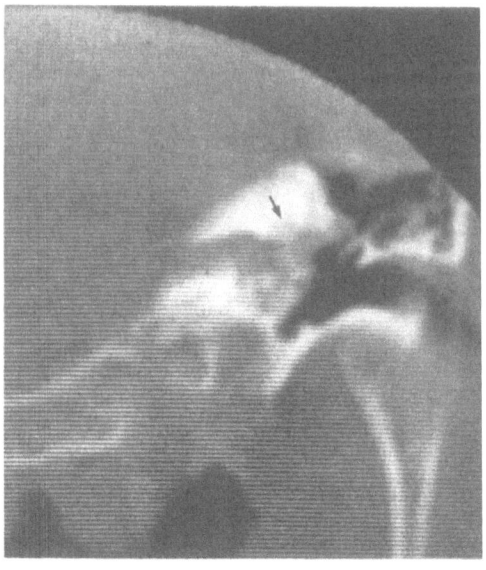

Fig. 10.4. Coronal CT section showing labyrinthine otosclerosis (otospongiosis). As well as rarefaction around the cochlea there is also decreased density in relation to the vestibule (*arrow*).

Fig. 10.5 a. A post-stapedectomy metal piston which protrudes too far through the oval window. There was associated vertigo in this case. b. Base CT showing a prosthesis that is too long.

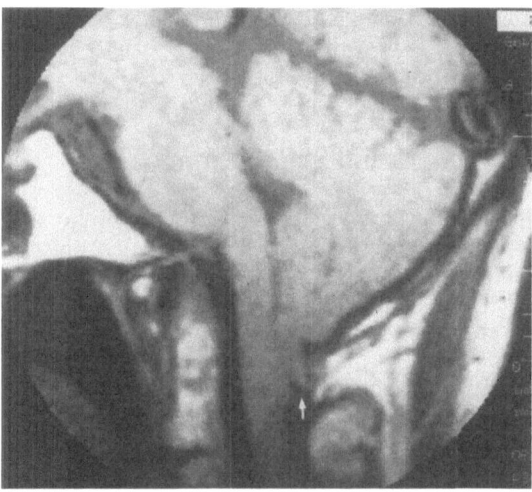

Fig. 10.6. Sagittal T_1-weighted MR scan (SE 700/26) showing slight protrusion of the cerebellar tonsils through the foramen magnum (Chiari malformation).

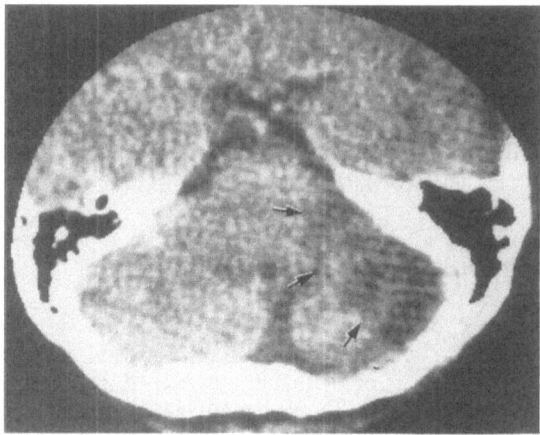

Fig. 10.7. CT scan of the posterior cranial fossa. There is an area of low attenuation in the cerebellar hemisphere and a small segment of the brainstem (*arrows*), representing infarction in the distribution of the posterior inferior cerebellar artery. The patient had multiple cranial nerve signs including deafness and disabling dizziness. This type of "stroke" does not usually create a problem in differential diagnosis from lesions of the petrous temporal bone.

Central Vertigo

A complete appraisal of the diverse pathological conditions affecting the central vestibular connections in the brain is beyond the scope of this book, but a brief consideration of central disorders causing dizziness and nystagmus is required. These may be difficult to discriminate from disorders affecting the peripheral labyrinthine system, and the patient may be referred, albeit mistakenly, to the ENT clinic.

1. Congenital skull base anomalies. The various Chiari malformations are characterised by herniation of the cerebellar tonsils into the foramen magnum (Byrd and Naidich 1988). This can give rise to various signs and symptoms, including nystagmus. The condition is now demonstrated easily by sagittal MR (Fig. 10.6)

2. Vascular disorders. Vascular insufficiency is a common cause of vertigo in patients over 50 years of age. Dobben and Valvassori (1984) have reviewed the assessment of hindbrain problems resulting from poor circulation in the vertebral arteries. These authors consider the dynamic CT study the most practical and available technique as it requires only a rapid intravenous injection of contrast. A normal graphic display comprises a "rapid increase" in density, followed by a rapid fall-off. The peak concentration is reached 15–20 seconds from the beginning of the injection.

When combined with electronystagmography and auditory brain stem response assessment, these flow studies can help to confirm that dizziness results from poor circulation to the central vestibular connections. However, in the future, these flow rates will be better studied by MR spectroscopy. The subclavian steal syndrome causes a variety of symptoms including vertigo. Angiography of appropriate vessels is the only radiological investigation of value in these cases.

Brainstem infarction or the lateral medullary syndrome occurs from occlusion of the ipsilateral vertebral artery or, more rarely, from occlusion of the posterior inferior cerebellar artery (Fig. 10.7). Such areas of brainstem and cerebellar infarction are best shown by MR (Fig. 10.8).

3. Multiple Sclerosis. Demyelination is a common cause of vertigo and should always be considered in the differential diagnosis. Magnetic resonance is now the investigation of choice to demonstrate plaques in the brainstem.

4. Neoplasms. Gliomas of the brainstem grow slowly and infiltrate the brainstem nuclei and tracts, producing multiple symptoms and signs. These tumours can be difficult to identify by CT early in their course because of their infiltrative character. However, MR scanning gives a much better demonstration (Fig. 10.9). Cerebellar neoplasms are usually silent until they press on the brainstem or cause obstructive hydrocephalus (Fig. 10.10).

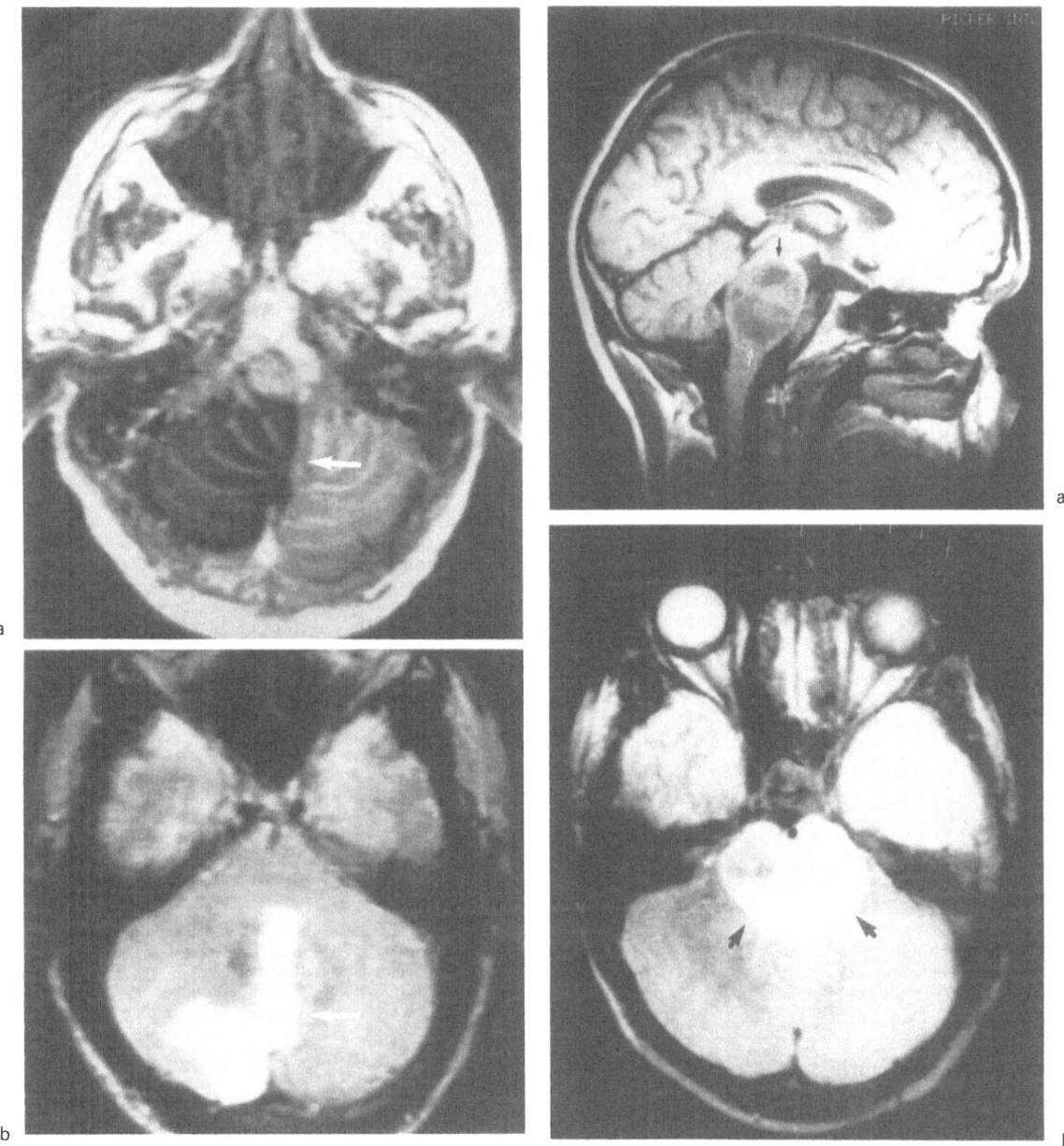

Fig. 10.8 a, b. Cerebellar infarct in a 38-year-old patient who presented with acute unsteadiness. a IR 2600/600; b SE 1500/80 base MR scans.

Fig. 10.9 a, b. A large brainstem glioma that presented with vertigo and unsteadiness. a IR 2800/800 sagittal; b SE 600/80 base MR scans.

5. Extra-axial masses. Acoustic neuromas, even if large, do not usually produce vertigo, but should always be considered in a dizzy patient. Other space-occupying lesions may cause central vestibular symptoms and signs (Fig. 10.11).

Cervical Vertigo

Cervical spondylosis is said to cause vertigo by disc degeneration and narrowing of the disc space, which affects nerves in close proximity, or by osteo-

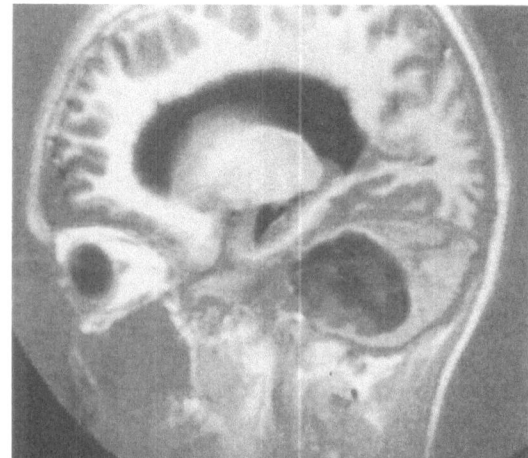

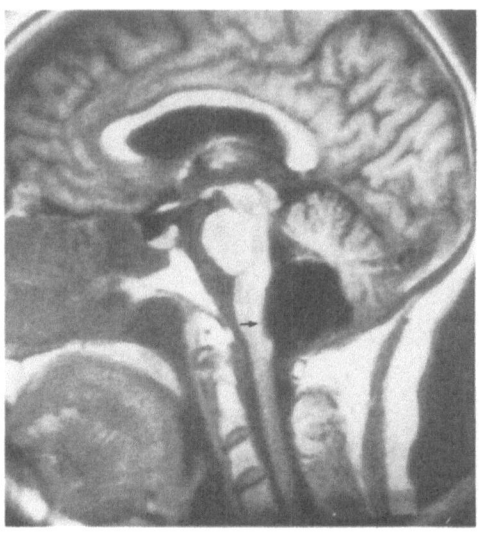

Fig. 10.11. Posterior fossa epidermoid (cholesteatoma). The same case as shown in Fig. 6.2. The sagittal IR 2600/600 section shows distortion and displacement of the cerebellum by the mass. Postural vertigo and nystagmus were the presenting features. Note also the pressure on the brainstem (*arrow*).

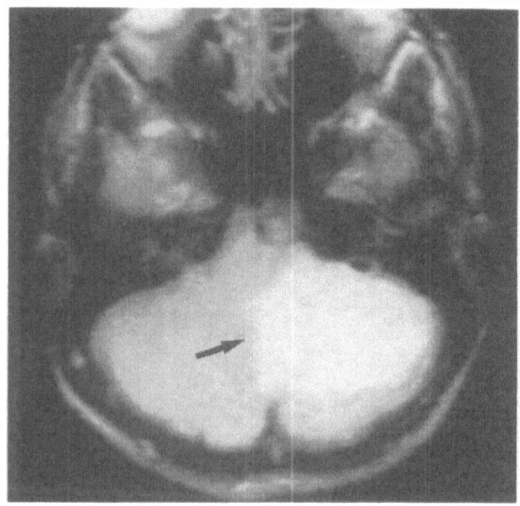

Fig. 10.10 a, b. Cerebellar astrocytoma in a 17-year-old patient who presented with headache, unsteadiness and papilloedema. **a** IR 3200·600 sagittal; **b** SE 1500/80 base MR scans.

phyte formation, which compresses blood vessels. Unfortunately, some degree of cervical spondylosis is almost always present in the elderly and in the authors' opinion, routine radiographs· of the cervical spine are not of value in dizzy patients.

References

Arenberg IK, Dupatrocinio I, Breisbach JM, Seibert C (1984) Radiographic classification of the vestibular and cochlear aqueducts: the paired correlation between normal and abnormal vestibular aqueduct and cochlear aqueduct anatomy. Laryngoscope 94: 1325-1333

Byrd SE, Naidich TP (1988) Common congenital brain anomalies. Rad Clin North Am 26: 755-772

De Groot JAM, Huizing EH (1987) Computed tomography of the petrous bone in otosclerosis and Ménière's disease. Acta Otolaryngol Suppl 434, 116

Dobben GD, Valvassori GE (1984) Role of the neurotologist in the diagnosis of brain ischaemia. Amer J Otol 5: 397-404

Emery PJ, Gibson WR, Lloyd GAS, Phelps PD (1983) Polytomography of the vestibular aqueduct in patients with Ménière's disease. J Laryngol Otol 97: 1007-1012

Hall SF, O'Connor AF, Thakkar CH, Wylie IG, Morrison AW (1983) Significance of tomography in Ménière's disease. Visualisation and morphology of the vestibular aqueduct. Laryngoscope 93: 1546-1550

Kraus EM, Dubois PJ (1979) Tomography of the vestibular aqueduct in ear disease. Arch Otolaryngol 105: 91-98

Montandon PB, Hausler R (1984) Relevance of otopathological findings in the treatment of dizzy patients. Ann Otol Rhinol Laryngol, Suppl 112

Sando I, Ikeda M (1984) The vestibular aqueduct in patients with Ménière's disease. Acta Otolaryngol 97: 558-570

Stahle J, Willbrand HP (1974) The vestibular aqueduct in patients with Ménière's disease. Acta Otolaryngol 78: 36-48

Valvassori GE (1969) Ménière's disease. Excerpta Med Int Congress Series, p 206

Valvassori GE (1988) Diagnosis of retrocochlear and central vestibular magnetic resonance imaging. Ann Otol Rhinol Laryngol 97: 19-22

Valvassori GE, Clemis JD (1978) Abnormal vestibular aqueduct in cochleovestibular disorders. Adv Otorhinolaryngol 24: 100-101

Valvassori GE, Dobben GD (1984) Multidirectional and computerized tomography of the vestibular aqueduct in Ménière's disease. Ann Otol Rhinol Laryngol 93: 547-550

Wilbrand HF, Stahle J, Rask-Andersen H (1978) Tomography in Ménière's disease: why and how. Adv Otorhinolaryngol 24: 71-93

11 Otosclerosis and Bone Dysplasias. Cochlear Implants

The otic capsule forming the bony labyrinth of the inner ear is composed of hard, poorly vascularised, endochondral bone which is metabolically inert and, therefore, relatively unaffected by systemic bone disease. Widespread bone disorders such as Paget's disease, hyperparathyroidism, rickets and osteogenesis imperfecta may eventually affect the labyrinthine capsule and cause sensorineural deafness but the periosteal bone, forming the remainder of the petrous temporal bone and base of skull, is affected first in these diseases. The rare congenital dysplasias which are present at birth or appear during childhood are considered in Chapter 4 although there is a considerable, if poorly understood, hereditary factor in the dysplasias considered here. Otosclerosis, the most common bone disorder causing deafness, affects only the labyrinthine capsule. Obliteration of relevant parts of the lumen of the labyrinth by otosclerosis or by labyrinthitis ossificans, which was described in Chapter 6, are relative contraindications for cochlear implants. This is the most important feature of the preoperative imaging assessment for implants which is discussed at the end of the chapter. A review of sensorineural hearing loss in bone dysplasias has been made by Booth (1982).

Otosclerosis

Otosclerosis is a localised disease of the bony labyrinth in which new bone, initially spongy and later denser, replaces the endochondral bone of the otic capsule and may cause ankylosis of the footplate of the stapes. The French term "otospongiose" is more descriptive.

Deafness is usually first noticed between 20 and 30 years of age, and otosclerosis accounts for about one half of the cases of bilateral conductive deafness in adults. It is twice as common in females as in males, and may be accelerated by pregnancy. There is a family history in about 50% of cases but the pattern of inheritance is obscure. The disease is unique to man and most common in the fair-haired races.

Although the aetiology of otosclerosis is unknown, the pathological process is fairly straightforward (Morrison 1979a). The hard avascular bone of the otic capsule becomes replaced by apparently normal healthy new bone in a localised area. This is immature woven bone of increased thickness, vascularity and cellularity, such as may be seen in healing fractures (Fig. 11.1). It has a lower radiographic density than the bone of the otic capsule. The focus becomes less active and more sclerotic with increasing maturity and, probably, also as a result of fluoride therapy.

The localisation of the otosclerotic process in the bony capsule of the labyrinth has been the subject of several histological studies. Generally, there is agreement with the findings of Nylen (1949) who examined the temporal bones of 74 patients with typical otosclerosis. Nylen found, in 90% of all cases, the localisation was in the oval window region, 50% being accompanied by stapes ankylosis: in 40% the process was localised to the round window region: the cochlear capsule was involved in 35%, the internal auditory canal region in 30% and the

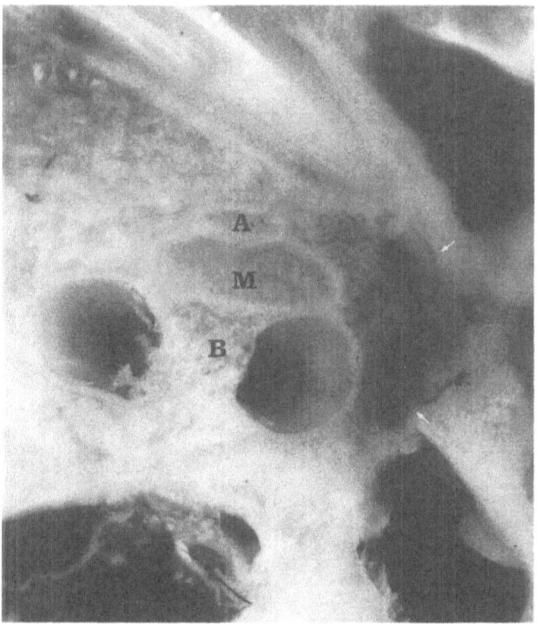

Fig. 11.1. Microslice of temporal bone showing large focus of otosclerosis (*arrows*) closely associated with the apical (*A*), middle (*M*), and basal (*B*) coils of the cochlea. (From Michaels L, *Ear, Nose and Throat Histopathology* with permission).

semicircular canal capsule in 15%. Incidence of lesions not affecting the windows did not, however, seem to accord with clinical practice and formerly three diagnoses of sensorineural otosclerosis were made for every 100 with stapes involvement (Morrison 1979a). Our recent work with CT densitometry would seem to confirm Nylen's findings and sensorineural deafness from cochlea otospongiosis appears much more common than is generally realised.

Fixation of the stapes or obliteration of the round window will cause a conductive type of deafness, but the mechanism by which otosclerosis produces a sensorineural hearing loss remains obscure. It may be a metabolic phenomenon associated with otosclerotic involvement of the endosteum of the spiral ligament. Parahy and Linthicum (1984) studied histologically 47 temporal bones with a clinical diagnosis of otosclerosis or cochlea otosclerosis. These authors considered that while otosclerosis and otospongiosis may coexist in the same bone, they develop independently. Hearing loss is worse when hyalinisation of the spiral ligament is present, when the lesion is active, and when the lesion is otospongiotic. Because hyalinisation occurs most often with otospongiosis and rarely

with otosclerosis, they suspect that toxic enzymes liberated by an active otospongiotic lesion cause the hyalinisation. They suspect that sodium fluoride slows or halts the progression of otosclerotic hearing loss by neutralising and inactivating the hydrolytic and proteolytic enzymes that are toxic to the hair cells, rather than by changing an active otospongiotic lesion to an inactive otosclerotic lesion.

Imaging Assessment

Sodium fluoride therapy for cochlear otospongiosis and the importance of the differential diagnosis for sensorineural hearing loss have made imaging for otospongiosis of the labyrinthine capsule more important than the demonstration of fenestral otosclerosis which has always been essentially a clinical diagnosis. Nevertheless for historical reasons, the latter will be considered first.

Fenestral Otosclerosis

Base sections of the petrous temporal do not adequately demonstrate the oval window. It can be shown in the coronal plane or even better in the semi-axial view with the patient's head rotated 20% towards the side to be examined. This brings the medial wall of the middle ear cavity, including the oval window, into the plane of the X-ray beam and enables the stapes footplate to be seen as a fine line crossing the oval window niche.

These appearances were described comprehensively in the days of polytomography (Rovsing 1974). Valvassori (1973) considered that there are four types of abnormality which may be apparent when the oval window is involved by otosclerosis:

1. Rarefaction of bone in the active phase of the disease gives the impression of a window that is wider than normal
2. Encroachment by more mature otosclerotic bone leads to narrowing of the oval window niche, the margins of which are poorly defined
3. There may be total obliteration of the window, the site of which cannot be recognised (Fig. 11.2). In such cases, it is important to be sure that there has been adequate coverage of the oval window niche by the tomographic sections
4. A thickened nodule of bone representing the footplate may be seen within the oval window margins (Fig. 11.3)

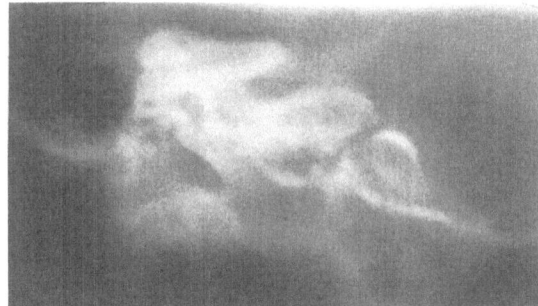

Fig. 11.2. Coronal section tomogram, vestibular cut, showing complete obliteration of the oval window by dense otosclerotic bone. The lumen of the basal turn of the cochlea is also markedly narrowed.

Although we do not think that otosclerosis affecting the oval window is any better demonstrated by CT, others (Swartz et al. 1984; Mafee et al. 1985) have described the CT appearances of abnormal body excrescences at or adjacent to the oval window.

We do coronal section CT to show the oval window after a base CT study with densitometry if there is a significant "air-bone gap". We have experimented with a histogram reading across the stapedial footplate to try to demonstrate a thickened footplate (Fig. 11.4) but have insufficient surgical confirmation yet to know if the technique is useful.

Cochlear Otospongiosis

The normal labyrinthine capsule is the densest bone in the body. We agree with Valvassori (1973) that it cannot become *more* radiopaque but only thicker

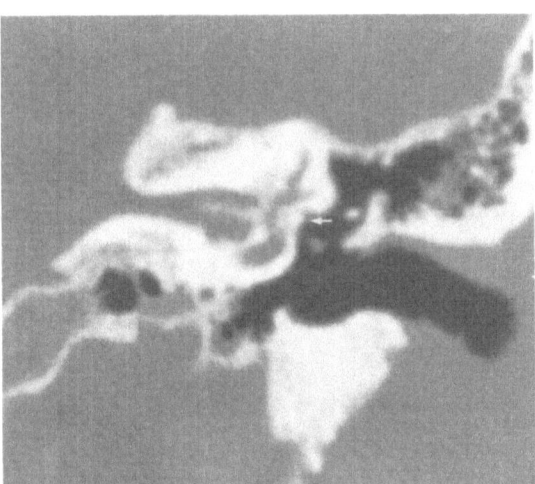

Fig. 11.3. Severe fenestral otosclerosis: a nodule of spongy bone is present in the oval window niche, the margins of which are poorly defined (*arrow*). Coronal CT section.

Fig. 11.4. A thickened stapes footplate. The histogram across the footplate gave a relatively constant reading of 500 HU. The figure itself has little meaning, being made up of various partial volume effects, but we record a lower figure for normals.

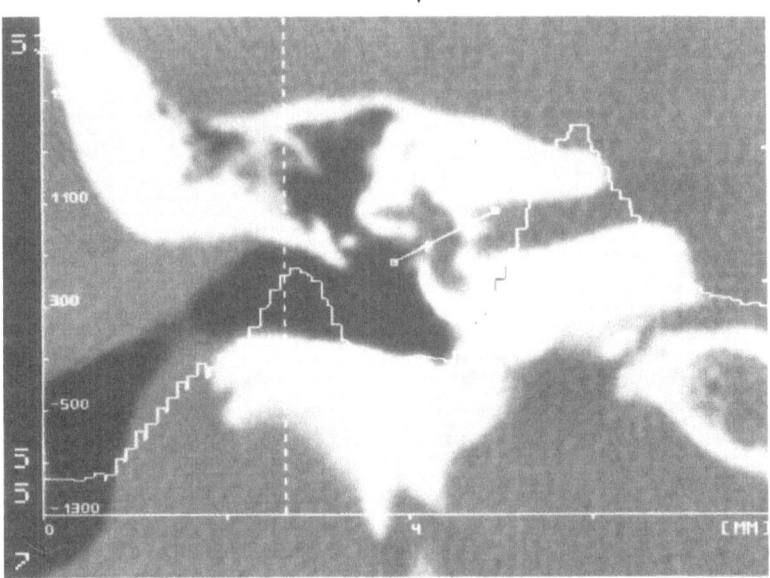

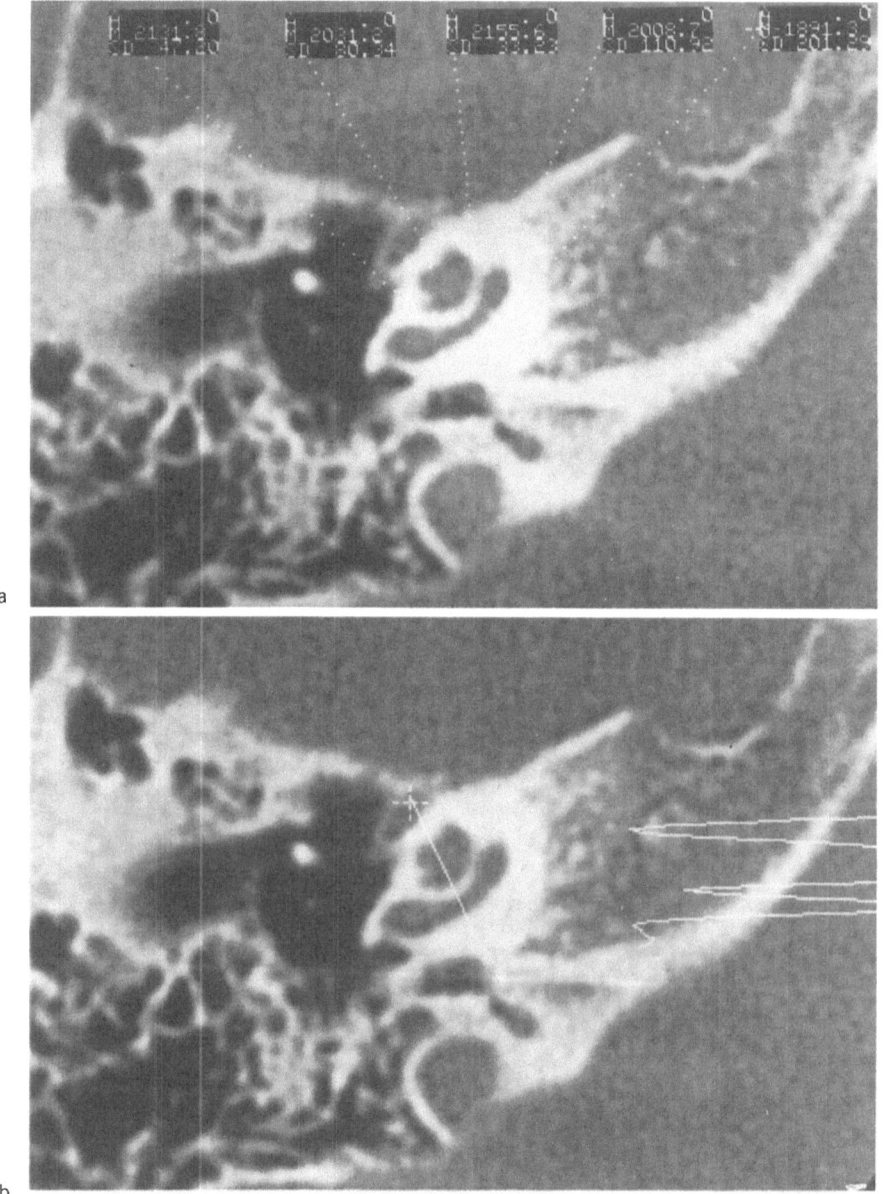

a

b

Fig. 11.5 a. The four points used with readings within the normal range of densitometric values with an extra reading in the region of the fissula ante fenestra. **b.** A normal histogram across the cochlear coils.

by apposition of otosclerotic bone. Thus the only way that imaging can demonstrate the sclerotic phase of the disease is by distortion of the normal outlines (Fig. 11.2).

It is a different matter for the more active spongiotic lesions which have been demonstrated as areas of rarefaction, not only of the cochlear capsule but also involving the semicircular canals and

fundus of the IAM. These were well shown by polytomography. However, high resolution CT has distinct advantages because of improved contrast resolution and the freedom from blurring which is inherent to multidirectional tomography from incomplete cancellation of structures outside the focal plane. Moreover, CT enables measurements of attenuation values to be made at various points in the labyrinthine capsule. These densitometry readings are most useful on two counts: (i) to confirm the diagnosis in mild cases where the areas of rarefaction are not convincingly evident on direct inspection of the images; (ii) as a quantitative and comparative assessment over a period of time to show increasing demineralisation, i.e., deterioration, or alternatively, remineralisation perhaps as a result of therapy (vide infra). The main difficulty is to obtain readings at constant and reliably reproduceable points. To cover the whole cochlear capsule on thin sectional imaging and thereby avoid missing a small focus of otospongiosis is both time-consuming and difficult. Partial volume averaging must be avoided at the edge of the capsule. Various protocols have been put forward for densitometric assessment, all of which involve sections 1.0 or 1.5-mm thick at 1-mm intervals in the base plane. Probably the best of these is the protocol described by Valvassori and Dobben (1985) for which two sections, one at the level of the round window and another high mid-modiolar section at the level of the oval window are used. Multiple measurements give two profiles around the coils of the cochlea. The most recent regime is that of De Groot and Huizing (1987) who attempt to define six reproducible points around the basal turn of the cochlea using four imaginary lines. Points 1 and 6 were too afflicted by partial volume averaging to be useful. They do, however, correctly stress the necessity for measuring the point of maximum density but, like us, have found no evidence that this is ever raised significantly above the figure in normals. These authors also correlated the bone density loss with the bone conduction hearing loss. They found the maximum correlation at Point 4 located between the first and second cochlear turns for the frequencies 100 and 2000 HZ.

Our Regime: We obtain a series of 1-mm HRCT sections through the cochlea in the base plane at 1-mm intervals. These are inspected for evidence of overt otospongiosis and then the section at the level of the round window niche is selected and magnified for the following densitometric assessment:

1. The maximum capsular density is measured by "high lighting" and increasing the window level until one point remains equivalent to the maximum density.
2. Four points, equivalent to Points 2, 3, 4 and 5 of the regime of De Groot and Huising, are depicted. Attenuation readings are obtained; a further refinement is to take the average of several readings at a particular point (Fig. 11.5a).
3. A histogram is drawn across the cochlear coils through the middle of the modiolus and central

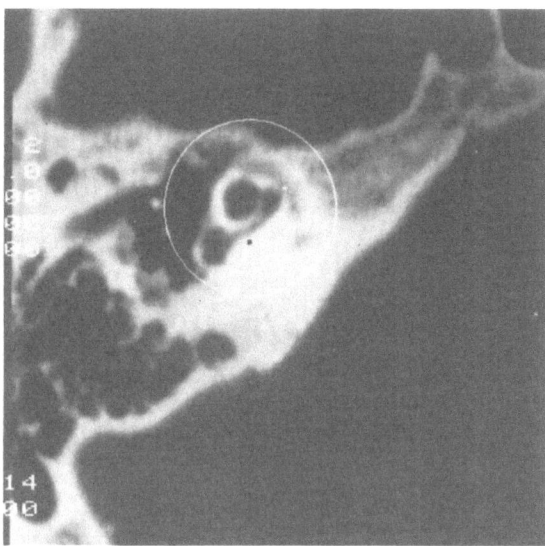

Fig. 11.6. Cochlear otospongiosis showing a zone of rarefaction. The white dot is one of the four points, M, 1193 HU. The black dot is the point of maximum capsular density, ME, 2414 HU.

bony spiral (Fig. 11.5b). This will show a "dip" for any zone of decreased bone density surrounding the cochlea which is the commonest feature of otospongiosis and readings below 1800 HU will be revealed at one or more of the four points (Fig. 11.6). Normal values appear to be 2300–2400 HU for the maximum capsular density; 1800–2200 HU for the four points; and below 1500 HU for severe otospongiosis. Thus the range 1500–1800 HU would seem to represent the critical level for mild loss of density not appreciated by the naked eye, although a small focus 1 mm or less in size would probably not be apparent.

Severe cochlea otospongiosis appears as a double ring effect (Fig. 11.7). This is due to confluent spongiotic foci within the thickness of the capsule (Valvassori and Dobben 1985). The ring may be incomplete or the lesions may be patchy (Fig. 11.8). If severe, the areas of demineralisation may extend to the region of the vestibule and semicircular canals (Fig. 11.9) and give rise to vestibular symptoms and signs (see Chap. 10).

Sodium Fluoride Therapy

Fifteen years ago Shambaugh and Causse (1974) proposed the use of sodium fluoride to promote recalcification and to reduce the activity of oto-

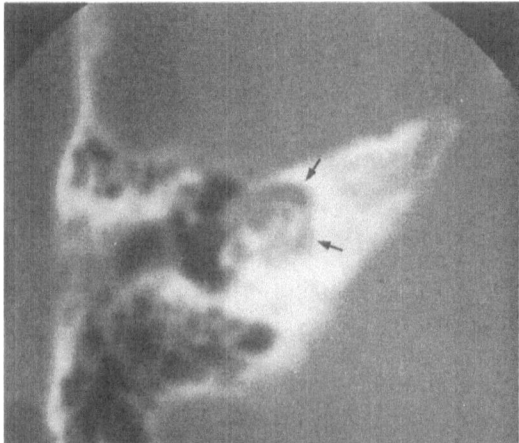

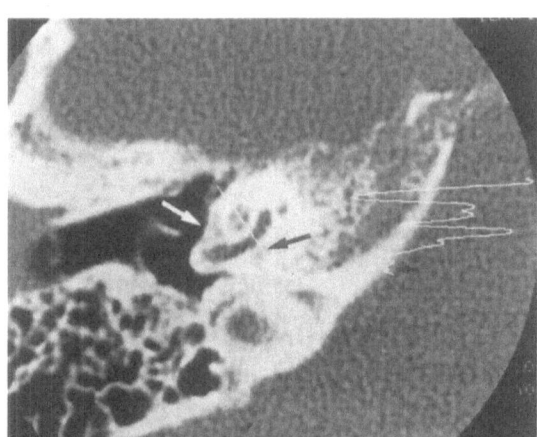

a

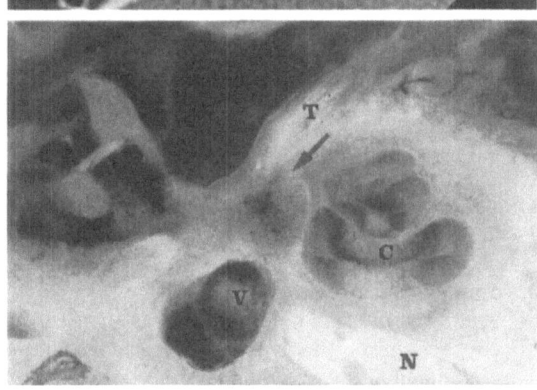

b

Fig. 11.7. The ring-like effect of severe otospongiosis shown by an older scanner.

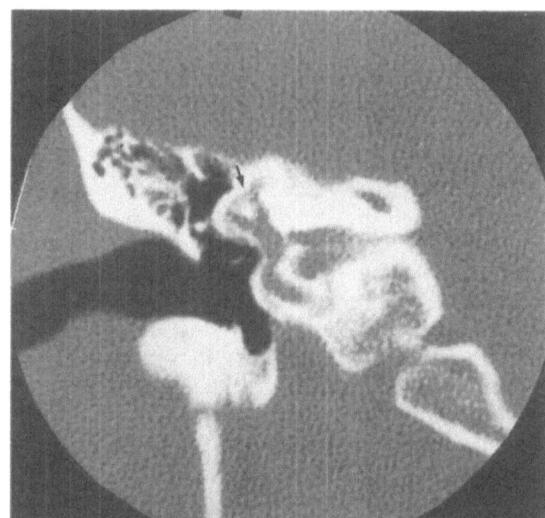

Fig. 11.9. Rings of otospongiotic rarefaction in the region of both cochlea and semicircular canals shown on this coronal section at the level of the oval window (*arrow*).

Fig. 11.8 a. The histogram confirms the presence of otospongiosis medial to the basal cochlear coil (*black arrows*) but also shown is a plaque anterior to the stapes (*white arrow*) in the region of the fissula ante fenestra. This is presumably causing footplate fixation accounting for the patient's mixed type of hearing loss. b. A histology section showing a plaque in a similar position (*arrow*). T, tensor tympani; C, cochlea; V, vestibule (from Michaels L, *Ear, Nose and Throat Histopathology*).

spongiotic bone. They discussed the safety and effectiveness as well as the proposed mode of action. They reported results of treatment in more than a thousand patients, but without adequate controls. Further reports (Cody and Baker 1978) have testified to the arrest of deterioration of hearing and even reversal of the hearing loss as a result of using sodium fluoride. These authors even show evidence of remineralisation on tomographic images. However, there was a similar lack of controls. More recently, Bretlau et al. (1985) studied the effect of sodium fluoride treatment in patients with otospongiosis evaluated blindly in a morphological and microchemical element analysis of otospongiotic specimens together with a prospective clinical double-blind, placebo-controlled study. The results show that using the calcium/phosphorus ratio as an indication for bone maturity, the sodium fluoride treatment can stabilise otospongiotic lesions in retaining calcium relative to phosphorus. The clinical double-blind, placebo-controlled study of 95 patients showed a statistically significant worse deterioration of the hearing loss in the placebo group than in the active treated (40 mg sodium fluoride daily) group, supporting the view that sodium fluoride can change otospongiotic, active lesions to more dense, inactive otosclerotic lesions. The authors postulated that the actual mechanism of the cochlear loss is toxic enzymes produced by histiocytes at the periphery of the microfoci, and it may be that sodium fluoride has some effect on these enzymes. Sodium fluoride therapy can only show longterm benefits but densitometric studies using equivalent sections and recordings at yearly intervals should demonstrate remineralisation. To our knowledge, none have so far been made.

Paget's Disease (Osteitis Deformans)

The clinical and radiological features of this common disease of old age are well known. The pathological changes are explained by simultaneous bone resorption and new bone apposition, greatly altering the normal bony architecture. There is not only variable rarefaction and sclerosis but the bone also becomes thickened and softened. When the skull base and petrous temporal bone are involved, Paget's disease may cause a severe degree of deafness, usually sensorineural but often with a conductive component. The hearing loss is fairly symmetrical and, as it occurs in an older age group, is not usually mistaken for otosclerosis. The cause of the deafness is uncertain and may be due to abnormal new bone formation infringing on neurosensory structures or to toxic changes in the labyrinthine fluids. It is thought unlikely to be due to narrowing of the IAM which undoubtedly does occur. Facial nerve function remains intact in Paget's disease of the temporal bone.

The radiological appearances of the petrous pyramids are pathognomonic. The periosteal bone is affected first and the extensive demineralisation that occurs makes the labyrinthine capsule stand out more clearly than normal in this initial osteoporosis circumscripta stage (Fig. 11.10) when shown by conventional imaging. The causation of the conductive component of the deafness seems to be involvement of the ossicles rather than stapes ankylosis and, occasionally, this may be shown tomographically (Fig. 11.11). Ossicular mobilisation and even stapedectomy may, occasionally, be used to try to close the air-bone gap.

The most satisfactory imaging is now by thin section, high-resolution CT which will show the abnormal "cotton wool" appearance of pagetoid bone in the skull base (Fig. 11.12). The encroachment on the labyrinthine capsule may be seen

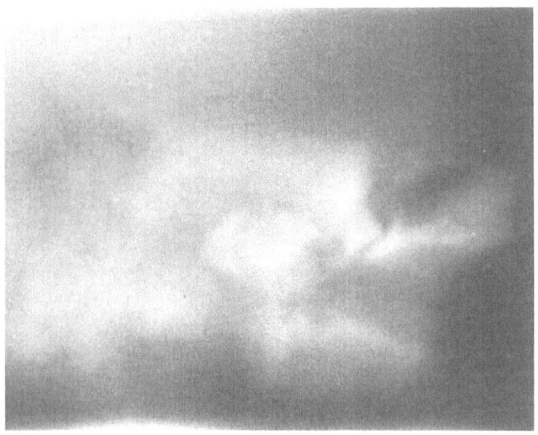

Fig. 11.10. Coronal tomogram at the level of the cochlea, showing typical Paget's disease encroaching upon the labyrinthine capsule. The "curl" of the modiolus of the cochlea is clearly seen but most of the cochlear capsule cannot be identified.

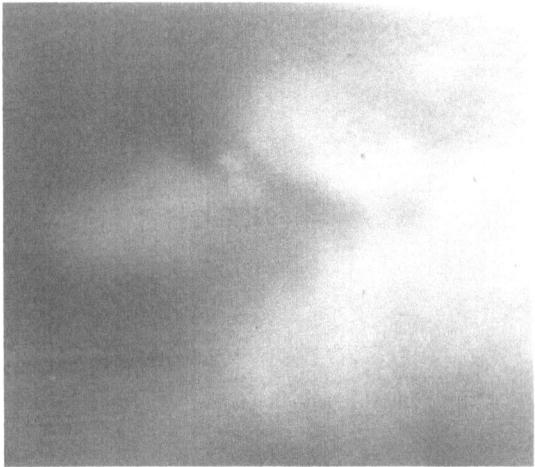

Fig. 11.11. Severe Paget's disease which is involving the ossicles. Few landmarks remain in the inner ear but parts of the cochlea can be identified.

clearly (Fig. 11.13). Distortion of the cochlea with osseous fractures between the basal and middle turns has been documented, and cochlear capsule demineralisation occurs frequently. Nager (1975) recognises three phases of the disease as shown by histology: (i) an initial phase of osteoblastic resorption; (ii) subsequent phase of osteoblastic regeneration of primitive bone, (iii) final phase of "mosaic" bone replacement. Benign and malignant tumour may occur, especially when the disease is widespread.

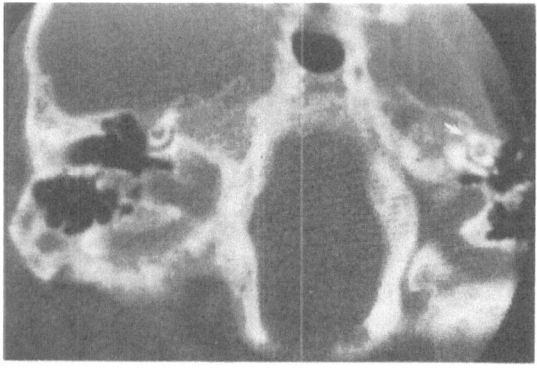

Fig. 11.12. Base CT showing typical Paget's disease of the skull base encroaching upon the most anterior part of the cochlea (*arrow*).

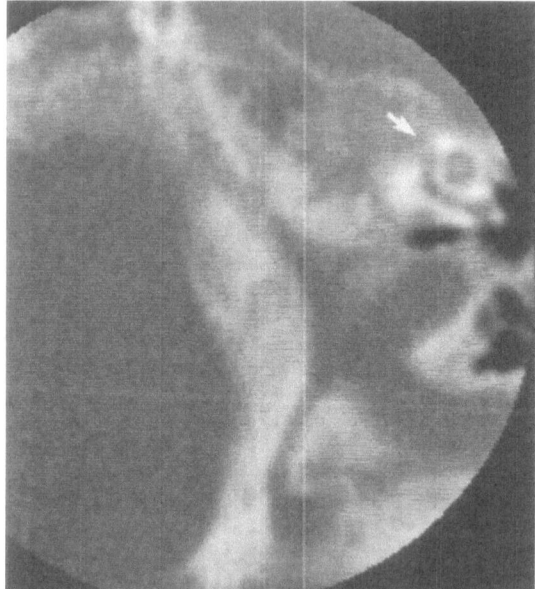

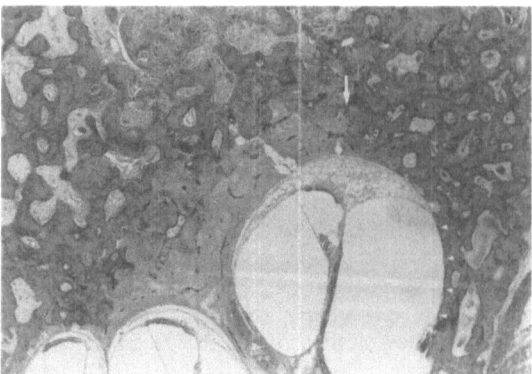

Calcitonin is advocated for Paget's disease of the petrous bone, to slow the progression of the hearing loss. The rationale is similar to the use of sodium fluoride in otospongiosis. Reports of the efficacy of calcitonin in reversing the progression of hearing loss are variable. Menzies et al. (1975) found no improvement in hearing in four patients treated whereas Morrison (1979b) showed audiograms with a definite hearing gain. Recently, calcitonin in combination with etidronate disodium an inhibitor of bone resorption, has been used on patients shown by CT to have Paget's disease of the petrous bone and subsequently monitored by alkaline phosphatase response curves (Sando et al. 1988).

Fibrous Dysplasia

A fairly localised disorder of bone which may be monostotic or polystotic fibrous dysplasia is characterised by abnormal proliferation of fibrous tissue with normal or immature bone. Skeletal aberrations and deformities occur and sometimes certain endocrinopathies and abnormal skin pigmentation form part of the entire disease process. The craniofacial skeleton is a common site but the petrous temporal bone only rarely becomes involved. The most comprehensive review of fibrous dysplasia affecting the temporal bone including the presenting and radiological features and differential diagnosis was by Nager et al. (1982). They found 69 cases reported in the world literature and described in detail three more. The usual presenting features were abnormal bone growth or presumed exostoses obstructing the external auditory meatus. Meatal stenosis and swelling of the temporal region were common.

Pathologically, fibrous dysplasia appears as a poorly circumscribed lesion replacing normal bone. Grossly it is soft and gritty in texture, and may appear white to red, depending on its vascularity. The expanded surrounding bony cortex may be thinned, but generally remains intact, maintaining a smooth outer contour. The transition between dysplastic and normal bone may not be distinct,

Fig. 11.13 a. Close-up of another case with extensive Paget's disease of the skull. The less dense pagetoid bone is affecting the coils of the cochlea. Compare with a similar histological section. **b.** Paget's disease involving the bony cochlea. The line of demarcation between pagetoid tissue and endochondral bone is shown by arrows. The *arrowheads* indicate where pagetoid tissue has reached the endosteum, and is therefore in contact with the cochlear lumen. (Courtesy of Dr. Christopher Milroy.)

since no true capsule exists at the margins of the lesion. Histologically, there is an array of fibro-osseous elements.

Smouha et al. (1987) have recently reported three patients with this disorder who presented with occlusion of the external meatus. Two patients developed external canal cholesteatomas medial to the obstruction, due to entrapment of keratin. The cases reported illustrate three surgical criteria necessary to manage these unusual cases successfully: (i) removal of sufficient diseased bone to create a patulous canal; (ii) resurfacing denuded bony areas with thin split-thickness skin grafts to prevent soft tissue contraction; (iii) an adequate meatoplasty.

Imaging Assessment

Three types of radiological appearance have been described for fibrous dysplasia: pagetoid, sclerotic and cyst-like (Nager et al. 1982). As with Paget's disease, softening of bone in the skull base may result in platybasia and an upward sloping external and internal auditory meatus. Generally, the expanded involved bone produces displacement of adjacent structures with preservation of the surrounding attenuated cortex. Pagetoid lesions are chacterised by alternate areas of density and radiolucency. Sclerotic lesions are homogeneously dense. Cyst-like lesions are spherical or ovoid, lucent, and have a dense boundary. On computerized tomography (CT), fibrous dysplasia typically has a non-homogeneous, ground-glass appearance (Fig. 11.14).

We have studied seven cases of fibrous dysplasia affecting the petrous temporal bone. Multi-directional tomography and high-resolution CT were used and the latter is now the imaging investigation of choice. We confirmed that narrowing or obliteration of the external auditory meatus is the most important feature of fibrous dysplasia affecting the petromastoid, usually with encroachment upon the middle ear cavity (Fig. 11.15). Two of our cases appeared to have narrowing of the IAM (Fig. 11.16) as did two of the cases reported by Nager (1982).

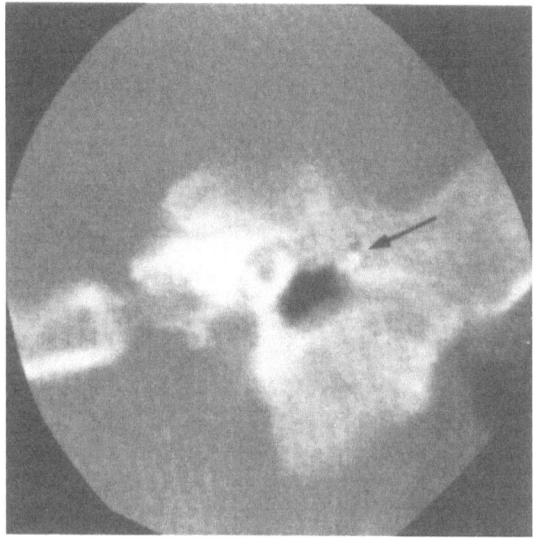

Fig. 11.15. Virtual obliteration of the external auditory meatus and reduction of the middle ear cavity so that the ossicles are "squeezed" in the attic (*arrow*). Coronal CT section of fibrous dysplasia.

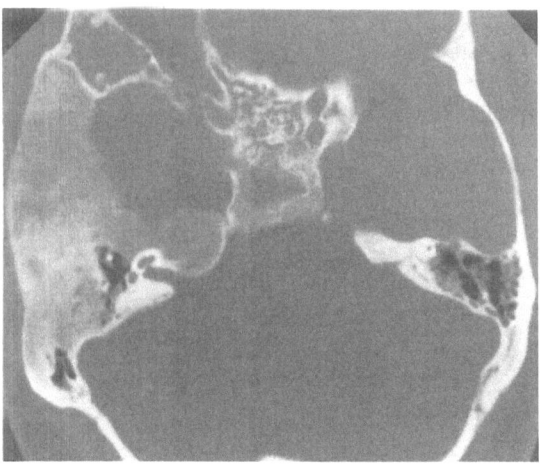

Fig. 11.14. Fibrous dysplasia of the side of the head involving the petro-mastoid and reducing the middle ear cavity. Note the "ground glass" appearance of the abnormal bone on this base CT section.

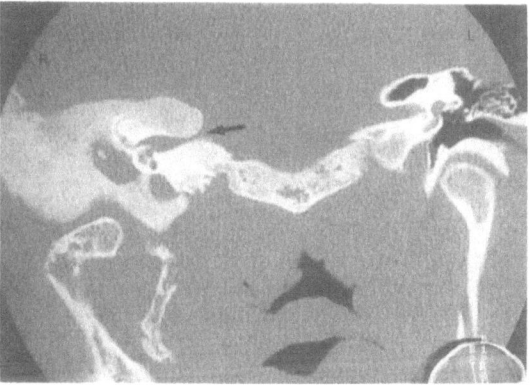

Fig. 11.16. Coronal CT of another case of fibrous dysplasia affecting the whole of the right petro-mastoid and the mandible. The right IAM is narrowed by the abnormal bone.

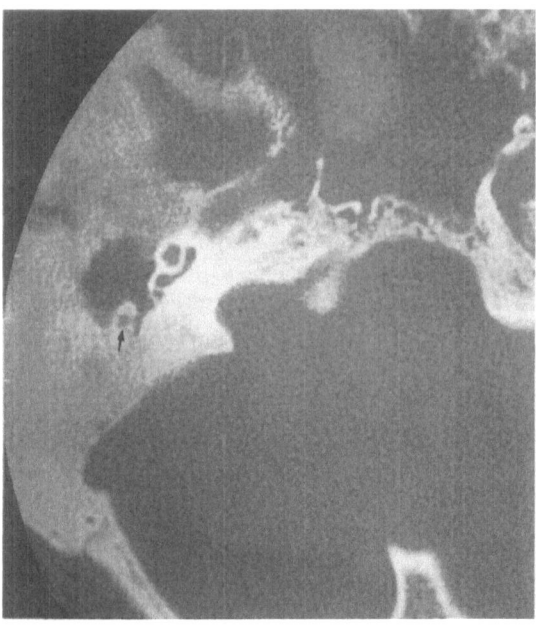

Fig. 11.17. Base CT showing fibrous dysplasia surrounding but *not* involving the cochlear capsule and the descending facial nerve canal (*arrow*).

We also agree that, in contradistinction to Paget's disease, the labyrinthine capsule is not affected by fibrous dysplasia, nor is there encroachment on the facial nerve canal (Fig. 11.17).

Cholesteatoma medial to an external meatal occlusion by fibrous dysplasia is the most important complication when the disease affects the petro-mastoid although, unfortunately, CT cannot confirm or exclude cholesteatoma when there is soft tissue opacification (see Chap. 6). In the two cases reported by Sharp (1970) the cholesteatoma developed after surgery to the external meatus.

Cochlear Implants

The recent development and progressive success of cochlear implants has shown the need for high resolution thin section imaging in the pre-operative, and to some extent, postoperative assessment of suitable candidates. Balkany et al. (1986) have described a systematic evaluation of the petrous temporal bone by CT:

1. The thickness of the parietal bone for seating the receiving device

2. The degree of pneumatisation of the mastoid
3. The measurement of the size of the facial recess
4. The description of the size and orientation of the round window niche
5. The patency of the basal turn of the cochlea

As most implants, both single and multichannel, are done through the facial recess and round window niche, the anatomical situation and relations of these structures must be fully assessed pre-operatively. This is best achieved by a base section through the round window niche which will also show the "hook" and full length of the basal turn of the cochlea. These structures are depicted in Fig. 1.23. Closely related air cells and a high dome of the jugular bulb also need to be identified. If possible, coronal sections to show the cochlea and oval and round windows should be obtained in addition.

Partial or total obstruction of the basal turn of cochlea or round window is common in severely deaf patients being assessed for implants. Harnsberger et al. (1987) screened 42 patients and showed labyrinthine ossification in 12 (28.6%), cochlear or fenestral otosclerosis (or both) in four (9.5%), and congenital cochlear malformation in two. This information provided by CT was used to exclude patients in whom implantation was likely to be unsuccessful and also to help select the best ear for implantation. We have found a similar high incidence of obliterative disease of the cochlea and round window niche (Fig. 11.18).

Although CT can show a normal calibre IAM and give a good demonstration of labyrinthine ossification, it does not adequately depict fibrous obliteration. Thus Valvassori (1987) advocates MR for the following reasons:

1. To show whether the cochlear lumen contains fluid or fibrous tissue. The normal fluid-filled cochlea will give a stronger signal, i.e. appear brighter, especially on T_2-weighted images
2. To show the acoustic nerve and possibly, in the future, to assess the degree of degeneration. In some congenital abnormalities with very narrow IAMs, there may be no acoustic nerve present but only a tract for the facial nerve
3. To reveal central pathology which will contra-indicate an implant

Unfortunately, for the nerve and cochlear assessments, the latest MR using high-field thin sections and surface coils is really required and so far MR has not been able to predict the size of the acoustic nerve (Harnsberger et al. 1987).

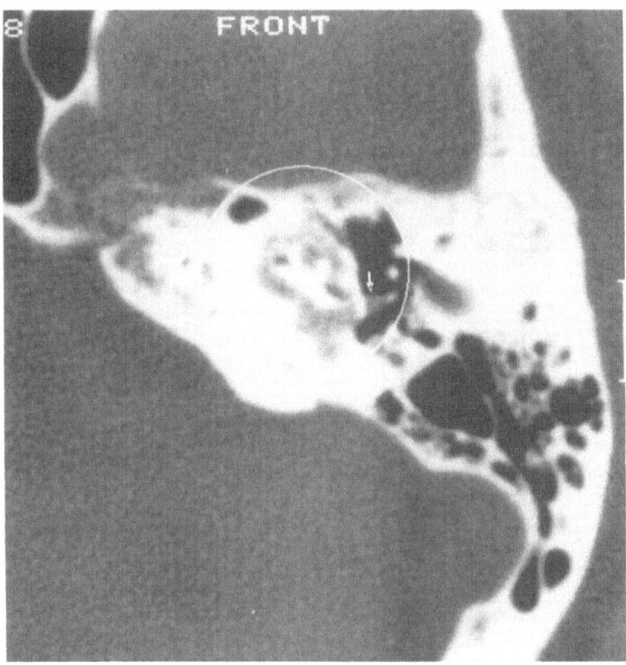

Fig. 11.18. Severe otospongiosis/otosclerosis narrowing and partially obliterating the coils of the cochlea in a severely deaf patient being assessed for a possible cochlear implant. There is abnormal bone in the round window niche and replacing the stapes superstructure (*white arrow*).

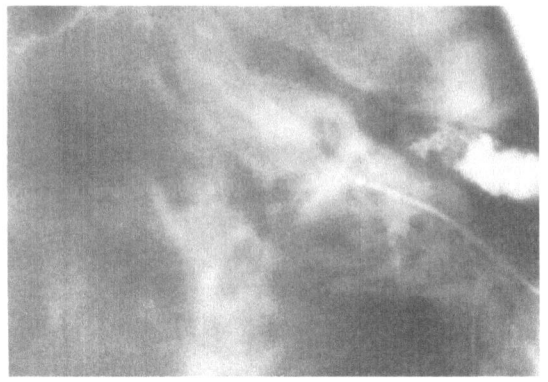

a

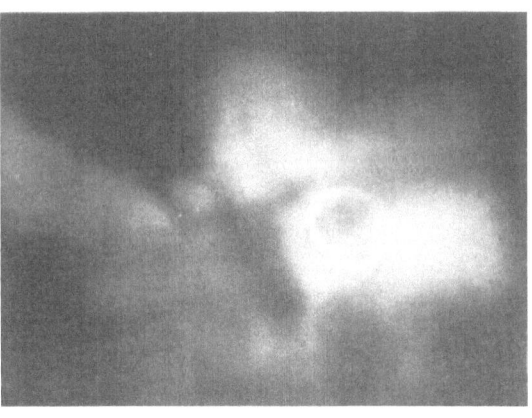

b

Fig. 11.19 a. Conventional tomography showing a single channel cochlear implant in the round window niche (from Scott Brown's Textbook of Otolaryngology, Vol 3). **b.** Coronal pluridirectional tomography showing a multichannel electrode in the cochlea.

Conventional imaging still has a limited place, mainly in the postoperative assessment (Fig. 11.19) as the metal structures in the implant degrade the CT image and would be affected by the magnetic field by MR. Qaiyumi et al. (1988) find multi-directional tomography in the coronal plane most useful for assessing the intracochlear location of their multichannel electrodes.

References

Balkany TJ, Dreisbach JN, Seibert CE (1986) Radiographic imaging of the cochlear implant candidate: preliminary results. Otolaryngol Head Neck Surg 95: 592–597

Booth JB (1982) Medical management of sensorineural hearing loss. Pt II Muscolo-skeletal system. J Laryngol Otol 96: 773–

795

Bretlau P, Causse J, Hansen HJ, Johnsen NJ, Salomon G (1985) Otospongiosis and sodium fluoride: a blind experimental and clinical evaulation of the effect of sodium fluoride treatment in patients with otospongiosis. Ann Otol Rhinol Laryngol 94: 103–107

Cody DTR, Baker HL (1978) Otosclerosis vestibular symptoms and sensorineural hearing loss. Ann Otol Rhinol Laryngol 87: 778–797

De Groot JAM, Huizing EH (1987) Computed tomography in otosclerosis and Ménière's disease. Acta Otolaryngol Supp 434

Harnsberger HR, Dart DJ, Parkin JL, Smoker WR, Osborn AG (1987) Cochlear implant candidates: assessment with CT and MR imaging. Radiology 164: 53–57

Mafee MF, Hendrikson GC et al. (1985) Use of CT in stapedial otosclerosis. Radiology 156: 709–714

Menzies MA, Greenberg PB, Joplin GF (1975) Otological studies in patients with deafness due to Paget's disease before and after treatment with synthetic human calcitonin. Arch Otolaryngol 79: 378–383

Morrison AW (1979a) In: Ballantyne J, Groves J (eds) Diseases of the Ear, Nose and Throat. 4th edn. Butterworths, London, p 425

Morrison AW (1979b) In: Ballantyne J, Groves J (eds) Diseases of the Ear, Nose and Throat. 4th edn. Butterworths, London, p 474

Nager GT (1975) Paget's disease of the temporal bone. Ann Otol Rhinol Laryngol 22 (Suppl): 1–32

Nager GT, Kennedy DW, Kopstein E (1982) Fibrous dysplasia: A review of the disease and its manifestations in the temporal bone. Ann Otol Rhinol Laryngol 91 (Suppl 92): 1–52

Nylen B (1949) Histopathological investigations on the loca-

lization number activity and extent of otosclerotic foci. J Laryngol Otol 63: 321–327

Parahy C, Linthicum FH Jr (1984) Otosclerosis and otospongiosis: clinical and histological comparisons. Laryngoscope 94: 508–512

Qaiyumi SAA, Hendricks L, Lasgig R, Battmar RD, Bochor E (1988) The value of conventional x-ray tomography in cochlear implant patients. Paper given at the XI International Congress of Head and Neck Radiology, Uppsala, Sweden

Rovsing H (1974) Otosclerosis: fenestral and cochlear. Radiol Clin North Am 12: 505–515

Sando M, Hoover LA, Finerman G (1988) Stabilization of hearing loss in Paget's disease with calcitonin and etidronate. Arch Otolaryngol Head Neck Surg 114: 891–894

Shambaugh GE, Causse J (1974) Ten years with fluoride in otosclerotic (otospongiotic) patients. Ann Otol Rhinol Laryngol 83: 635–642

Sharp M (1970) Monostotic fibrous dysplasia of the temporal bone. J Laryngol Otol 84: 697–707

Smouha EE, Edelstein DR, Parisier SC (1987) Fibrous dysplasia involving the temporal bone: report of three new cases. Am J Otol 8: 103–107

Swartz JD, Faerber EN, Wolfson RT, Marlowe FI (1984) Fenestral otosclerosis: significance of preoperative evaluation. Radiology 151: 703–707

Valvassori GE (1973) Otosclerosis. Otolaryngol Clin North Am 6: 379–389

Valvassori GE (1987) Workshop: surgical anatomy and radiographic imaging of cochlear implant surgery. Am J Otol 8: 195–200

Valvassori GE, Dobben GD (1985) CT densitometry of the cochlear capsule in otosclerosis. Am J Neuroradiol 6: 661–667

Subject Index